Infectious diseases in Europe

A fresh look

World Health Organization
Regional Office for Europe
Copenhagen
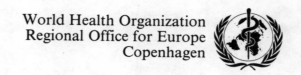

Infectious diseases in Europe

A fresh look

B. Velimirovic

Regional Officer for Communicable Diseases
WHO Regional Office for Europe
Copenhagen, Denmark

In collaboration with

D. Greco, N. Grist, H. Mollaret,
P. Piergentili & A. Zampieri

Printed in England

Contents

Acknowledgements

The author wishes to thank the following: Dr F. Assaad for encouragement; Mrs K. Estewes, Mrs A. Wiedersheim and Mrs A. Müller for help in preparing the tables; Dr F. Fuglieni, Dr M. Pasquali, Mrs M.A. Stazi, Mr M. Panatta and Dr F. Forastiere for help in writing the computer programs and producing the graphs; Mr M. Curianó for help in collecting data; Dr A. Weber, Dr J.-P. Jardel, Dr I. Carter and Dr P. Pasquini for reviewing parts of the manuscript; and Dr S. Moles and Mr F. Theakston for their patient and painstaking editing of the text.

Preface

Europe has achieved remarkable success in both the surveillance and the control of a number of infectious diseases (a term the authors prefer to communicable diseases, for reasons set out in the book). It is widely believed that the vast improvements in the living conditions of people in general and the immense strides that medical science has made in this century have reduced infectious diseases to a problem of minor importance. This belief is helped by the method of classifying infectious diseases in a way that obscures their importance.

In fact, as the book shows very clearly, infectious diseases are as prevalent and as important as ever. Except for influenza, they do not on the whole manifest themselves in great epidemics, nor do they cause such high mortality as they used to, because of the medical advances referred to above. But they cause an immense amount of morbidity and economic loss and play a role in the health care systems of countries that is seriously underestimated at present. Furthermore medical science is constantly turning up new evidence to show what consequences long-past infection may have on health in later life.

In this volume some examples of the notification systems, and the information obtained from them and elsewhere, have been collected to present, albeit incompletely, a picture of facts, figures, trends and achievements, as well as of the problems encountered with selected infectious diseases in the European Region.

Epidemiological surveillance is the cornerstone of work on the control of infectious diseases, and their prompt reporting at the national level and to WHO might put the focus on problem areas, old and new. Under-reporting, particularly at the primary health care level, is an area where more effort is needed. Increased surveillance, as part of better epidemiological services, and better control efforts can only be to the advantage of the countries themselves. It is timely today to realize, 100 years after the first effective bacterial vaccine was developed, that the current effort in surveillance and control by immunization is still not commensurate with the needs and possibilities we have.

The time is therefore ripe for a fresh look at infectious diseases in Europe, and this volume seems to me to provide ample food for thought in health administrations and among health personnel of all kinds. Nor is its value limited to the European Region; the problems it describes are prob-

lems that other regions in the world are faced with, however different their conditions may be. It is to be hoped that this volume will meet with the acclaim it deserves, not only in Europe but also further afield. It is also to be hoped that it will encourage countries to improve the gathering of data on infectious diseases and cooperate internationally in dealing with them.

Leo A. Kaprio
WHO Regional Director for Europe

1

Does Europe have a communicable disease problem?

B. Velimirovic

The aim of this publication is to survey the situation of communicable diseases in Europe. The most recent surveys are more than a decade old and, because of delay in the consolidation and publication of statistics, usually deal with the situation 15–20 years ago. Moreover, information on communicable diseases, even from countries that have comprehensive health services, does not provide a picture of the situation in Europe as a whole.

To avoid duplicating other WHO publications, *subjects discussed by Regional Office working groups during the period 1979–1981 have been omitted*, even though they are particularly important and would have given additional emphasis to the field under discussion. These are: the classical and second-generation sexually transmitted diseases, acute respiratory infections, hospital-acquired infections, echinococcosis, yersiniosis and Legionnaires' disease. Also omitted are subjects in the 1982/83 programme of the Regional Office: prenatal and perinatal infections, the role of molecular biology in infectious diseases, the immunization of certain high-risk groups, and mycotic infections. It is anticipated that WHO publications will be issued on all these subjects in the near future.

Most of WHO's efforts in the past decade towards controlling communicable diseases have been devoted to the developing countries, where communicable diseases are major health problems and furnish half or more of the principal causes of death. WHO has sought to help countries to make use of existing knowledge to reduce mortality and morbidity and to foster research into treatment and the development of control strategies. Examples of its efforts are the Expanded Programme on Immunization, the global diarrhoeal diseases control programme, and the tropical diseases research programme.

In Europe the sharp decline of most of the major classical communicable diseases, particularly those for which immunization is available,

1

shifts in the demographic structure, changes in the environment, advances in technology, and rising living standards have led to changes in the pattern of mortality, an increasing proportion of deaths from chronic degenerative diseases, cardiovascular diseases, malignant neoplasms, and such external causes as accidents, violence, and suicide. The treatment and prevention of the latter have directed attention away from communicable diseases, which until very recently were considered almost on the verge of extinction and were relatively neglected. As a consequence it is difficult to obtain a comprehensive picture of their present importance. This volume, on problems of communicable diseases, is a status inventory, a plea for better surveillance, and hopefully also a new point of departure in the reorientation of our approach to infections. In any effort to understand what lies ahead, as much as what lies in the past, the role of infections and their changes cannot be left out of consideration. McNeill (1) has said:

> Ingenuity, knowledge and organization alter but cannot cancel humanity's vulnerability to invasion by parasitic forms of life. Infectious disease which antedated the emergence of humankind will last as long as humanity itself, and will surely remain, as it has been hitherto, one of the fundamental parameters and determinants of human history.

Medical professionals, particularly after the Second World War and in the euphoric 1950s, were more than optimistic about the future. Sir MacFarlane Burnet (2) wrote in 1953 about the changing problems of medicine:

> Infectious disease will always be with us, and there will always be room for further refinement in prevention and treatment; but as a major cause of death in the years of youth and maturity it is becoming relatively unimportant. Though it may seem an inappropriate remark for one whose whole professional life has been concerned with infectious disease, I believe that, provided the established mechanism of preventive medicine, medical care and drug production continued to function, fundamental work on the nature of micro-organisms and on the diseases they produce could stop today without influencing the current process by which all the main infectious diseases except poliomyelitis are disappearing. This is of course an overstatement: as long as the human race exists there will be long-term changes and sudden new episodes of infectious disease that will need intelligent investigation and appropriate action to counter them. My point is only that it is extremely unlikely that any new principles will be needed to maintain our present very effective control of infectious disease: in that sense fundamental research is not called for by an expressed human need.

Here it should be stated that not everybody shares Sir MacFarlane Burnet's opinion about the reasons for the decline of infections. Many agree with McKeown (3–5) who in all his writings, but particularly in *The role of medicine: dream, mirage or nemesis?* (6), assigns a rather modest role to medical science. McKeown's views have implications not only for the infectious diseases field but also for health policy generally, as reflected, for example, in some national health programmes (7) that have influenced WHO. However, McKeown's arguments have flaws "which make full acceptance of this conclusion unlikely" (*8*), and have been justly criticized. Although large parts are now viewed rather as a philosophy of medical care than as epidemiologically valid inferences, his influence has been and will still be felt.

McKeown's argument is as follows: "Many medical scientists believe that the control of bacterial infections is based on knowledge of infectious diseases derived from basic research and applied largely, although by no means exclusively, through immunization and therapy". He arrives at a quite different conclusion, namely, "that these measures had little effect on the [mortality] rates before 1935 and since that time have been less important than other influences". On the basis of evidence from England and Wales, he concluded that BCG vaccination had little or no influence on the decline of mortality in tuberculosis. In pneumonia, chemotherapy had a moderate effect on morbidity in the age groups 0–14 and 45–64 years, but the effect on deaths at all ages was not large and was certainly not the main reason for the continued decline of the death rate, which was well established from the beginning of the century. Mortality from measles and pertussis fell to a low level without effective immunization or treatment. "The usefulness of immunization is now being assessed by the effect on morbidity ... the results so far are not very impressive". His conclusion is not "that immunization or treatment were of no value; on the contrary they are probably effective in all the diseases listed above. But their impact on mortality and associated morbidity was small in relation to other influences". Diphtheria and smallpox were the only common infections in which a specific measure, immunization, may have been the main reason for their decline. "In the other common ones, tuberculosis, pneumonia, measles, whooping cough, typhoid and typhus (and scarlet fever may be added), mortality had fallen to a relatively low level before effective medical intervention was possible. In other diseases — smallpox, syphilis, poliomyelitis and tetanus, in which specific measures are generally regarded as the main reason for their decline ... taken singly or collectively [they] made only a small reduction in infectious deaths".

McKeown pointed out that the decline in deaths from infectious diseases preceded by more than a hundred years the discovery of microorganisms. The trends in the last two centuries indicated that deaths were declining before effective procedures became available, falling to a small fraction of their earlier level without medical intervention, and they suggest that had none been available they would have continued to decline, if not quite so rapidly in some diseases. In a number of infectious diseases there have been considerable advances in immunization and therapy, but their mortality was decreasing prior to the introduction of such treatment, which in the present century had little observable impact on the continuing downward trends. The exceptions to this, he considers, are streptomycin therapy for tuberculosis and poliomyelitis vaccine.

Among the causes of the decline in mortality from infectious diseases he places nutrition as the most important: increased food production, the use of fertilizers, the provision of safer water, food refrigeration, better hygiene, behavioural influences, and other scientific developments of a

3

non-personal kind that owe little or nothing to the biomedical sciences and would have been introduced even if health was not brought forward as an argument in their favour. The reduction in exposure to infection had some effect on mortality in the nineteenth century and the impact of the medical procedures of immunization and therapy was delayed until the twentieth century.

McKeown is less categorical about and more appreciative of medical science and laboratory research when it comes to the present day. In his view about three quarters of the decline in morbidity is associated with the control of infectious diseases, the remainder with conditions not attributable to microorganisms. In his last book, admitting that medical sciences contributed to the "extension and refinement of methods of preventing the spread of infectious diseases" he suggests that, without abandoning the laboratory sciences, medical research should pay greater attention to health intelligence and epidemiology. With this last point we are all in agreement. As for his main thesis, however, *audi partem alteram* and his prominent contemporaries have other views.

Perhaps because McKeown has not been actively engaged in patient care during most of the past four decades, during which clinical medicine has altered beyond recognition (9), he is unfamiliar with present-day therapy, downgrades antimicrobial therapy, regards the evaluation of therapeutic procedures from a curious perspective, and pays insufficient attention to the importance of advances in the caring and curing services that enable individuals to receive a high level of care and treatment during illness (10). He does not mention the highly successful vaccination against yellow fever, tetanus and diphtheria. He is sceptical about the value of vaccines against whooping cough and measles, although his data seem in keeping with the conclusion that their introduction coincided with a decline in the incidence of both diseases (9). More important are the methodological objections raised against his views. What is the point of calculating the effect of specific anti-tuberculosis therapy on the number of deaths from tuberculosis since 1898, when the first effective drug came into use long afterwards (9)? The death rate from tuberculosis has been reduced by 51% since the introduction of specific chemotherapy. McKeown seems to have been victim of "the fallacy of the stretched abscissa" (9, 11); tracing mortality from a particular cause further back than unreliable diagnoses should permit and extrapolating, for example in tuberculosis, must be suspect (8).

Foremost among the problems that have drawn criticism is his use of mortality figures as the principal index of health and his virtual neglect of morbidity (12–14). "This narrow focus seems to indicate McKeown's basic contention that personal medical diagnosis and treatment has played a relatively small part in the improvement of 'health'. For health certainly means more than prolonged life, and in the public mind, at least, many of the most striking achievements of modern medicine have to do not only with saving life, but with the relief of serious suffering. The impact of antibiotics on painful and disabling infectious diseases is a case in point" (14). The assumption that standardized mortality ratios can be a measure

4

of morbidity and thus of the need for health care leads to the neglect of infections that affect people without always causing death, for example sexually transmitted diseases and influenza. "McKeown seems to give some credence to a widely held and fallacious belief that expenditure could be reduced in the short term by prevention of chronic degenerative disease" (8). Emphasis on mortality alone tends to obscure the importance of lengthening survival in an incurable or recurrent disease such as diabetes or pneumonia, where the age at death is significant (12). "Few persons would disparage medicine's ability to provide years of additional productive life to individuals who may eventually succumb to a disease they have borne" (14).

While the already well recognized influence of external, environmental and social factors on health has been rightly emphasized, it has been used by a number of non-medical writers for often very readable attacks on medicine which have been taken up by the media and also adopted by some institutions. They say that modern medicine concentrates on disease to the exclusion of the wholeness of the sick person. The malady is seen as somehow separate from the sufferer. The treatment of the disease as apart from the patient is widespread, and this is taken as a crime. "It is clearly bad science to conceive of illness in terms of specific diseases caused by specific agents; ...the notion of disease comes from those who have a vested interest in the continued viability of the notion of specific disease entities. By concentrating on diseases a form of medicine has developed, which beside being mechanical, is conceived as a rescue or repair service ... by thinking of illness in terms of diseases one has been led to believe that diagnosis leads to cure. The whirligig of disease identification goes round on and no one seems anxious to stop it, or get off" (15).

The critics of modern scientific medicine usually give ambiguous examples that lend themselves to various interpretations and are not necessarily accepted as disease entities in the strict sense; among them are mental conditions, dissatisfaction, frustration, barrenness, homosexuality, stress from overwork, depressive moods, the consequences of social isolation or alcoholism, and diet-related habits. There is, however, very little vagueness in the term infectious illness, although it can manifest itself in various forms or even reach an equilibrium with the organism. Since the discovery of the tuberculosis bacillus a century ago, the importance of such factors as the susceptibility of the host has been well recognized and the concept of human ecology has entered medical science.

Infectious diseases are nosological entities, caused by invasion of the body by various pathogenic microorganisms. The diseases may be affected by stress, nutrition, fatigue, and social and environmental factors, but without the pathogens there would be no infectious disease at all. This does not mean that the ill person as such, with his fears, feelings, perceptions and reactions, is not to be considered as a whole. Obviously it is necessary to create economic and social conditions conducive not only to the absence of disease but also to maximum wellbeing. Physicians concerned with infectious diseases do not dissociate themselves from political and social action to improve health. They were the first to promote prevention, first

5

to think about solving problems before they occurred as against the emphasis on curative medicine alone, and also first to realize the need for international cooperation; it was for infections that this started years before WHO was created.

Beginnings of a reappraisal

In *Man adapting* Dubos (*16*), under the heading "the so-called conquest of microbial diseases", says about the optimistic 1950s:

> A very large percentage of the microbial agents of disease had been isolated, identified, and cultivated in artificial media or in tissue cultures; bacteriological cleanliness of the food and water supplies had been improved through technological advances; practical procedures had been worked out for the large-scale production of killed or attenuated bacterial and viral vaccines; highly effective drugs had become available for the treatment of bacterial and parasitic infections; a variety of pesticides had been synthesized and had proven their usefulness for the control of insect vectors.
>
> In many places, economic prosperity and social organization have now made it possible to translate into practice the scientific achievements of the microbiological era. As a result, the mortality rates of infectious diseases have been brought down to a very low level, particularly among children and young adults, and the life expectancy at birth has soared to unprecedented high levels.

Most clinicians, public health officers, epidemiologists and microbiologists felt justified therefore in proclaiming during the 1950s that the conquest of infectious diseases had finally been achieved (see Fig. 1).

> Surprisingly enough, this euphoria has not yet been dampened by the fact that the morbidity rates of infection have not decreased significantly, and in some cases have actually increased. Despite so much oratory on the conquest of microbial diseases, the paradox is that the percentage of hospital beds occupied by patients suffering from infection is now as high as it was fifty years ago. Today, as in the past, moreover, disorders of the respiratory and digestive tracts with a microbial etiology constitute the most frequent causes of absenteeism from school, office, factory, or from training in the armed forces.

The same applies in Europe and other developed regions.

One of the first sobering warnings came from Sabin (*17*) in 1969, showing that in the United States the problem of infectious diseases is still present and that it produces many deaths and illnesses, and is a considerable cost to the economy. In the special volume as tribute on his 80th birthday to the Nobel prizewinner in immunology Sir MacFarlane Burnet, whose contribution to infectious disease research is inestimable, one of his closest collaborators, Fenner (*18*), himself one of the world's leading microbiologists, commented on Burnet's upsetting many of his colleagues from about the mid-fifties by playing down the importance of research on infectious diseases and later by his attack on molecular biology in terms of its value to society (*19*). "The events since suggest that he overstated the case in considering the 'conquest' of infectious diseases by considering only mortality and not morbidity and by not recognizing the enormous potential of DNA recombinant research for understanding nature, and for its potential contribution to human wellbeing".

6

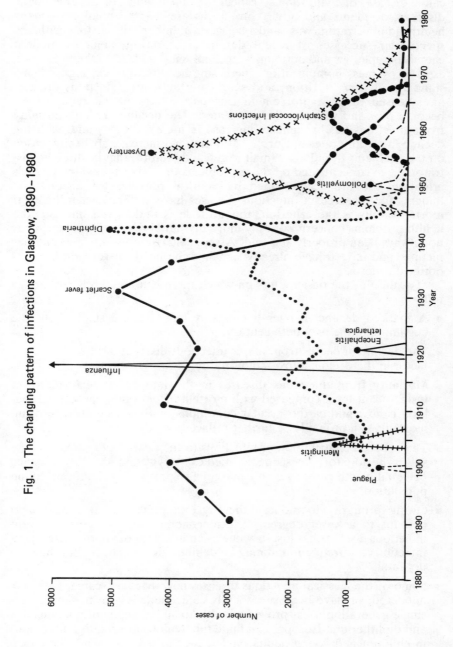

Fig. 1. The changing pattern of infections in Glasgow, 1890–1980

As one by one the major infections disappeared from the ten top ranking diseases in the mortality lists of countries, to be replaced by the so-called diseases of civilization — cancer, cardiovascular diseases, metabolic diseases, accidents and other chronic diseases — the opinion of many health administrators was, and of a good number still is, that with the spectacular successes of recent decades, the development of modern chemotherapeutics and antibiotics, technological advances, the protection assured by mass immunization, increasing health coverage, higher living standards, better nutrition, and safe water supplies, infectious diseases have ceased to be a problem in Europe, and those that remain have become rare and will soon be eradicated. The decline in child mortality from infections has brought an increase in life expectancy and, with the decline in fertility rates in Europe, attention has increasingly been focused on the problems of old age. Small wonder, therefore, that health administrators have concentrated on those problems that have gained the public's attention and are accompanied by political pressure for action. The budgets for research in infectious diseases have suffered accordingly. If mortality only is the criterion, this attitude is understandable. But the health problems concern not only mortality but also morbidity, which has not always been properly assessed. Assessments of morbidity give another picture, and indeed have already signalled the need for revision of over-optimistic views.

To sum up, the basic points on which there is no disagreement are as follows.

- A marked decline in overall mortality has occurred since about the beginning of the twentieth century.

- The decline in deaths from major infectious diseases has been the main factor in the decline in overall mortality.

- Mortality from infectious diseases in the late 1970s declined to an insignificant level compared with mortality from other causes, particularly cancer and cardiovascular conditions, and as a percentage of all mortality can probably be further reduced.

- The reduced contribution of infections to the death rates cannot be the sole criterion for the scope of medical services in the future, since personal health care, even in a marginal role, is vitally significant to the population.

- Owing primarily to modern therapy and preventive measures, and perhaps to a lesser degree to socioeconomic factors, mortality from infectious diseases has lost its value as an indicator of importance. Many infections are frequent and may be debilitating and costly, but they are not fatal.

- Some of the classical infectious diseases have become scarce, have disappeared, or have been successfully controlled. Within the space of a single generation it has proved possible to all but wipe out poliomyelitis and diphtheria in Europe, eliminate tuberculous meningitis and tetanus in children and young adults, and reduce tuberculosis and many bacterial infections. On the global level, for the first time in history one of the most serious diseases, smallpox, has been eradicated. Diagnosis and therapy have become more precise and effective in reducing the case fatality. Scientific progress has made it possible to influence microorganisms and to modify positively the response of the human organism.

● Society cannot neglect the single patient or the small group affected by a serious disease, who will continue to depend on scientific medicine. Considering all the various bacterial and viral infections to which man is, and will continue to be, exposed until better control methods are to hand, such people are not in the minority. Not only deaths from but also the prevalence of communicable diseases can further decline in Europe, and indeed many diseases may disappear; but some will continue and cannot be eradicated simply by bureaucratic changes to statistical categories or professional competences.

A vital necessity: better information

Accurate information on the morbidity and mortality of disease is difficult to obtain, but in many parts of Europe more is available than in most parts of the world. All recent analyses have used two sources of information from countries in all WHO regions: one is the list of diseases considered by governments as major public health problems, the other the list of principal causes of death.

Information for the decade of the 1960s shows that, except in Europe, North America and a few other countries, infectious diseases and malnutrition constituted nearly all of the first ten major public health problems, and from about a third to a half of the ten principal causes of death. In the European Region[a] (except for Algeria, Morocco and Turkey) the situation was different. Only two infectious diseases were mentioned as public health problems (tuberculosis and venereal diseases) and two as principal causes of death (tuberculosis and respiratory infections). Infectious diseases accounted in Europe for between about 5% and about 17% of the total causes of death.

It is difficult to construct a table of the top ten public health problems from the information provided by Algeria, Morocco and Turkey, but all of the five clear priorities in public health were communicable diseases, and three of the ten main causes of death were also communicable diseases. These three countries therefore differ considerably from the others in the European Region.

The country reviews and statistics (for 1974–1977) of European countries in the latest edition of *Health services in Europe* (*20*) record the infections of importance as influenza, hepatitis, mumps, rubella, varicella, scarlet fever, meningococcal conditions, dysentery, salmonellosis and other food

---

[a]The European Region is the geographical area from Greenland to Vladivostok in the USSR and from the North Pole to North Africa. It includes 33 countries with a population of approximately 800 million. Algeria, Morocco and Turkey come within the European Region but are included in WHO statistical tables under "North Africa and the Eastern Mediterranean".

infections, tuberculosis, and sexually transmitted diseases. However, the picture for Europe as given in the usual WHO tables is not a true reflection of the situation. The respiratory diseases, though in the list of main causes of death, are not among the principal health problems. Only a few countries have included pneumonia and influenza among the group of communicable diseases, yet they are of great importance as causes of morbidity, disability and absenteeism and are thus of great economic importance. Their not being included points perhaps to a lack of adequate notification and recording. Similarly, hepatitis, non-classical venereal diseases and hospital infections are not mentioned but are relatively important. In one country of the European Region about 800 cases of diarrhoeal disease were notified in a year. However, 1800 patients with dysentery alone were hospitalized in that year, up to 120 000 cases of diarrhoeal diseases of all kinds occurred per month, and the national epidemiologist estimated that about 1.2 million cases occurred every year.

Although all countries of the European Region have general statistical information about certain major infectious diseases (see Chapter 3), not all have systems assessing preventive services, for example vaccination coverage, diagnostic procedures, and other measurements such as those relating to the environment and the social background. Most information is derived from hospitals, little from the primary care services except in eastern Europe. It is difficult to imagine how it is possible to plan for health services, assess health needs, or deploy health resources without information from the primary community level. The picture is certainly distorted by the evaluation of effectiveness and of trends on the basis of information from inpatient facilities, which account as a maximum for 10% but usually much less of total illnesses; this leads to a serious underestimation of outpatients or community episodes of disease. "The term 'statistics' is now wholly inadequate without an indication of the specific uses to which they will be put for clinical, planning, evaluation, or epidemiological surveillance purposes. This poses questions about the information that should be collected and at what level" (21).

WHO in Europe plans its programmes according to the wishes of its member governments as expressed before the programmes are finalized. WHO provides a brief situation analysis and the programme perspectives, objectives, targets, and approaches for the different sectors, and governments are requested to give their comments on whether they consider the proposed targets relevant to the regional programme, and to suggest alternative targets and assign to each individual activity "high", "medium" or "low" priority. There is substantial subjective disagreement about such expressions, which inevitably are value judgements depending on the professional positions and attitudes of the reviewers. In the field of infections it is difficult to plan exactly for a period years ahead (although it is possible to plan for services) as the stated choices are often overruled by the changing situation. A single outbreak or the importation of even one dangerous pathogen may change the priorities. Whatever the situation, the replies by governments will probably be based on an imperfect information system. Far from being useless such information could, in spite of its

10

Table 1. Official numbers of cases of (and deaths from) some infectious diseases in Europe as reported to WHO between 1973 and 1977, illustrating the gross underreporting of these diseases

Disease	1973	1974	1975	1976	1977
Influenza	6 938 030 (32 959)	4 286 720 (15 489)	6 233 666 (8 487)	4 533 901	2 686 258
Hepatitis	331 350 (2 417)	282 878 (1 884)	268 517 (976)	233 723	207 577
Salmonella infections	20 406 (214)	16 053 (128)	60 115 (3)	81 586	47 282
Other gastrointestinal diseases	143 422 (196)	123 791 (211)	162 384 (3)	605 556	583 056
Sexually transmitted diseases	480 580	478 783	394 110	439 003	213 660
Tuberculosis	343 010 (33 892)	309 409 (23 769)	268 226 (5 828)	178 315	107 712
Diseases involving the CNS	13 898 (1 648)	12 387 (1 274)	18 056 (235)	25 534	17 822
Measles	935 534 (1 000)	712 975 (511)	688 742 (85)	614 308	305 027
Mumps	363 824 (34)	445 588 (29)	633 483 (4)	382 379	438 398
Pertussis	64 111 (279)	71 579 (135)	55 256 (8)	56 578	45 639
	1 363 469 (1 313)	1 230 142 (675)	1 377 481 (97)	1 053 265	789 064
Total	9 634 165 (72 639)	6 740 162 (43 430)	8 782 565 (1 562)	7 140 883	465 241

Source: World health statistics quarterly.

11

subjectivity, be an element in assessing what is considered important in the field of infections. A major disadvantage is that there is no proper balance between, for example, communicable diseases, chronic diseases, accidents, mental health, manpower planning and environmental health in relation to the resources proposed.

How can the importance of infections be assessed? The classical assessment is on the basis of reports of infectious diseases as prepared and sent by governments to WHO. An analysis of the pattern of notification in Europe shows that the reports are incomplete and unreliable. Nevertheless, an attempt has been made in Chapter 3 to deduce trends from this information. Table 1 presents the official figures for ten selected infectious diseases. It shows that in the years 1973–1977 a *minimum* of 37 million Europeans suffered from selected infections, and even those were vastly underreported. This brings us to the International Classification of Diseases (ICD).

What does the ICD tell us?

In 1855, William Farr, the medical statistician of the General Register Office of England and Wales, submitted to the International Statistical Congress in Paris a proposal for a classification of causes of death arranged under five groups: epidemic diseases, constitutional (general) diseases, local diseases arranged according to anatomical site, developmental diseases, and diseases that are the direct result of violence.

This arrangement was used as the basis for an international list of causes of death from 1864, and proved so durable that ICD in its ninth revision retains the same basic structure. By and large, Chapter I of the ICD includes the main communicable diseases (with the notable exceptions of pneumonia and influenza, which are in Chapter VIII), while localized infections are classified with other diseases of the organ concerned (eye and ear infections in Chapter VI, skin infections in Chapter XII, etc.). This last group is becoming more and more important in Europe. Throughout the various revisions of the ICD the content of Chapter I has changed little, and the diseases notified under it and other chapters have become important indicators of public health in comparisons between developing and developed countries.

The introduction to the ICD in 1977 describes the difficulties in selecting criteria for the classification of diseases: "...efforts to base a statistical classification on a strictly logical adherence to any one axis have failed in the past. The various titles will represent a series of necessary compromises between classifications based on aetiology, anatomical site, circumstances of onset, etc., as well as the quality of information available on medical reports". It quotes William Farr's statement a century ago as valid today: "Classification is a method of generalization. Several classifications may, therefore, be used with advantage; and the physician, the pathologist, or the jurist, each from his own point of view, may legitimately classify the diseases and the causes of death in the way he thinks best adapted to facilitate his inquiries, and to yield general results". The ICD is a valuable, indeed indispensable work. Although it gives many possible choices, that made in Chapter I does not show the importance of communicable diseases if the health administration does not exercise the freedom of choice. Thus any statistics on communicable or infectious diseases should refer not only to the 001–139 categories of the ICD but also to other specified parts; this may be possible, at least in Europe where computers are widely used for statistics.

The ICD three-digit list includes infectious pharyngitis among acute respiratory infections (460–466) but among infectious and parasitic diseases only if it is caused by streptococci. Bacterial and viral pneumonia and influenza (480–487) are not included among infectious and parasitic diseases, nor is pleurisy (511) or abscess of the lung (513). Bacterial meningitis (320), meningitis attributable to other organisms (321), meningitis of unspecified cause (322), and encephalitis (323) are under diseases of the nervous system and sense organs. Only meningococcal infection (036) is under infectious and parasitic diseases. Acute rheumatic fever with or without heart involvement (390,391) is under diseases of the circulatory system. Infections of the kidney (590) are also not under infections in the basic list of the ICD, which everyone uses, but under diseases of the genitourinary system. This is also the case for cystitis (595), the most common hospital infection; inflammatory diseases of the female genital organs (614–616), a most common consequence of sexually transmitted disease or other infections; infective and parasitic conditions in the mother classifiable elsewhere but complicating pregnancy, childbirth, and the puerperium (647); infections of the skin and subcutaneous tissue (680–686); osteomyelitis, periostitis and other infections involving bone (730); and infections specific to the perinatal period (771). Supplementary classifications of factors influencing health status and contact with health services use V01–V007 codes for contacts and carriers or the need for vaccination, but are not used for assessing the importance of diseases.

The tabular list of inclusions and detailed four-digit subcategories, a more comprehensive extension of the three-digit list, also excludes acute respiratory infections and the other above-mentioned infectious diseases. This list is little (if at all) used in practice. The ICD has been brought to near perfection and is very valuable in the classification of malignancies or accidents, but it is tied to classification by organ and manifest conditions, in which the etiology of diseases is often lost; and the dual code is of little help in practice. Some of the inconsistencies have been recognized. But the ICD is revised only about once in ten years and until the next revision the classification will not take the etiology into consideration or group bacterial, viral and parasitic diseases adequately. The basic problem is that the ICD assumes that epidemiological surveillance systems are primarily to collect data on deaths from classical infections excluding, for example, respiratory infections. This has been justified on the grounds that diagnosis for some can be confirmed, but for others it is possible in probably a very small proportion of cases only, since many countries do not have enough facilities for virus identification. Terms like "flu", "influenza" and "grippe" are very loosely used, both in epidemic and non-epidemic periods, and separation of the diagnosis of influenza from that of other upper respiratory infections is, in many instances, artificial. For these rather strange reasons transferring influenza to Chapter I has always been opposed and repeatedly rejected during successive ICD revisions; but it appears that acute respiratory infections (460–466) will be included there in the next revision. The usefulness of the ICD for infectious diseases in Europe is limited; as it is applied it is an obstacle to the proper evaluation of infections.[a]

Efforts to modify the ICD are not lacking, but seem to be mostly in relation to impairment and disability rather than etiology and pathology. In an interesting innovative approach WHO (22) suggests that impairments, disabilities and handicaps should be classified according to the principle that classification is subordinate to the purpose of assessing the consequences to the individual. But this has nothing to do with the ICD, which should theoretically help in obtaining an exact knowledge of what is happening in the community in terms of the relationship between host, agent and environment. To obtain a total count of infectious and parasitic diseases involves a question of definition that is not easy to resolve. There are two possible approaches: either a clear and logical etiological classification or a purely organ-oriented (anatomical) classification with etiological subgroups. In either there will be problems when the etiology is not known or specified, or when infections affect many organs. Tables 2 and 3 illustrate some possible definitions of deaths due to infectious and parasitic diseases classified outside Chapter I of the ICD. In Table 2, based on the eighth revision of the ICD, the definition is in terms of the categories of list A; the ratio of deaths from diseases outside Chapter I to those in Chapter I varies from over 20:1 (England and Wales) to under 2:1 (Yugoslavia). Overall, about 81% of deaths due to infection are not counted as being due to infection! Table 3, based on the ninth revision of the ICD, has two different definitions, one in terms of the detailed four-digit list (see also Annex 1), the other in terms of categories of the basic tabulation list. This clearly shows how vastly the infectious diseases are underestimated.

During the preparation of the ninth revision of the ICD, requests were made that certain manifestations of infectious disease classified in Chapter I should appear in the anatomical chapters. These requests were met by introducing a dual classification for these conditions and differentiating the two categories by means of a dagger symbol and an asterisk. Thus tuberculous meningitis is classified in two places: 013.0† and 320.4*. In all such cases the code with a dagger is the primary classification and that with the asterisk secondary. For the tenth revision it might be appropriate to insert in Chapter I some secondary categories for infectious and parasitic diseases classified primarily in other chapters, using two different symbols to differentiate them. A simpler solution would be to tabulate the data

---

[a] In fact studies carried out in France, in November 1982, showed that there is a considerable artificial decline in mortality from infectious diseases in infants when the ninth revision of the ICD is used. This is due to classifying deaths from infection according to Chapter XV (document U. 164, INSERM, November 1982).

14

Table 2. Deaths in Europe, 1974–1978, from infectious diseases, according to the eighth revision of the ICD

Country	ICD-8 chapter	1974	1975	1976	1977	1978	Average 1974–1978
Austria	Chapter I	781	743	728	654	566	695
	Other chapters	5 482	6 667	6 062	4 532	4 992	5 547
Belgium	Chapter I	890	916	967	875		
	Other chapters	3 504	4 284	4 469	3 153		
Bulgaria	Chapter I	1 127	1 061	987	941	907	1 004
	Other chapters	7 681	10 273	8 082	9 016	7 497	8 509
Czechoslovakia	Chapter I	1 363	1 230				
	Other chapters	11 249	11 526				
Denmark	Chapter I	283	247	249	232	238	249
	Other chapters	3 243	2 783	3 705	2 494	2 634	2 971
Finland	Chapter I	470	512	492	464		
	Other chapters	2 723	2 824	3 166	3 062		
France	Chapter I	8 069	8 030	8 243	7 940		
	Other chapters	18 544	18 723	19 320	16 063		
German Democratic Republic	Chapter I	1 538	1 586	1 453			
	Other chapters	8 991	10 518	9 521			
Germany, Federal Republic of	Chapter I	6 399	6 589	6 033	5 234	5 290	5 909
	Other chapters	26 910	33 394	27 657	24 203	26 085	27 649
Greece	Chapter I	1 386	1 306	1 331	1 301	1 115	1 288
	Other chapters	3 666	4 759	3 627	4 379	2 759	3 838
Hungary	Chapter I	2 148	1 969	1 971	1 720	1 715	1 904
	Other chapters	4 064	5 409	4 428	4 272	6 383	4 911
Iceland	Chapter I	13	13	17	13	10	14
	Other chapters	139	155	147	139	156	147
Ireland	Chapter I	350	311	325	334		
	Other chapters	3 095	2 792	3 097	2 510		
Italy	Chapter I	5 997	5 462	4 729	4 124		
	Other chapters	24 127	28 634	23 988	23 284		
Luxembourg	Chapter I	30	20	27	22	24	25
	Other chapters	152	121	146	72	103	119

continued

15

Table 2. (contd)

Country	ICD-8 chapter	1974	1975	1976	1977	1978	Average 1974–1978
Malta	Chapter I	25	23	19	21		
	Other chapters	84	69	80	48		
Netherlands	Chapter I	736	756	624	590	578	657
	Other chapters	4 675	4 724	4 918	3 901	4 447	4 533
Norway	Chapter I	277	351	287	297	290	300
	Other chapters	3 816	4 000	3 934	3 589	3 444	3 756
Poland	Chapter I	6 442	6 444	6 417	6 439	6 113	6 371
	Other chapters	13 134	16 385	14 438	14 214	14 860	14 606
Portugal	Chapter I	2 564	2 188				
	Other chapters	7 920	6 877				
Romania	Chapter I	3 783	3 446	2 768	2 847	2 477	3 064
	Other chapters	17 229	18 902	19 189	17 318	16 589	17 845
Spain	Chapter I	5 953	5 853	5 846	5 616	5 697	5 793
	Other chapters	25 294	24 275	21 538	19 928	18 221	21 851
Sweden	Chapter I	671	670	653	609	557	632
	Other chapters	4 093	4 362	5 060	4 240	4 788	4 509
Switzerland	Chapter I	692	617	543	523	451	565
	Other chapters	2 304	2 566	3 205	2 191	2 300	2 514
United Kingdom: England & Wales	Chapter I	3 063	3 008	2 670	2 450	2 401	2 719
	Other chapters	58 959	59 986	73 712	62 438	63 295	63 478
United Kingdom: Northern Ireland	Chapter I	155	125	119	111	96	121
	Other chapters	1 451	1 090	1 267	1 137	1 222	1 234
United Kingdom: Scotland	Chapter I	447	412	427	344	329	392
	Other chapters	4 152	4 189	5 378	4 333	4 818	4 574
Yugoslavia	Chapter I	5 013	5 080	4 477	4 149	4 014	4 547
	Other chapters	8 913	11 158	9 539	7 443	8 100	9 031

[a] Defined as the following categories of list A: A72, A78, A80, A81, A89, A90, A91, A92, A95, A99, A100, A107, A116, A119, A123.

16

Table 3. Deaths in the United Kingdom, 1979–1980,
from infectious diseases,
according to the ninth revision of the ICD

ICD-9 chapter	England & Wales	Scotland	
		1979	1980
Chapter I	2 273	285	292
Other chapters[a]	78 064	6 236	6 107
Other chapters[b]	66 406	4 865	4 898

[a] Defined as in Annex 1, Group B.

[b] Defined as the following categories of the basic tabulation list: 220, 233, 240, 250, 251, 303, 310, 311, 312, 314, 320, 321, 322, 342, 351, 371, 372, 373, 392, 436.

according to the basic tabulation list in the ninth revision and extract the infectious categories as presented in Annex 1. Here the relations are shown in the relative position of the two broad groups using the basic tabulation list grouping instead of the detailed four-digit categories.

Some experts using the ICD feel that the transfer of *all* the infectious and parasitic diseases to Chapter I would bring advantages but also the loss of some useful health indices. The correctness of those indices may be, and indeed is, contested. Such experts assume sophisticated services and epidemiological interest, more work by persons tabulating the disease, and also perhaps a certain detachment from the day-to-day realities of health institutions and from the ways tabulation is actually carried out. This question will be discussed by ICD committees in the future but, in the mean time, national health authorities should use their freedom of choice and include, as some already do, all bacterial, viral and parasitic diseases among infectious diseases, regardless of where they are classified at present.

Other approaches to assessing the importance of infections

Another way of assessing the importance of infections is by consulting specialists in the field who advise WHO on activities needed. Such a consultation was held at the WHO Regional Office for Europe in June 1979,[a] on the basis of a yearly questionnaire sent to governments. This indicated that the areas of primary concern should be: respiratory infections, hepatitis, diarrhoeal diseases, bacterial and viral foodborne infections, bacterial meningitis, hospital infections (bacterial and viral), sexually transmitted diseases of the first and, in particular, of the second generation, rabies, and imported diseases (especially malaria). Among related problems, the areas of primary concern were: vaccination practices, laboratory-acquired infections, plasmid-transferred resistance and

[a] Unpublished WHO document ICP/ESD 005, Copenhagen, 1979.

17

genetic engineering, interferon and antiviral drugs, the dissemination of epidemiological information, and the availability and breeding of non-human primates in Europe for medical research, particularly for vaccine development. However, such experts may have all the scientific knowledge but not necessarily an appreciation of the magnitude of the problem — for example, herpes vaccine has been developed, but how can it can be used?

A third way of assessing the importance of infectious diseases is to ask countries. This method implies value judgements, but might show where improvement in the delivery of health care can be made. In 1981 a questionnaire containing some 39 items was sent to the national officers responsible for communicable diseases and preventive health measures in 34 European countries, asking them to indicate what they thought should be considered by WHO in Europe in future, and to rank the subjects in order of priority. They were also invited to make suggestions about subjects not mentioned in the questionnaire. This addition is without scientific rigour and may include purely personal views — areas in which a particular officer lacks up-to-date information or for which he would like to have a more comprehensive regional picture. However, the assumption was that such areas are those regarded by the people responsible for national guidelines, rules, and regulations and the formulation and implementation of control strategies (and so eventually the evaluation of the situation at the national level) as being particularly important or as presenting problems. Disregarding answers from four countries that had not provided the ranked list, the priorities were as follows (listed according to frequency when indicated by more than five countries).

1. *New vaccines:* utilization; results; quality control; new developments in immunology.

2. *Epidemiological surveillance systems:* improvement of present national systems and practices; need to integrate data from laboratories and from special community investigators; trials and epidemiological studies to obtain a better picture of epidemiological happenings; assessment of trends; role of communicable diseases surveillance centres; harmonization of lists, forms and codes for notification of diseases; dissemination and exchange of information.

3. *Immunizable diseases:* reassessment of present policies and programmes; evaluation of delivery and coverage; surveillance of undesirable effects and sequelae.

4. *New diseases:* unusual diseases; uncommon diseases caused by dangerous pathogens of recent appearance and their management; procedures from clinical suspicion to etiological diagnosis; role of opportunistic pathogens.

5. *Serological epidemiology:* assessment of circulating pathogens; silent infections and antibody prevalence; results of immunization activities.

6. *Training in communicable diseases:* improved specific training for epidemiologists and primary health physicians.

18

Priorities 7–10 were of equal rank and have been arbitrarily placed in the following order.

7. *Handling of data:* computers and other automatized techniques.

8. *Imported diseases:* increasing importance of the importation of diseases that are at present rare, especially of tropical diseases.

9. *Change in emphasis:* need for reorientation and institutional adjustment to the changing ecology and pathology of infectious diseases.

10. *Economic and social aspects of infectious diseases:* cost of preventive measures, treatment, invalidity, social outlays, absenteeism, and social conditions contributing to the occurrence, spread or maintenance of infections.

Many countries requested discussion of specific diseases of particular national concern such as tuberculosis, hepatitis, rabies, meningitis, streptococcal infections, hospital infections, zoonoses, foodborne and waterborne infections, sexually transmitted diseases, tick-borne meningoencephalitis, haemorrhagic fevers and influenza. Special subjects not included in the WHO check list but brought forward were:

- epidemiological aspects of the influence of modern technology on the risk of infectious disease: intensive care units, dialysis procedures, catheters, ventilation and air-conditioning systems, new farming and food-chain techniques, irrigation projects and urbanization

- relationships and cooperation with the mass media in outbreaks or epidemics of various infectious diseases and the need for full discussion

- access to reference material on specific infections or epidemiological problems.

It should be noted that the priorities as seen by the administrators responsible for infectious diseases were remarkably similar to those proposed by the experts.

Expectations and realities

Some of the forecasts made in the United Kingdom in 1970 for the period up to 1990 (*23*) proved correct, others did not. In bacterial infections it proved correct that the range of available antibiotics would continue to increase and that they would in many cases be more specific. But the development of resistance has been equally impressive. It is doubtful whether we have achieved the early diagnosis and control of urinary infections expected to be routine by the 1980s. Progress has been made in understanding the process of intracellular survival of bacteria and the biochemical bases of the hypersensitivity and autoimmune processes that accompany long-term persistence of bacteria and their products in the tissues. We are still at the beginning of the development of substances that may enhance man's natural resistance to infections generally. Progress has been achieved in health measures to prevent the transfer of organisms between species, and in the typing of the pathogens responsible for outbreaks of infections.

Although some progress has been made, we are still far from the predicted development of vaccines against sexually transmitted diseases.

In virus infections progress has been made in the development of vaccines, for example hepatitis B vaccine, and is expected to continue, for example with hepatitis A vaccine. Research on effective antiviral drugs for prophylactic and therapeutic use (amantadine, rimantadine, ribavirin) is encouraging, but the predictions half way to 1990 for other than RNA viruses (influenza and respiratory syncytial viruses) have so far failed. It was also hoped that by 1980 a way would have been found to stimulate the body's own production of interferon. This has not happened. Developments have made it possible for larger quantities of leukocyte and fibroblast interferon to be produced in laboratories, and experiments in the preventive and therapeutic use of interferon started in 1981. While broad-spectrum antiviral compounds safe enough to be used against minor infections are expected to be available by 1990 and perhaps earlier, it is feared that resistance to them will by then begin to emerge as a problem similar to that of antibiotic resistance.

An unprecedented success was that of the global eradication of smallpox. The eradication of measles, thought to be possible by about 1975, has not yet been achieved, and rubella vaccination, expected to be routine by that time, is carried out in only a few European countries. An effective mumps vaccine has become available as predicted, but its application is not general and it meets with little enthusiasm.

Influenza vaccines have not, as was hoped, been added to routine child immunization programmes. The forecast that improved inactivated vaccines would be available by the early 1970s and safe attenuated vaccines by 1980 is more or less correct, but the frequent antigenic mutations of the influenza virus still present difficulties and make necessary a very careful selection of virus strains for the production of vaccines, particularly live vaccines. We still have to wait for the predicted effective multiple oral vaccine against rhinoviruses. No usable vaccine to prevent respiratory syncytial virus infections is as yet available, but work is progressing.

By 1980 viruses were expected to have been identified as causal agents in a number of tumours. So far progress has been slow, although in at least three instances there is very strong evidence to support the hypothesis: transformation induced by herpesvirus type 2, nasopharyngeal carcinoma due to Epstein-Barr virus, and primary liver cancer (the chances of developing hepatoma are 200–300 times greater in HBsAg carriers).

Information systems on morbidity are not adequate and have not in general improved. A population-based approach to assessing the importance of infections, particularly respiratory and enteric infections, has only sporadically been attempted because of the overtaxing of the health services. WHO and all the governments of Europe place emphasis on primary care, for which there is as yet no suitable and agreed international classification, and at this level the reporting of infections is the most deficient.

20

By the very nature of his discipline, the clinical or laboratory worker in infectious diseases tends to concentrate on new diagnostic methods, drugs, the antigenicity of vaccines, biochemical research or parasitic taxonomy, rather than on trend assessment, perspectives and ecological changes in the infections he is dealing with, or on the public health importance of infections in general and the options he will have to face in the future. Indeed, comments on the newer historical perspective are rare at scientific meetings or in journals of infectious diseases. On the whole, more effort has been invested in recent decades in laboratory work than in the synoptic and constructive epidemiology of infectious diseases.

The latest WHO report on the world health situation (24) states:

> Data on morbidity are even less reliable than those on mortality. It appears, though, that there has been a significant increase or resurgence of certain communicable diseases, schistosomiasis being an example of an increase and malaria of a resurgence. Little progress can be reported with regard to tuberculosis or sexually transmitted diseases, though the conquest of smallpox appears to have been completed during the period under review.[a] ... The leprosy problem has not declined to any great extent over the past 15 years. ... During the period 1973–1977, a rise in morbidity from epidemic cerebrospinal meningitis was observed in many European countries. ... There have been increases in the incidence of zoonoses and in the risk factors associated with poor food hygiene. It is expected that in future years the increasing populations of man, livestock, pet animals, and man-associated wildlife will cause an exponential increase of zoonotic and foodborne diseases in rural and urban areas if the development of those activities of veterinary services with a bearing on human health goes on at the present pace. ... Although some countries managed to free themselves of cholera, the disease spread to 15 cholera-free countries or areas in all regions except the Americas during the 5-year period [1973–1977]. ... The resistance of gonococcal strains to penicillin and other antibiotics continued its upward trend, particularly in areas where non-observance or absence of national drug control regulations fostered the misuse of antibiotics. ... Since 1975 an increasing number of countries have reported an impressive increase in syphilis transmission. ... The epidemic trend of gonococcal infections has been declining in some countries after reaching a peak in about 1974–1975, but this decline has often been more than compensated for by an increase in the incidence of nongonococcal genital infections — the latter being now more common in nearly all countries. Particular attention is being paid to certain serotypes of *Chlamydia trachomatis* which are associated with 35–50% of all cases of nongonococcal urethritis and cervicitis.

---

[a] Eradication of smallpox has since been confirmed. However, 32 cases of monkeypox were recorded in humans in 1982 and a further 5 up to 13 May 1983. The current total of such cases is 88. During 1982 there were 5 episodes in which human transmission could be presumed, including one instance where it was thought that, for the first time, a third generation of cases had occurred. The revised estimate for unvaccinated household contacts is about 15%. Reports from the field suggest that the greater number of monkeypox cases detected is due not only to better surveillance but also to a real increase. It is impossible to say whether this trend will continue or whether it is only part of a regular cyclic fluctuation. It is, however, a matter of greater concern than had originally been anticipated, and intensive surveillance continues in Zaire. *Weekly epidemiological record*, **58**: 149–154 (1983).

Globally, dengue has raised its head again, expanded in Asia, and caused, for example in 1981, over 100 000 cases of disease and a number of deaths in one small Caribbean country alone.

In spite of all the successes, morbidity from many infectious diseases in Europe is still very high. "New" infectious agents and diseases have emerged and new challenges have been created by the importation of diseases into Europe. Unexpected problems have arisen from resistance, new technology, or the public attitude to preventive measures. In fact, a 1982 consultation in Geneva on the surveillance of microbial resistance has said that in recent years the risk of serious bacterial infections has actually increased among many groups of patients in the developed countries.

Since the heralded conquest of infectious diseases, Lassa, Marburg and Ebola fevers and a few other haemorrhagic diseases have made their appearance, and unexpected epidemics of Rift Valley fever, formerly thought to be of little or no relevance to man, have broken out. New agents of disease, *Legionella pneumophila* and the agent of Pontiac fever, have been identified. *Yersinia enterocolitica* and *Campylobacter* infections have become major new infections in man. Most importantly, new forms of non-A non-B and delta agent hepatitis have been discovered as new nosological entities in the hepatitis complex, and hepatitis B has been linked etiologically with primary liver cancer. Acquired immune deficiency syndrome (AIDS) and Kawasaki disease have entered the list of suspected new infections. Rotavirus has been discovered and identified as a major cause of diarrhoea in children and Norwalk agent newly identified as an entero-pathogen. Pseudomembranous ulceronecrotic colitis of the newborn has been demonstrated to be an infectious disease, a number of sudden infant deaths have been linked with common respiratory infections and botulism, the role of cytomegalovirus has proved to be equal to or more important than that of rubella in its damaging consequences to the newborn, the staphylo-coccal toxic shock syndrome has appeared as a new disease, and chlamydiae have been identified as the cause of a wide range of clinical diseases. Epidemic outbreaks of cholera, dysentery and typhoid fever, some causing hundreds of cases, are again happening, and salmonellosis is everywhere on the increase. Pediculosis and scabies have reappeared in the affluent countries of Europe after more than 20 years of extreme rarity, giardiasis has become a common disease and mycoses are becoming more common.

Moreover, the so-called residual health problems attributable to infections have refused to disappear and some have increased. With changes in ways of living, international travel, and medical technology and therapy, new problems have arisen. Infectious and parasitic diseases are imported; tourists die of imported malaria, and in one country of the Region this disease has become a major public health problem. Opportunistic pathogens, organisms of low virulence that cause clinically significant disease in man, particularly in hospitals, are of increasing importance. Patients and personnel working in transfusion and renal dialysis units are at risk and increasingly victims of certain viral infections; patients with systemic diseases such as diabetes mellitus, leukaemia, aplastic anaemia, advanced cancer or Hodgkin's disease, and those treated with immunosuppressive drugs or who have received transplants, are particularly vulnerable. However, nosocomial infections (often caused by organisms with plasmid-mediated resistance to antibiotics) are unfortunately not statistically numbered among the communicable diseases.

Infectious diseases and primary health care

At the International Conference on Primary Health Care at Alma-Ata in September 1978, a Declaration (25) was accepted by the countries of the world, European countries among them, that will shape health policies in the years to come. It has been extensively discussed and written about and WHO has made it the cornerstone of its philosophy and a base for the formulation of strategies for health for all by the year 2000.

Before Alma-Ata, primary health care was regarded as synonymous with "basic health services", "easily accessible care", "first-contact care", "services provided by generalists", "family physician care", "first physician care", "non-specialist, non-hospital care", "immediate care", "care that can be provided most economically", "immediate care for disease and trauma", "care that satisfies the need of the population", "care for common conditions, triage, and referral", "what most people use most of the time for most of their health problems", "majority care", etc. (26). The definition in the Declaration of Alma-Ata is:

> Primary health care is essential health care ... made universally accessible to individuals and families in the community through their full participation and at a cost that the community and country can afford. ... It forms an integral part both of the country's health system, of which it is the central function and main focus, and of the overall social and economic development of the community.

The aim, given in the Declaration's ten points, is to achieve an acceptable level of health that will permit all people of the world to live a socially and economically productive life in a spirit of social justice; the points also set out the moral principles and philosophy that motivate the Declaration and how to achieve the policy. The main operative point, in VII.3, states that primary health care includes at least:

> education concerning prevailing health problems and the methods of preventing and controlling them; promotion of food supply and proper nutrition; an adequate supply of safe water and basic sanitation; maternal and child health care, including family planning; *immunization against the major infectious diseases; prevention and control of locally endemic diseases; appropriate treatment of common diseases* and injuries; and provision of essential drugs [our italics].

It is clear that the control of infection is an essential part of the primary health care concept.

WHO recognizes that it can be difficult at this stage to specify well-defined objectives and targets and incorporate them into national policies and strategies. "However, in spite of the complexities involved, it is important to attempt to specify national, regional and global targets such as those adopted by the World Health Assembly when it resolved to

23

provide by 1990 immunization for all the children of the world against the main infectious diseases, and safe drinking-water and sanitation for the entire population" (*27*).

In WHO documents the countries of Europe have been divided into four groups (*28*) according to child mortality and the respective health situation (only the parts referring to infections are quoted):

Group I. Tuberculosis mortality rates less than 5 per 100 000 population and deaths from infectious and parasitic diseases under 10 per 100 000.

Group II. Tuberculosis mortality rates less than 10 per 100 000 population and infectious and parasitic diseases mortality rates 20 per 100 000 or lower.

Group III. Tuberculosis mortality rates over 20 per 100 000 population and infectious and parasitic diseases mortality rates rising to over 35 per 100 000.

Group IV. Countries facing a large number of health problems ranging from communicable and parasitic diseases through high infant mortality to unsatisfactory sanitary conditions and poor nutrition (these represent about 10% of the Member States).

When mortality was the only criterion it was assumed that countries in the first two groups had few problems in relation to infectious diseases and that primary health care as conceived by the Declaration of Alma-Ata was fundamentally different in such countries. While health problems in the developed part of Europe are much more complex and infections are only a part of them, infections still have great relevance, although they can be masked by the present system of notification of diseases and their importance cannot be measured by mortality rates. The health care systems in any country are shaped by a certain set of points of emphasis influenced by consumer pressure, which is dependent on expectations about the role of the system as a whole and of the health profession in particular. While in the past the major emphasis was on physical diseases, the situation in Europe at present is less simple. With rising expectations in all domains of life, claims are being made for the treatment of ailments without disease, of physiological processes such as aging experienced as illness, of the psychological stress of everyday life also perceived as illness, and of the emotional problems of personal and social relations and interactions. These are often experienced as vague somatic symptoms and increasingly subject to ever-expanding interventions, not necessarily by the medical profession. If the means are plentiful and the cost irrelevant, there is no limit to the expansion of care for such sociocultural and psychological constructs, care that was given formerly by families, friends, churches and schools. The more sober definition of primary health care given by WHO deals with the prevention and care of real diseases, biologically important because they occasion suffering, disability and death.

The problem is not whether the treatment, control, and prevention of infectious diseases are part of primary health care in Europe, as they obviously are, but rather how best to integrate them in an overall programme for a comprehensive health service. In order to make public health care effective greater participation by the communicable disease sector is required. This means the establishment of cooperation with other services or agencies to identify priorities or population groups for action, for example pockets of poverty, migrant or special-risk groups, ethnic minorities and age groups at risk, and the creation of incentives for community and professional participation and of structures and facilities for effective epidemiological surveillance. In many countries vertical programmes for the control of some communicable diseases exist, but no satisfactory procedures have yet been established for their necessary, but difficult, integration into primary health care structures.

The problem cannot be solved until the boundaries of primary health care and the functions of each level of care have been defined and the providers' role more specifically delineated, which will obviously need a certain period of discussion and negotiation in each individual society to decide which group of people should receive primary health care and for what purpose. Treatment of infections is an essential part of such care, so essential as to be taken for granted and neglected if, at present, mortality is a measuring rod. Notifications are predominantly for serious and mostly acute diseases, not for all the microbial, viral or parasitic diseases primary health care physicians see in their daily consultations. Up to 40% of all primary contacts with the health services in the winter months in northern and central Europe are occasioned by respiratory infections, and in summer in southern Europe by enteric infections, and most of them remain unnotified. The largest number of primary contacts of children with the health system are for the prevention of infectious disease; at least 16 million primary immunization procedures are carried out yearly. Outpatient attendance for sexually transmitted diseases in the United Kingdom alone in 1981 was over 500 000 (29). It shows that there is undernotification in other countries since it is more than the total number of reported cases for the whole of Europe (all 31 countries) for any year. The data from the German Democratic Republic (30) probably apply to most countries: each year one third of all work absenteeism, two thirds of school absenteeism, and 80% of absences from day-care centres (crèches) are due to acute respiratory virus infections and enteric infections. A prospective study (two years) showed that 77.9% of diagnoses in children's outpatient clinics in that country were due to infectious diseases (H. Maahs & U. Peter, personal communication, 1982). Data of this kind affect the appraisal of the health situation in Europe and should be considered in the assignment of priorities. Towards the periphery information becomes more and more incomplete and is most deficient at the primary health care level.

Thus the establishment of primary health care and the monitoring of its performance imply not only the creation or modification of organizational structures at central and peripheral levels where necessary (decentralization, regionalization, referral) but also an improvement in information systems and networks for the production of primary data for epidemiological analysis.

There are good reasons for the lack of information from the primary level. One is the lack of time in overburdened health centres for precise etiological diagnosis and notification, particularly if the disease does not appear to be serious. Moreover, even if the primary health physician is willing to embark upon more precise diagnosis requiring more than a physical examination, he probably does not have easy access to laboratories. And if laboratories were accessible and costs not a constraint, the time required for a reply would make them of little use. Improvement of the diagnosis, better treatment, and reliable notification of diseases depend *inter alia* on conditions that are rarely fulfilled at the primary level. They are:

● Immediate microbiological and biochemical examination by direct methods of the necessary specimens for either a presumptive diagnosis or selection of patients for further laboratory testing. Most physicians may have forgotten how to carry out such examinations, or lack the time to do so, and the younger generation may never have been given a proper chance to practise them. However, non-professional staff can be rapidly and effectively trained to carry them out.

● Development of simple rapid diagnostic techniques. As more sophisticated techniques for hospital or special laboratory use started appearing, rapid and simple diagnostic techniques for bacterial and rickettsial diseases, a promising development in the 1940s, were neglected until recent years and until the emphasis on primary health care. Rapid diagnostic techniques for viral diseases are new and very promising but are at present available for use only in big hospitals, require highly specialized staff or sophisticated equipment or both, and need a regular supply of antigens, which must be either brought from outside or produced by the laboratory itself. The question of a regular supply of antigens might eventually be solved, in Europe at least.

Counting the dead is not enough

Analysis of mortality from selected infectious diseases has been carried out in Europe only rarely: by WHO in 1974, 1978 and 1982 for respiratory diseases (see Annex 1) and by Peruzy & Coppi (*31*) for urogenital and respiratory diseases for the period 1968–1972. Peruzy & Coppi used the 150 disease code, taking the selected countries with the highest and lowest mortality rates, and included bronchitis, emphysema and bronchial asthma (Tables 4 and 5). In Europe the average age at death from acute respiratory infections was 47.7 years, ranging from 67.3 in Finland to 14.5 in Romania. For deaths from urogenital infections the average age in Europe was 69.8 years with a much less pronounced range: from 75.1 years in Sweden to 60.2 years in Poland. Urogenital infections are therefore one of the most important causes of mortality in old age. Acute respiratory infections (rate 14.8 per 100 000 population) and pneumonia (average rate 87.2 per 100 000) cause death primarily in the age groups 0–4 years and over 55 years (8.3 and 135.8 per 100 000 respectively), while the proportion

Table 4. Mortality from infections of the respiratory system in selected European countries, 1969–1971 (per 100 000 population)

Acute infections of the upper respiratory system		Influenza		Other types of pneumonia		Empyema and pulmonary abscess		Bronchitis, emphysema and asthma	
Spain	6.8	Spain	17.4	England & Wales	83.3	Austria	2.4	Romania	74.3
Austria	5.7	Bulgaria	17.3	Romania	77.3	Romania	2.3	Ireland	65.7
Germany, Federal Republic of	5.6	Switzerland	13.2	Bulgaria	70.2	Hungary	1.5	England & Wales	63.1
Italy	4.5	Italy	7.8	Italy	37.1	England, Wales & Scotland	0.5	Italy	36.8
France	0.8	Netherlands	6.2	Denmark	20.8	Italy	0.5	Norway	13.9
Norway	0.6	Denmark	5.8	Netherlands	20.8	Ireland	0.2	Sweden	12.9
Romania	0.5	Sweden	3.5	France	19.3	Northern Ireland	0.1		
				Hungary	15.7				

Source: **Peruzy & Coppi** (31).

27

in the age group 5–54 years is insignificant. The mortality is greater in males, a trend that increases with age (*32*).

The analysis shows that, in spite of generally available vaccines for influenza and antibiotics and other drugs, infections of the respiratory tract and urogenital system are still an important cause of death in early childhood and older age groups in all countries of Europe, with the relative exception of Denmark, the Netherlands and Sweden.

In the most comprehensive review ever published by WHO (*32*) using the latest available years, 1970–1973, it was found that in Europe the mortality from acute respiratory diseases by groups (all ages) for those years (as a percentage of all acute respiratory infections) was:

Acute upper respiratory tract infections	12 002 (5.8%)
Influenza	24 075 (11.5%)
Viral and bacterial pneumonia	173 518 (82.7%)

The mortality from chronic respiratory diseases by groups (as a percentage of all chronic respiratory diseases) was:

Tuberculosis	32 893 (16.7%)
Chronic bronchitis, asthma, emphysema	163 977 (83.3%)

The mortality from acute respiratory infections as a percentage of that from all respiratory diseases in Europe was 51.6%.

The review of acute respiratory infections showed that for the years 1970–1973 the mortality rate for all ages for Europe (28 countries) was 45.3 per 100 000 population (a total of 209 054 deaths) with an excess mortality attributable to influenza of 13%. The overall mortality from acute respiratory infections, including influenza, as a percentage of all causes of death was 4.4%.

In relation to the mortality from acute respiratory infections in 1970–1973, that for the age group 0–14 years was:

< 1 year	28 376 (390.3 per 100 000)
1–4 years	4589 (15.3 per 100 000)
5–14 years	1580 (2.1 per 100 000)

For those of 55 years of age and over, the mortality in 1970–1973 was:

55–65 years	14 390 (30.8 per 100 000)
65–75 years	40 026 (107.7 per 100 000)
⩾ 75 years	108 727 (380.4 per 100 000)

The mean mortality rate for infants and children taken together was 30.7 per 100 000 population. The percentage of all causes of death due to acute respiratory infections in children 0–14 years was 15.1%. As mortality rates in the older age groups rise, deaths in these groups tend to become increasingly prominent as a percentage of the total number of deaths from acute respiratory infections in all age groups. There is a drastic increase, particularly in Europe, from 6.9% to 51.9%. The mean mortality rate for the age group 55–75 years and over was 145.1 per 100 000 population.

In spite of the incompleteness and the poor comparability of data for all ages, these data indicate that respiratory infections are a most important

Table 5. Mortality rates from infectious diseases in Europe, 1969–1971

Country	Mortality per 100 000 population	Mortality as a percentage of deaths from all causes
Austria	112.9	8.5
Belgium	80.7	6.51
Bulgaria	147.7	15.65
Czechoslovakia	119.9	10.37
Denmark	69.6	7.06
Finland	84.8	8.37
France	56.8	5.18
Germany, Federal Republic of	96.4	7.87
Greece	75.9	9.23
Hungary	62.3	5.37
Ireland	151.1	13.44
Italy	91.3	9.34
Netherlands	61.9	7.41
Norway	93.4	9.31
Poland	70.4	8.48
Romania	165.2	17.04
Spain	92.8	10.67
Sweden	70.7	6.92
Switzerland	67.2	7.21
United Kingdom		
England & Wales	168	14.30
Northern Ireland	125.9	11.72
Scotland	121.9	10.23
Yugoslavia	66.8	7.42
Europe	97.7	9.40

Source: **Peruzy & Coppi** (31).

cause of mortality in Europe, a true public health problem with infants, young children and elderly people as the critical age groups.

A comparison of mortality from infectious diseases in Europe and its percentage of mortality from all causes has been made only once (Table 5). The difference between mortality from infectious disease (ICD-8) according to Chapter I of the ICD and according to other chapters is shown in Table 2.

In one of the developing countries of the Region, Algeria, 24% of deaths in children under 5 years of age were due to intestinal infections, 9% to measles, 7% to pneumonia, 4% to meningitis, 3.2% to other respiratory infections, and 2.4% to other infections. A special survey on mortality carried out in part of the city of Algiers and in two rural communes in 1974–1975 showed that 50% of all deaths in children in this age group were due to infections (33). In infants aged 1–11 months infectious diseases were responsible for 82% of all deaths, 43% from diarrhoeal diseases alone.

The fallacy of indicators

In 1965, a President's Commission on Heart Disease, Cancer and Stroke, after analysing mortality data in the United States, found that 71% of all deaths in that country were caused by heart disease, cancer and stroke, and stated: "Compared with them, all the other enemies of man — the great range of infectious diseases, accidents, congenital and nutritional disorders — fade into relative insignificance". While the statistics were no doubt correct, the Commission's views were challenged by analyses indicating that competing claims for health resources for programmes to reduce mortality needed to be evaluated primarily in terms of age-specific mortality. As Stickle (*34*) pointed out:

> 80% of those who died from these causes were at least 60 years of age. In contrast, only 49% of the deaths from all other causes occurred in persons aged 60 and over. ... The death of male infants represents an average loss of 67 years of life, including the entire reproductive period, and over 50 years of economic productivity; the death of a man at age 60 on average represents a sacrifice of only 16 years of life and even fewer years of economic productivity. On the basis of years of life lost and future income sacrificed, deaths from heart disease, cancer and stroke still appear to be major public health problems, though not nearly of the same relative magnitude as is indicated by a simple comparison of the absolute number of deaths from these and other causes.

Infant deaths alone, Stickle pointed out, about 105 000 as against about 1 163 000 deaths from the three "big killers", accounted for only 10% fewer years of life than the loss due to heart diseases, for 61% more than the number of years lost as a result of cancer, and for 254% more than the number of years of life sacrificed as a result of strokes. The death of infants in terms of future productive capacity exceeded by 3% death from cardio-vascular diseases, by 99% death from cancer, and by 404% death from stroke.

It is indeed in the area of infant mortality that a reduction can add to life expectancy at birth. Although the infant mortality rate is already low in some European countries, for example Sweden, in many it can be reduced further, and a range of 5–10 deaths per 1000 may be expected for the end of the century. In the age group 1–15 years influenza and pneumonia play an important role in mortality, particularly in those aged 1–5 years, and this suggests that further reduction is feasible. Prenatal and perinatal virus infections contribute to abortion (both spontaneous and induced), still-birth, malformations and/or crippling invalidity, which for cytomegalovirus infections alone is 1 per 1000 births. "The dead or malformed have few advocates, but the publicity sponsored programmes aiming at reducing the death rate from the three 'big killers' find immediate and often vociferous response among persons at greatest risk of death from these causes. ... Heart disease and stroke are primarily diseases of increased longevity. As our expectation of life rises, so will the proportion of deaths due to those conditions. The most fruitful approaches to the achievement of improved life expectancy have come, and will continue to come, from reduced mortality in infancy and childhood" (*34*).

30

In a review of the importance of cancer, Hansluwka (35) discusses the limitations of various indices used to measure the dimensions of the disease and their implications for public health.

Black & Pole [36] have developed five indices of the burden of illness as a basis for establishing priorities in biomedical research: inpatient days; out-patient referrals; consultation in general or primary family practice; sickness benefit days; and years of life lost to premature death. Rice [37] carried out some pioneering work in this area in the early 1960s and has since refined her methodology. The eight indices used by Rice are: potential years of life lost; inpatient days; primary care visits; sickness benefit days; bed disability days; persons limited in their major activity; impact of selected chronic conditions; and economic costs. On this basis she concluded (for the United States of America) that the burden due to cancer is less clear-cut than, for instance, that due to diseases of the circulatory system. Cancer ranks second in only one of these eight indices, namely, potential years of life lost; in all other indices it is not among the top three. The low prevalence of cancer — a result of its high fatality — depresses its ranking with respect to measures such as inpatient days, sickness benefit days, etc.

Cancer, a disease that often causes death within a relatively short time after diagnosis and has a relatively high case fatality, fares rather poorly in terms of indicators used to measure the impact of disease, such as hospital inpatient days, primary care utilization and limitation of activity. On the other hand, respiratory infections would rank high in importance by some of these indicators. Even perfunctory examination of the reasons for which people use the health services shows how important are other indicators for assessing the dimension of disease.

"Cancer is a good example of the dangers associated with an indiscriminate application of a cost/effectiveness and cost/benefit approach. In view of the vast resources spent on cancer research and cancer control activities throughout the developed (and developing) world, the results so far achieved are not necessarily convincing or up to expectation from a mere cost/benefit point of view" (36). On the other hand, cost/effectiveness and cost/benefit analyses would appear to give positive results in the control of infectious diseases.

*   *   *

Data provided in accordance with the ICD are submitted to politicians and decision-makers, who are unable to go into detail, and the decisions made are inevitably influenced by them. The ICD data are used for international comparison and in connexion with the allocation of funds and priorities not only by the country concerned but also by international bodies. Scientists use them in the analysis of health situations, as a basis for the formulation of health policies, and in projections of global needs.

Governments in Europe know well that it is necessary to make a permanent commitment of resources to the prevention of infectious diseases. However, if measurement of health effects is made only on the basis of mortality from disease, the services dealing with infectious diseases

31

will always rank low in the priority lists and those diseases will not appear among the top health problems.[a]

The officials responsible for communicable diseases in Europe therefore concluded, at a meeting in April 1982 in Copenhagen, that: "The currently used International Classification of Diseases (ICD) fails to document the frequency and importance of infections. Therefore mechanisms should be worked out with the aim of achieving a more realistic picture of infectious diseases in terms of both morbidity and mortality".

References

1. **McNeill, W.** *Plagues and peoples.* New York, Doubleday, 1976.
2. **Burnet, F.M.** The future of medical research. *Lancet,* **1**: 103–108 (1953).
3. **McKeown, T.** *Medicine in modern society.* London, George Allen & Unwin, 1965.
4. **McKeown, T. & Lowe, C.R.** *An introduction to social medicine.* Oxford, Blackwell, 1974.
5. **McKeown, T.** *The modern rise of population.* London, Arnold, 1976.
6. **McKeown, T.** *The role of medicine: dream, mirage or nemesis?* London, Nuffield Provincial Hospitals Trust, 1976.
7. **Lalonde, M.** *A new perspective on the health of Canadians.* Ottawa, Government of Canada, 1974.
8. **Godber, G.** McKeown's "The role of medicine": comments from a former Chief Medical Officer. *Health and society,* **55**: 373–378 (1977).
9. **Beeson, P.** McKeown's "The role of medicine": a clinician's reaction. *Health and society,* **55**: 365–371 (1977).
10. **Holland, W.** McKeown's "The role of medicine": a view of social medicine. *Health and society,* **55**: 383–388 (1977).
11. **McDermott, W.** *Perspectives in biology and medicine.* Chicago, University of Chicago Press, 1976.
12. **Lever, A.F.** Review of "The role of medicine". *Lancet,* **1**: 352–353 (1977).
13. **Ingelfinger, F.** Review of "The role of medicine". *New England journal of medicine,* **296**: 448–449 (1979).
14. **Green, R.** Beyond the role of medicine — McKeown as medical philosopher. *Health and society,* **55**: 389–403 (1977).
15. **Kennedy, J.** *The unmasking of medicine.* London, George Allen & Unwin, 1981.
16. **Dubos, R.** *Man adapting,* 7th ed. New Haven, Yale University Press, 1971, pp. 163–164.
17. **Sabin, A.** Control of infectious diseases. *Journal of infectious diseases,* **121**: 91–94 (1970).

---

[a] If mortality is classified according to etiology, the rates increase almost 10 times, as an analysis in the German Democratic Republic has shown (S. Dittmann, personal communication, 1982).

18. **Fenner, F.** *Burnet and infectious diseases.* Melbourne, Walter and Eliza Hall Institute of Medical Research, special volume, Annual Review, 1978–1979.

19. **Burnet, F.M.** Men or molecules? A tilt at molecular biology. *Lancet*, **1**: 37–39 (1966).

20. *Health services in Europe*, 3rd ed. Copenhagen, WHO Regional Office for Europe, 1981, Vol. 2.

21. **McLachlan, G., ed.** *The planning of health services: studies in eight European countries.* Copenhagen, WHO Regional Office for Europe, 1981.

22. *International classification of impairments, disabilities, and handicaps.* Geneva, World Health Organization, 1980.

23. *Medicine in the 1990s: a technological forecast.* London, Office of Health Economics, 1979.

24. *Sixth report on the world health situation.* Geneva, World Health Organization, 1980, Part I.

25. *Alma-Ata 1978: primary health care.* Geneva, World Health Organization, 1978 ("Health for All" Series No. 1), p. 9.

26. **Parker, A.** *In:* Corey, L. et al., ed. *Primary care, definition and purpose in medicine in a changing society.* Saint Louis, Mosby, 1977.

27. *Formulating strategies for health for all by the year 2000.* Geneva, World Health Organization, 1979 ("Health for All" Series No. 2).

28. **Kaprio, L.A.** *Primary health care in Europe.* Copenhagen, WHO Regional Office for Europe, 1979 (EURO Reports and Studies, No. 14).

29. *Communicable disease report No. 81/47.* London, Public Health Laboratory Service, 1981.

30. **Dittmann, S. et al.** Zur actuellen und zukunftigen Bedeutung von Infektionskrankheiten in der DDR. *Gesundheitswesen*, **34**: 2515–2553 (1979).

31. **Peruzy, A.D. & Coppi, R.** Mortality for some infectious diseases in Europe. *Minerva medica*, **69**: 4017–4027 (1978).

32. **Bulla, A. & Hitze, K.** *Bulletin of the World Health Organization*, **56**: 481–491 (1978).

33. *Morbidité infantile et juvénile en rapport avec les tendences de la fécondité.* Geneva, World Health Organization, 1980.

34. **Stickle, G.** What priority, human life? *American journal of public health*, **55**: 1692–1699 (1965).

35. **Hansluwka, H.** Cancer mortality in Europe, 1970–74. *World health statistics quarterly*, **31**: 159–194 (1978).

36. **Black, D.A.K. & Pole, J.D.** Priorities in biomedical research. *British journal of preventive and social medicine*, **29**: 222 (1975).

37. **Rice, D.** *Estimating the cost of illness.* Washington, DC, US Public Health Service, 1966 (Health Economics Series No. 6); The economic cost of illness revisited. *Bulletin of social security*, February 1976, p. 21; *Economic cost of cardiovascular diseases and cancer.* Washington, DC, US Public Health Service, 1962 (Health Economics Series No. 5).

2

Why we don't know:
an incomplete system

B. Velimirovic

With the commitment of all States to attaining the basic regional goals in health, greater emphasis is placed on international cooperation and better exchange of data among countries. Increased travel and trade, the movement of labour across frontiers, declining levels of vaccination, the importation of exotic diseases, and awareness that the magnitude of infections cannot be correctly assessed have raised interest in the different mechanisms existing in countries for the notification of diseases. The question of the adequacy of present information regarding infections needs to be examined bearing in mind that:

— there is no ideal notification system

— there is no universally applicable system

— there is no ideal cooperation in notification between the parties concerned

— there is a vast underestimation of the magnitude of infections in Europe.

Notification of infections was based in the past on the occurrence of traditional communicable diseases in epidemic form, and this system has influenced profoundly the development of statistical systems and legislative measures for notification. In Europe at present most of the classical epidemic communicable diseases play little part and there have been profound changes in the disease pattern; moreover in principle most infectious diseases can be controlled, the ICD emphasis on mortality rather than morbidity thereby relegating those diseases to a minor role. As a consequence, a closer analysis of epidemiological happenings is not made and the view is widespread that infections are no longer a problem in Europe. This is an erroneous view. "If we think that infectious disease has ceased to matter, one shall find that it will be neither understood nor effectively controlled. Ignorance favours infections, promotes panic and is wasteful of human effort and resources" (*1*).

35

The background

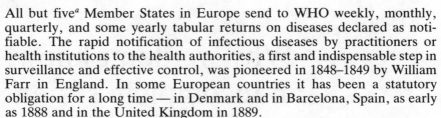

All but five[a] Member States in Europe send to WHO weekly, monthly, quarterly, and some yearly tabular returns on diseases declared as notifiable. The rapid notification of infectious diseases by practitioners or health institutions to the health authorities, a first and indispensable step in surveillance and effective control, was pioneered in 1848–1849 by William Farr in England. In some European countries it has been a statutory obligation for a long time — in Denmark and in Barcelona, Spain, as early as 1888 and in the United Kingdom in 1889.

The listing of what used traditionally to be called communicable diseases has been attempted twice in the past by the WHO Regional Office for Europe, on the basis of the situation in 1962 and 1969 respectively, with some amendments in 1972.[b] Both lists are out of date, but represent a stimulating attempt to provide such information, which is available only to WHO for the whole of Europe. Unfortunately the *World health statistics annual* published by WHO contains even less information than that given in national returns, as it tries as briefly as possible for the purposes of comparison to present the notified diseases most commonly reported by all countries.

There is no absolutely logical way of listing diseases; it has been done in alphabetical order, by order of organs affected, or according to etiology. In this review, for want of a better system (apart from the diseases subject to the International Health Regulations, which constitute a separate class) the alphabetical order of bacterial, viral, rickettsial and parasitic subgroups has been arbitrarily chosen. For the sake of convenience some respiratory, enteric and venereal diseases have been placed in separate groups. Two groups concerning other situations also reported are included. The corresponding number in the ICD is appended. Additional information about countries and diseases reported by fewer than two countries has been included as footnotes in order to simplify Tables 6–8, which summarize the morbidity statistics of notifiable diseases available in various countries in Europe.

WHO, the final link in the notification chain, obviously cannot give an opinion about the functioning of the system in each country or about the geographical area covered, the degree of completeness of notification or its regularity, the time gaps, the quality of the information, the accuracy of the diagnosis, or the capacity of the national services for handling the available data. Additional information exists in countries in special reports and official and scientific publications, which often give a more reliable

---

[a] Albania, Bulgaria, Morocco (which started sending annual reports for the first time in 1982), San Marino and the USSR. Some countries (Andorra, the Holy See and Liechtenstein) have not declared their position to the WHO Regional Office for Europe. Gibraltar sends reports to WHO in Geneva but not to the Regional Office. The USSR provided yearly information on diseases under the WHO Expanded Programme on Immunization in 1979 and 1980.

[b] Unpublished WHO document EURO 1002, Copenhagen, 1974.

picture of the epidemiological situation than official reports. The picture presented here is therefore that seen from an international perspective on the basis of official reports that should, but may not necessarily, reflect the national situation. It is used as a basis for answering the frequent requests from countries to WHO for information. At present several countries in Europe are revising and updating their systems or converting them to computer-assisted handling, the details of the changes not yet being available. The examples used are from countries with good notification systems.

Evaluation of the reports received

Of the 33 European Member States 26 (76.7%) send weekly or monthly notification returns to WHO. Of these, 10 (38.4%) also include narratives or comments. The length of the reports varies from 1 to 32 pages. Four countries (15.3%) include a map of the country with administrative divisions, which permits rapid identification of the locality of any occurrence. In 1980 and 1981, Algeria and Italy started revising their notification systems and transferring to computer-assisted handling, which is already in operation in Denmark, the Netherlands, Norway and Sweden and perhaps in other countries.

The number of infectious diseases reported ranges from 8 to 64 (average 32). Two countries have open-ended notification systems, diseases being included according to the reports received so that the number of columns varies from month to month. The diseases reported are listed in Tables 6–8. Owing to differences in the terminology used and in the combination of categories in some of the reports, errors could have been made in Table 7 for individual countries where no ICD numbers were included in the original report. Twelve countries in the Region send weekly reports to WHO, one a report every 10 days, and one a fortnightly report. A monthly report is sent by 15 countries. Two countries send quarterly reports; in one country this is additional and in another (Algeria) it is the only report available on a national scale.

Annual reports are forwarded to WHO from 7 countries only (26.9%). These usually take time to produce, up to 2½ years, although some countries such as the German Democratic Republic make their reports available much earlier.

Laboratory surveillance reports are received from Sweden and from the United Kingdom (one covering England & Wales, another Scotland). Special reports on influenza or on selected diseases are available from Austria, Finland, France, the German Democratic Republic, the Federal Republic of Germany and Italy. A separate and well prepared report on animal diseases is received from Yugoslavia. The average postal delivery time of all reports is about 10 days. In rare special cases information is provided to (or from) WHO by telex or, more frequently, by telephone.

The Regional Office is unable to answer the quite common requests for information about the legislative provisions regulating the notification of

Table 6. Diseases reported in the WHO European Region

Disease	Albania	Algeria	Austria	Belgium	Bulgaria	Czechoslovakia	Denmark	Finland	France	German Dem. Rep.	Fed. Rep. Germany	Greece	Hungary	Iceland	Ireland	Italy	Luxembourg	Malta	Monaco	Morocco	Netherlands	Norway	Poland	Portugal	Romania	San Marino	Spain	Sweden	Switzerland	Turkey	USSR	UK – England & Wales	UK – Northern Ireland	UK – Scotland	Yugoslavia
Diseases subject to the International Health Regulations																																			
Cholera		+		+	+		+				+	+				+					+			+			+						+	+	
Plague				+	+		+					+				+					+			+			+						+	+	
Smallpox				+	+		+					+				+					+			+			+						+	+	
Yellow fever				+	+							+				+					+			+			+						+	+	
Bacterial diseases																																			
Anthrax		+		+			+		+		+	+	+		+	+	+	+			+			+	+		+	+		+			+	+	
Botulism		+	+	+		+	+		+		+	+	+		+	+	+	+		+	+	+	+	+			+	+	+	+			+	+	+
Brucellosis		+	+	+		+			+		+	+	+	+	+	+					+			+			+	+	+				+	+	
Clostridium perfringens				+		+		+			+			+				+			+				+									+	+
Diphtheria		+	+	+		+	+	+	+	+	+	+	+	+	+	+	+	+		+	+	+	+	+	+		+	+	+	+		+	+	+	
Erysipelas			+			+	+	+			+		+	+									+					+	+						
Glanders														+				+			+													+	+
Legionella				+			+		+	+	+ (1)	+		+	+	+	+	+		+	+	+	+	+	+		+	+	+			+	+	+	
Leprosy		+							+	+	+ (3)	+		+	+	+	+				+	+	+				+	+	+			+	+	+	
Leptospirosis	+ (1)		+	+		+	+	+	+	+	+ (2)	+	+	+	+	+				+	+		+	+	+		+		+				+	+	
Listeriosis														+		+					+ (1)		+	+				+ (1)						+	
Meningitis		+		+		+	+ (1)	+	+	+	+ (5)	+	+	+	+	+	+	+		+	+	+ (1)	+	+	+		+	+	+			+	+	+	
Meningococcal septicaemia			+ (1)			+						+		+		+							+				+ (1)		+			+	+	+	+
Pertussis		+		+		+						+		+		+				+	+	+	+	+	+		+		+			+	+	+	+
Puerperal fever						+						+		+		+																+	+	+	
Relapsing fever		+ (2)		+		+	+ (1)		+	+	+ (3)	+	+	+		+											+ (1)					+	+	+	
Scarlatina						+								+															+					+	+
Septicaemia		+ (2)		+		+		+ (1)			+ (3)			+		+				+		+ +		+				+		+			+	+	+
Staphylococcus												+										+ +													

continued

Table 6. (contd)

Disease	Albania	Algeria	Austria	Belgium	Bulgaria	Czechoslovakia	Denmark	Finland	France	German Dem. Rep.	Fed. Rep. Germany	Greece	Hungary	Iceland	Ireland	Italy	Luxembourg	Malta	Monaco	Morocco	Netherlands	Norway	Poland	Portugal	Romania	San Marino	Spain	Sweden	Switzerland	Turkey	USSR	UK – England & Wales	UK – Northern Ireland	UK – Scotland	Yugoslavia
Bacterial diseases (contd)																																			
Streptococcus		+ +												+								+			+							+			+
Tetanus		+	+	+ +		+	+ + + + +	+	+ +	+	+	+ +	+			+	| + + +	+ +		+ +	+ +	+	+	(1) +	+		+	+	+			+	+ +	+	
Tuberculosis		+														+	+	+						(2) +								+ + +		+	
Tuberculosis/pleurisy			+				+										+	+		+ +				+										+	
Tuberculosis (non respiratory)		+	+				+	+	+		+					+	+					+ +		+				+ +							
Tuberculosis/meninges/CNS																					+ +	+ +													
Tularaemia																																			
Yersiniosis																																			
Virus diseases																																			
Cytomegalovirus						+					+			+		+						+	+					+	+			+	+	+	+
Herpes zoster		+ +	+	+ +		+ + + +	+ + +		+ (1) +	(1) (1)	+ + +	+ +	+	+ +	+	+ + + +	+	+		+	+ +	+ + + +	+ + +	+	+		+	+ +	+ +	+		+ +	+ +	+	+ + + +
Hepatitis A						+ + +	+ + +		+		+ (3)	+ +	+ + +	+ + +	+ +	+ + + +	+	+		+	+ +	+ + +	+ + +	+	+		+	+	+	+		+ +	+ + +	+ +	+
Hepatitis B			+						(1)	+	(3)	+ +	+ + +	+ + +		+ + +		+			+ +	+ +	+	+				+	+	+		+	+	+	+
Hepatitis (not specified)							(2)									+						(2)	(1)	+				+	+			(1)	+		+
Influenza-like diseases		+	+			+ +	+		+	+	+	+		+ + + +		+ +						+ +	+ +					+ +	+ +				+	+	+
Lassa fever																																			
Measles			+			+ + +	+		(3)	+	+	+	+ + +	+ + +	+ +	+ + + +				+	+ +	+ +	+					+	+			(1)	+		
Mononucleosis									+																							+			
Meningoencephalitis				+												+						(2) +	(1)	+				+	+				+		
Meningitis serosa (leptomeningitis)																+					+ +	+ +	+	+					+						
Meningitis			+	+		+ +	+		+	+ +	+	+	+ + +	+ + + +		+				+	+	+ +	+ +					(1)	+ +				+ +	+ +	+
Parotitis		+																									(1)	(1)							
Poliomyelitis (paralytic)																																			
Poliomyelitis (non paralytic)																																			

continued

Table 6. (contd)

Disease	Albania	Algeria	Austria	Belgium	Bulgaria	Czechoslovakia	Denmark	Finland	France	German Dem. Rep.	Fed. Rep. Germany	Greece	Hungary	Iceland	Ireland	Italy	Luxembourg	Malta	Monaco	Morocco	Netherlands	Norway	Poland	Portugal	Romania	San Marino	Spain	Sweden	Switzerland	Turkey	USSR	UK – England & Wales	UK – Northern Ireland	Yugoslavia	UK – Scotland
Virus diseases (contd)																																			
Poliomyelitis (not specified)	+	+	+	+	+		+	+	+		+	+	+			+	+	+		+	+	+	+	+			+	+		+					+
Psittacosis (ornithosis)		+		(1)					+		+	+	+		+	+	+				+			+	+		+	+	+	+				+	+
Rabies		+	+	+	+	+	+	+	+	+	+	+	+			+	+			+	+	+	+	+			+	+		+				+	+
Rubella		+		+	+	+	+	+			+	+	+	+		+		+			+	+	+				+							+	
Trachoma		+	+													+								+			+								
Varicella (chickenpox)						+	+	+				+				+																			
Viral encephalitis												+				+					+		+	+			+						+	+	+
Viral haemorrhagic fever				+	+		+									+																	+	+	+
Rickettsial diseases																																			
Boutonneuse fever		+								+	+	+	+			+		+					+	(3)				+	+					+	+
Q fever		+								+	+	+	+			+					+		+	+			+	(2)	+				+	+	+
Typhus exanthematosus												+																							
Typhus murinus												+																							
Parasitic diseases																																			
Amoebiasis	(3)	+	+	+		+					+	+	+			+		+						+			+								
Ancylostomiasis		+	+	+		+										+								+			+	+							
Bilharziasis		+		+												(1)								+											
Leishmaniasis		+		+		+			+		+	+			+	(2)				(1)				+			+	+		+					
Malaria		+	+	+	+	+										+					(1)			+			+	+		+		+		+	+
Mycosis/dermatophytosis		+				+						+				+		+						+			+								
Pediculosis						+						+				+								+						+					
Taeniasis						+			+	(3)		+	+			+								+						+					
Toxoplasmosis						+	+	+	+				+			+					+	+		+			+			+					
Trichinosis																+						+	+	+				+	+						
Scabies																+				+	+		+						+						
Hydatidosis/echinococcosis	+														+	+												+							

continued

Table 6. (contd)

Disease	Albania	Algeria	Austria	Belgium	Bulgaria	Czechoslovakia	Denmark	Finland	France	German Dem. Rep.	Fed. Rep. Germany	Greece	Hungary	Iceland	Ireland	Italy	Luxembourg	Malta	Monaco	Morocco	Netherlands	Norway	Poland	Portugal	Romania	San Marino	Spain	Sweden	Switzerland	Turkey	USSR	UK – England & Wales	UK – Northern Ireland	UK – Scotland	Yugoslavia
Respiratory infections																																			
Bronchitis																																+ +			
Pneumonia	+									+		+		+ (1)								+										+			
Upper respiratory infections		+						+		+				+								+													
Enteric infections																																			
Colienteritis	(4)		+	+		+		(2)		+											+	+						+							
Diarrhoeal disease	+	+	+	+	+	+	+	+	+	+	+	+	+	+	+	+	+				+	+	+	+	+		+	+	+	+			+	+	+
Dysentery bacillus (shigellosis)				+		+	+		+	+	+		+	+	+	+	+				+	+	+	+				+	+			+	+	+	+
Foodborne disease										+	+										+	+	+					+				+	+	+	+
Gastroenteritis (children under 2 years)																					+	+	+					+							
Paratyphoid fever			+	+		+	+			+	(4)	+	+	+		+	+				(2)	+	+	+	+		(2)	+	+			+	+	+	+
Salmonelloses, other	+		+	+		+	+	+	+	+	(5)	+	+	+	+	+	+				(2)	(3)	+	+	+			+	+			+	+	(1)	+
Typhoid fever	(5)	(5)	+	+		+	+	+	+	+	+	+	+	+	+	+	+	+		+	+	+	+	+	+		+	+	+			+	+	+	+
Venereal diseases																																			
Gonorrhoea		+	+	+			+	+				+				+	+			+	(4)	(4)		+				+	+				+	+	+
Lymphogranuloma venereum																+	+			+	+			+				+							
Ophthalmia neonatorum																+					+			+											
Syphilis		(2)	+				+					+				+	+			+	+			+			+		+					+	+
Syphilis (congenital)																					+	+										+			
Ulcus molle (chancroid)																																			
Other diseases																																			
Pemphigus neonatorum														+							+	+													
Poisoning (bacterial)				+ +			+																												
Other situations notified																																			
Animal bites						+ +							+ +			+ +																			
Conjunctivitis																				+								+ + +							+

41

Notes to Table 6

ALGERIA

The report includes narratives. The reporting of 30 diseases is obligatory. The reporting of some diseases is optional: streptococcal infections (erysipelas and impetigo), acute respiratory infections (influenza, acute pneumonia, etc.), diarrhoeas (enteritis and other diarrhoeal diseases), other intestinal parasitoses, and trachoma (obligatory in Adrar, Bechar, Laghouat, Biskra, Djelfa, Ouargla, Tamarasset, Saida).
(1) Other forms of meningitis reported separately.
(2) Scarlatina and tonsillitis reported together.
(3) Amoebiasis and bacillary dysentery reported together.
(4) Colienteritis and diarrhoeal disease reported together.
(5) Typhoid and paratyphoid fever reported together.

AUSTRIA

Only a table. Animal bites are reported on a separate form.
(1) Puerperal fever after normal birth and after abortion reported separately.
(2) Syphilis and gonorrhoea, no obligatory notification.

BELGIUM

The report includes narratives. Rickettsiosis is reported as a separate disease.
(1) Ornithosis and psittacosis reported as separate diseases.

CZECHOSLOVAKIA

Only a table. Some diseases are reported according to occurrence. Apart from the diseases reported in Table 1, Czechoslovakia also reports helminthiasis, ascariasis, stomatitis, mastitis and other exanthematic diseases.

DENMARK

The report includes narratives.
(1) Pertussis if vaccinated with 1 or 2 doses reported separately.
(2) Influenza reported separately for complicated or uncomplicated disease.

FINLAND

Only a table. Instead of separate columns for the three diseases subject to the International Health Regulations (formerly quarantinable diseases) a mention of their absence is put as a footnote. The report also indicates whether the disease was imported. A separate report on influenza is sent.
(1) Scarlatina and tonsillitis reported together.
(2) Colienteritis and diarrhoea reported together.
Finland also reports *Diphyllobothrium latum* infections.

FRANCE

Only a table. The report has empty spaces for some diseases, which are only mentioned if they occur.
(1) A separate report on influenza is sent.

GERMAN DEMOCRATIC REPUBLIC

Only a table.
(1) A separate table on influenza is sent.

FEDERAL REPUBLIC OF GERMANY

The report includes narratives.
(1) Leptospirosis reported separately for Weil's disease and for other forms.
(2) Meningitis/encephalitis reported in four forms: meningococcal meningitis, other bacterial meningitis, viral meningoencephalitis, and other forms.
(3) Only fatal cases reported.
(4) Paratyphoid fever: it states whether it is A, B or C.
(5) Salmonellosis and other forms reported separately.

GREECE

Only a table. Imported disease is indicated. Greece also has columns for dengue fever and sandfly fever (Pappataci fever).

HUNGARY

Only a table. Mentions if diseases are imported, and gives the median of the past five years and the previous year for comparison.

ICELAND

Only a table. The last report received was in 1978.
(1) Pneumonia reported as follows: viral pneumonia, pneumococcal pneumonia, and various other unidentified pneumonias. Also reports myositis.

IRELAND

Only tables. Space is left to include diseases according to occurrence.

ITALY

The report includes narratives.
(1) Leishmaniasis reported separately for the cutaneous and the visceral forms.
(2) Dermatophytosis and other mycoses reported separately. The report also mentions complications of vaccination, *Hymenolepis* infestation, venereal ulcers and rheumatic heart disease.

42

LUXEMBOURG	Only a table. Space is left for diseases when they occur.

LUXEMBOURG   Only a table. Space is left for diseases when they occur.

MALTA   Only tables. Space is left for diseases when they occur.

MOROCCO   No report received after 1970 till 1982, when one was received for 1979 and 1980.

NETHERLANDS   The report includes narratives in Dutch and English.
(1) Malaria reported, together with the country from which it was imported.
(2) Salmonellosis reported on a separate paper stating the type.

NORWAY   The report includes narratives.
(1) Meningitis following pertussis and other types reported separately.
(2) Measles in those vaccinated reported separately.
(3) Newport and Heidelberg salmonellosis reported separately.
(4) Gonorrhoea reported separately if it occurs in patients under 18 years of age.
Norway also reports acute poisoning (presumed chemical).

POLAND   Only a table.
(1) For meningitis there are three lines according to the etiology: meningococcal, other bacterial, and viral. For encephalitis too there are three lines according to the etiology: arbovirus, other herpes, and non-specified viruses.
Poland also reports chemical and mushroom poisoning.

PORTUGAL   Only a table. In addition to the national report there are also separate comprehensive reports, one for Lisbon and Oporto and another for the Azores and Madeira.
(1) Tetanus reported separately for postpartum and puerperal forms.
(2) Silico-tuberculosis reported separately.
(3) Q fever and other rickettsioses reported separately.
Portugal also reports rat-bite fever.

SPAIN   The report includes narratives.
(1) Relapsing fever transmitted by tick or louse.
(2) Typhoid and paratyphoid fever reported together.
Spain also reports rheumatic fever.

SWEDEN   The report includes narratives.
(1) Meningitis and meningococcal septicaemia reported together.
(2) Typhus and recurrent fever reported together.
Sweden sends a separate report from laboratories of all viruses isolated by type (adenovirus, *Coxiella burnetii*, coxsackie A and B, cytomegalovirus, cytopathogenic agents, echovirus, enterovirus, HBs antigen, herpes simplex, influenza A, influenza B, measles, parainfluenza, parotitis, poliovirus, reovirus, respiratory syncytial virus, rotavirus, rubella, varicella).
In addition Sweden reports *Campylobacter* infections, parapertussis, pneumococcal infections, all the salmonelloses by type, *Chlamydia trachomatis*, mycoplasmal infections and filariases.

SWITZERLAND   The report includes narratives.
Switzerland also reports dysentery, malaria, listeriosis, poliomyelitis and pertussis.

TURKEY   Only a table.

UNITED KINGDOM   The report includes narratives.

   England & Wales   (1) Primary encephalitis and post-infectious encephalitis reported separately.
Under others the United Kingdom reports typhus, rabies and viral haemorrhagic fever.
The report also mentions if disease is contracted abroad.

   Northern Ireland   Only a table.

   Scotland   The report includes narratives.
(1) Paratyphoid A and B reported separately.

YUGOSLAVIA   Only a table. It also provides separate lines for the federal republics and the median for five years and data from the previous year for comparison.

disease in individual countries. Changes in notification systems are forwarded to WHO and published in the *International digest of health legislation*, but these do not give a comprehensive picture of the system. An information system is being developed at present.

No information is available on the completeness of notification. Notifications are not absolute measures of disease frequency, although they may reflect changes in frequency if the pattern of notification remains the same. They do not if the pattern changes because, for example, of increased or decreased interest in a disease, publicity, an epidemic, changes in oganizational structure, or greater incentives. Some national officials claim completeness, others admit the information to be fragmentary. Rubella, for example, is notifiable in five English cities and brucellosis in one (2). Only a small proportion of cases of whooping cough are notified and there is considerable undernotification even of illnesses such as acute pyogenic meningitis. Eleven health authorities do not notify the most common infectious diseases such as measles or influenza, either because they do not want to be swamped by reports they cannot handle, or in the case of influenza because such diseases are included in the ICD not under infections but under diseases of the respiratory tract (2).

The greatest number of notifiable diseases common to all countries are in the classical group: diphtheria, pertussis, scarlatina, dysentery, typhoid and paratyphoid fevers, and hepatitis as an undivided group. The smallest common group contains perinatal and maternal, parasitic, and mycotic infections. Echinococcosis is not infrequent in at least eight countries of Europe, but it is reported by three only. No country except the United Kingdom (Scotland) routinely reports hospital infections, an increasing and serious problem everywhere, although several countries have established hospital surveillance schemes. Only one country reports *Mycoplasma* infections. Only four countries report the quite common clostridial infections. Following the ICD pattern, upper and lower respiratory infections are reported from only a few countries, and tuberculosis is found in the list of notifiable diseases in only 11 countries, although obviously some separate mechanism for its registration exists in every country, as may also be the case for venereal diseases.

Reporting in general raises the question of whether data are generated for epidemiological and control action or for statistical evaluation. If the latter, weekly or monthly reporting is of little concern when no specific control action is possible or intended. Infections, too, vary from the trivial to the serious; thus reports have different degrees of relevance for health administrations.

Sources of reports, quality of data, and structure of reporting

Rapid identification and notification of infectious diseases by practitioners or health institutions are sought by all European countries. Administrative procedures and legislation for notifiable diseases, the urgency attached to them, and the frequency of notification vary considerably, depending on

Table 7. Number of countries reporting diseases to WHO

ICD-9 code	Disease	No. of countries reporting
001	Cholera	12[a]
020	Plague	10[a]
050	Smallpox	10[b]
060	Yellow fever	9[a]
022	Anthrax	15[a]
005.1	Botulism	6
023	Brucellosis	18
005.2	*Clostridium perfringens* infection	4
032	Diphtheria	25
035	Erysipelas	7
024/025	Glanders	2
NOS 041.9	*Legionella* infection	2
030	Leprosy	12
100	Leptospirosis	16
027.0	Listeriosis	3
036	Meningitis	28
036.2	Meningococcal sepsis	6
033	Pertussis (whooping cough)	27
670/659.3	Puerperal fever	7
087	Relapsing fever	9[a]
034	Scarlatina	26
038	Sepsis	3
041.1	Staphylococcal infection	4
034	Streptococcal infection	3
037	Tetanus	18
010	Tuberculosis	13
011	Tuberculosis/pleurisy	9
014/018	Tuberculosis (non respiratory)	7
013	Tuberculosis/meninges/CNS	4
021	Tularaemia	11
NOS 041.9	Yersiniosis	3
078.5	Cytomegalovirus infection	2
053	Herpes zoster	2
070.0	Hepatitis A	7
070.2	Hepatitis B	8
070.9	Hepatitis, non-specified	27
487	Influenza-like diseases	16
078.8	Lassa fever	5[a]
055	Measles	21
075	Mononucleosis	5
062.9/049.9	Meningoencephalitis	16
049.0	Meningitis serosa	2
047	Meningitis (viral)	8
072	Parotitis, epidemic (mumps)	13
041.1	Poliomyelitis (paralytic)	5
045.2	Poliomyelitis (non-paralytic)	4

continued

[a] Some countries report this disease only when there is a case but have no column in the reporting forms.

[b] Smallpox has been eradicated but some countries still include it in their reporting forms.

45

Table 7. (contd)

ICD-9 code	Disease	No. of countries reporting
045/049	Poliomyelitis (not specified)	19
073	Psittacosis (ornithosis)	11
071	Rabies	15
056	Rubella	16
076	Trachoma	9
052	Varicella (chickenpox)	8
063/323.4	Viral encephalitis	4
065	Viral haemorrhagic fever[c]	7[a]
082.1	Boutonneuse fever	3
083.0	Q fever	10
080	Typhus exanthematosus	20
081.0	Typhus murinus	3
006	Amoebiasis	6
126	Ancylostomiasis	5
120	Bilharziasis	5
085	Leishmaniasis	5
084	Malaria	20
110	Mycosis/dermatophytosis	3
132	Pediculosis	3
123.3	Taeniasis	3
130	Toxoplasmosis	5
124	Trichinosis	8
133.0	Scabies	5
122	Hydatidosis/echinococcosis	3
466	Bronchitis	2
480	Pneumonia	4
465	Upper respiratory infections	5
007	Colienteritis	11
009	Diarrhoeal disease	6
004	Dysentery (bacillary, shigellosis)	28
005.9	Foodborne disease	13
009.0/009.2	Gastroenteritis (children under 2 years)	5
002.1/9	Paratyphoid fever	24
003	Salmonelloses, other	18
002	Typhoid fever	28
098	Gonorrhoea	14
009.2	Lymphogranuloma venereum	8
372.0	Ophthalmia neonatorum	3
091	Syphilis	15
090	Syphilis (congenital)	2
099.0	Ulcus molle (chancroid)	5
684	Pemphigus neonatorum	3
978	Poisoning (bacterial)	3
E906.0	Animal bites	3
372	Conjunctivitis	4

[a] Some countries report this disease only when there is a case but have no column in the reporting forms.

[c] Including Marburg virus disease.

Table 8. Frequency of reporting and number of diseases reported to WHO

Country	Frequency	No. of diseases
Albania	—	—
Algeria	3-monthly	33 obligatory, 5 optional
Austria	monthly/yearly	21 + animal bites
Belgium	weekly/monthly	49
Bulgaria	weekly	6
Czechoslovakia	weekly/monthly	42
Denmark	weekly/yearly	45
Finland	monthly + influenza report	30
France	weekly + influenza report	17 + according to occurrence
German Democratic Republic	weekly/yearly + influenza report	20
Germany, Federal Republic of	3-monthly/yearly	47
Greece	monthly	44
Hungary	monthly/yearly	33
Iceland	monthly	31
Ireland	weekly	13
Italy	monthly	63
Luxembourg	weekly/monthly	18 + according to occurrence
Malta	monthly	14
Monaco	—	—
Morocco	yearly (not received before 1982)	22
Netherlands	weekly/4-weekly	45
Norway	weekly/yearly	36
Poland	2-weekly	38
Portugal	monthly/yearly	43
Romania	monthly	15
San Marino	—	—
Spain	weekly	18
Sweden	weekly	33 (58 with laboratory reports)
Switzerland	monthly	25
Turkey	monthly/yearly	13
USSR	—	—
United Kingdom		
England & Wales	weekly	24
Northern Ireland	weekly/quarterly	27
Scotland	weekly	32
Yugoslavia	weekly/monthly	23

the organization and maturity of the health services and the degree of cooperation achieved between the health professionals and the health authorities (Fig. 2). Reporting to WHO depends in turn on those factors.

In all countries the basic data are collected at local level, usually as a report of cases (confirmed clinically and/or in the laboratory), and are forwarded to the next hierarchical level (district, province, region) or directly to the central authority. Collective reports may be sent according to the government's requirements, without any individual identification of outbreaks or as the result of epidemiological investigation of epidemics or serological or other surveys. The collecting of information varies in design, extent and timing according to the facilities available. The primary health contact, usually the physician, is generally responsible, but other professional workers such as nurses, veterinarians, or laboratory or administrative staff in the centres, hospitals or other institutions may do the work, according to the regulations or practices in the country. Notification is compulsory or optional, or a combination of both. An individual record is often prepared and used only for those diseases for which the health services conduct case-control activities, where the diseases have caused death, or where specific epidemiological and control measures are indicated. The authorities in most countries complain in general that it is very difficult to obtain the active participation of physicians, particularly private practitioners, in reporting, even when the legislative requirements are explicit. Reluctance to report is not the same for all diseases, being least for acute children's diseases and most for venereal diseases. It depends not only on the amount of data the physician is expected to record, the simplicity of the return and the existence, if any, of a financial incentive, but also on the time available to the physician, his feeling of responsibility, his views on the usefulness of the return, and the feedback to him by the health authorities. Even if only minimal basic data are required — name of the patient, age, sex, residence, diagnosis, place and date of report, and name of person reporting — and even if a nominal reimbursement is made for each report (as for example in the United Kingdom) collaboration in notification is extremely difficult to obtain. As a general rule the system is better accepted as being useful when the feedback is prompt and accompanied by comments and trend analyses; in this way the procedure is not just looked upon as bothersome bureaucratic form-filling. "Resistance to notification is higher [and thus the use of statistics more deceiving] if the disease is frequent and benign"(3). The main problem is to get the right balance between securing the recorder's sustained collaboration in producing regular, complete and accurate reports on the one hand, and an appropriate degree of sophistication in the data on the other. If the demands relating to quality are severe, quantity may be reduced to a point where it becomes too sparse and unrepresentative to be interpretable. This is a problem not solved satisfactorily in any European country.

The volume of unrecognized infection is unknown; while for example 90% of measles cases could theoretically be notified because the clinical illness is obvious, it would be possible to notify only about 1% of Epstein-

Fig. 2. Morbidity reporting

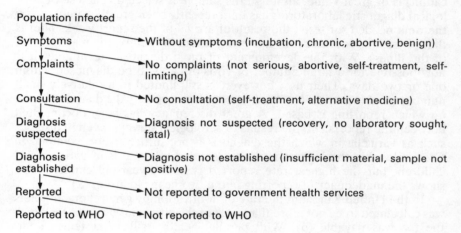

Population infected
Symptoms → Without symptoms (incubation, chronic, abortive, benign)
Complaints → No complaints (not serious, abortive, self-treatment, self-limiting)
Consultation → No consultation (self-treatment, alternative medicine)
Diagnosis suspected → Diagnosis not suspected (recovery, no laboratory sought, fatal)
Diagnosis established → Diagnosis not established (insufficient material, sample not positive)
Reported → Not reported to government health services
Reported to WHO → Not reported to WHO

Barr infections even by the best possible system. The underreporting of infectious diseases is a fact that should be taken into account by all health administrations. Although this is readily admitted, it also seems accepted as being in the nature of things. In some countries, such as Denmark, the weekly list of notifiable diseases has been drastically reduced to eight in an attempt to secure the collaboration of physicians in detailed reporting; the monthly reports, however, include 44 diseases. It is generally assumed that morbidity reports from general practitioners are more representative of what is happening in the country, although less diagnostically precise, than those based on laboratory- or hospital-referred samples. It is precisely at the level of primary health care that the systems are most deficient. Special arrangements are required to give more accurate information, and several approaches have been attempted in Europe, for example in the Netherlands and the United Kingdom; in addition to regular notification, there is a special sample system of well-motivated, randomly distributed sentinels whose "spotter" notifications will, it is hoped, provide a better idea of national trends and the degree of undernotification. A similar sentinel system exists for influenza in Finland, France and the German Democratic Republic. In France special surveys were conducted in selected *départements* (*4*) in which sample families were questioned directly over a limited period of time, and a sample of 267 school classes (6863 children in 22 cities) was instituted by the Institut national de la Santé et de la Recherche médicale in 1975 for influenza surveillance. In other places, returns from selected practitioners indicated the threshold of diseases that should have been notified. In some countries, such as Spain, Sweden and the United Kingdom, the system is complemented by special reports by laboratories with precise etiological classifications of the infections occurring, for example on the incidence of viral infections during a particular period.

The role of laboratories in the notification system, when precisely

49

defined and integrated (precautions being taken to avoid double notification) is of great value, although the sample is selected. The use of virological diagnostic laboratories has until recently been greatly hampered by the time needed for tests; the result of arrival of the report weeks later is that physicians consider it as not being useful in therapeutic management of the illness. With the development of rapid diagnostic techniques it is now possible for a large number of virus diseases to be diagnosed within one or two days. Their use, however, is still limited to a relatively small number of laboratories. National reports do not specify the diagnostic level on which reporting is based. A great discrepancy has been documented between the reports and the results of serological surveys, even in diseases such as varicella in which the diagnosis is not difficult. For example, in Czechoslovakia the highest infection (serological) rate is in two-year-old children, but the highest rate reported is in 3–4-year-old children; this shows the inadequacy of reporting in the two-year-old group (5).

In the United Kingdom the rate of notification by general practitioners was calculated to be not more than 22% of the infectious diseases for which the fee was payable (6). With parallel health delivery systems, a fair amount of multiple reporting is likely to occur for some diseases when the service suspecting the diagnosis is not the same as that making the final diagnosis or even providing the treatment and follow-up. In some countries no correction is made for suspected cases notified when the laboratory diagnosis fails to confirm the original diagnosis.

Do infections occur only in Scotland?

Every week the Communicable Diseases Surveillance Unit at the Ruchill Hospital, Glasgow publishes a report of about 12–15 pages, which includes not only notifications of infectious diseases from practitioners and clinicians from all areas in the country, but also data on the isolation of infectious pathogens from 72 laboratories (see Fig. 3). The report gives the exact etiological classification of notified infections according to the list of notifiable diseases, and contains an appreciation of the role of infectious agents in diseases not always included among communicable diseases according to the ICD, such as bacteraemias in nephritis, pyrexias of unknown origin, cholangitis, urinary diseases, peritonitis, leukaemias and burns, as well as a precise identification of the causes of alimentary and respiratory infections, pharyngitis, bronchitis, conjunctivitis, viral myalgias, myositis, pericarditis, stomatitis, genital and other herpetic lesions, respiratory diseases, otitis and skin lesions. Often more infections are reported in the weekly report from Scotland than in the monthly, and sometimes yearly, reports from a number of the other countries in the European Region. Scotland has one of the best organized health services in Europe and a high standard of living; obviously therefore these reports do not show a higher incidence of infection in Scotland (it is in fact much lower than in most countries) but instead a greater awareness by physicians and a greater effectiveness of the surveillance system. When WHO is asked whether a particular new disease or atypical syndrome not usually reported

50

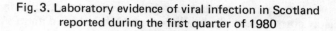

Fig. 3. Laboratory evidence of viral infection in Scotland
reported during the first quarter of 1980

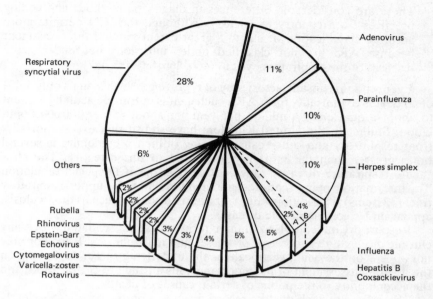

by the countries occurs in Europe, the report from Scotland is consulted
first as it is of invaluable assistance in the epidemiological assessment of
circulating infectious pathogens in general.

Examples of the misleading state of affairs

Respiratory infections

Deaths from acute respiratory infections (ARI) — upper respiratory
infections, influenza, and viral or bacterial pneumonias — in Europe
account for 51.6% of deaths from all respiratory diseases according to the
WHO returns, which are compiled on the principle that it is better to have
something reasonable to pick holes in than nothing at all.[a] This is a highly
unsatisfactory way of appreciating the importance of disease. Morbidity
data on ARI are available from very few countries. Mortality data from
respiratory diseases are available from 28 countries in Europe, but should
be taken into account only with caution for the following reasons.

— The data are not necessarily representative.

---

[a]**Hitze, K.L.** *WHO's global programme in acute respiratory infections.* Unpublished
document VIR/56L79.4 presented to the WHO Scientific Group on Virus Respiratory
Diseases, Geneva, 2–6 April 1979.

— In only a few countries is there a regular system of notification of deaths precisely correlated with the clinical and laboratory data.

— There are considerable differences in diagnostic methods and coding practices from country to country. Although the ICD permits more accurate classification, it has to a great extent vitiated the assessment because ARI are not classified under infections but under acute diseases of the respiratory system (460–466,480–483,487).

Even with this unsatisfactory way of reporting, which assigns only 4.4% of all deaths to mortality from ARI, such deaths in Europe actually amount to about a quarter of a million per year, or about 45 per 100 000 population. Studies in the United Kingdom have shown that excess mortality from respiratory and other causes during influenza epidemics is several times greater than the mortality attributed to this category. The class "acute respiratory diseases" does not exist in the ICD special tabulation list, information being scattered under diseases of the upper respiratory tract (32 items); in addition a few respiratory diseases, such as tuberculosis, appear under communicable diseases.

Respiratory infection is a common terminal event associated with many chronic diseases, degenerative processes and malignancies. It may or may not appear on the death certificate as the underlying cause, depending on the doctor's assessment of its importance, his attitude to certification, and the acceptability to the public of certain causes of death.

The order in which doctors record diagnoses on the certificates clearly determines whether a death is entered under one code or another. Analyses of deaths in which acute respiratory death was recorded as a direct or contributory cause, as well as of those in which it was recorded as the underlying cause, would give a more complete picture of the role of ARI as the cause of death.

Even in Sweden, a country with one of the highest standards of notification and diagnostic accuracy, analyses and multiple-cause codes reveal a large number of cases of acute respiratory death not included in the published statistics, as in the following for 1974:

Disease	ARI recorded as underlying cause of death	ARI not recorded as underlying cause of death
Influenza	234	81
Pneumococcal pneumonia	176	160
Bronchopneumonia	1312	8354

Thus it seems that acute respiratory death is very often recorded as a direct or contributory rather than as an underlying cause, and it is therefore not included in the national statistics.

The same applies to morbidity reporting. In only a few countries is the number of attendances at points of primary health care assessed, although ARI are responsible for up to 47% of all contacts with primary health care in the winter months. It is thus difficult to understand claims to the effect that infectious diseases are no longer a problem. The inaccuracy of these claims is even better demonstrated by analysis of claims for social security benefits, for sick leave from work (even if it refers to the employed population only, those usually least liable to respiratory infections) or school absenteeism. School absenteeism, according to the information available to the author, is monitored in Czechoslovakia, England & Wales, Finland, France and the German Democratic Republic.

Over five million cases of acute respiratory infection were reported in the German Democratic Republic in 1981, and this is considered a level probably applicable to many other countries. Finland, one of the least populated countries but with a high standard of notifications, reports over 300 000 cases a year (390 000 in 1980) or more than the whole of Europe for a three-year period (1970–1973). Some 900 000 cases of influenza are recorded yearly. These figures clearly show how infections are underestimated. The danger of relying too much on data from all countries in official WHO statistics is best seen in the data for the so-called "other gastrointestinal infections". The German Democratic Republic, with climatic conditions unfavourable for enteric infections and with a high standard of living, accounted in 1981 alone for 568 121 cases, almost the same number as is usually reported for all other countries together; this again is an example of undernotification in other countries. Romania reported in 1980 over half a million cases of viral pneumonia and over five million ARI of the upper respiratory tract while Spain reported over two million ARI in 1982. If the ICD is followed they will not appear under communicable diseases.

Special surveys to determine the incidence of illness below the threshold where notification is required, covering the people in the community who are a source of spread, are only in exceptional circumstances carried out. They are usually the only means of relating the illness to the personal characteristics of patients and the factors in their social environment that may identify high-risk groups. The most useful laboratory reports usually refer to selected hospital samples with an uncertain denominator.

Specific studies in France
A study carried out for eight months in 1975–1976 in Vaucluse (4) demonstrated that infection from eight common diseases was 10–100 times higher than was notified. The yearly incidence estimated per 100 000 persons for pertussis was 68–283 (only 9 cases were notified), for hepatitis 56–263 (8 notified), for measles 475–900 (43 notified) and for intestinal infections 300–1000 (12 notified). Among diseases where notification is optional, the incidence estimated for parotitis was 465–900 (40 notified), for rubella 150–430 (17 notified), for varicella 530–1000 (47 notified) and for influenza 3500–4300 (253 notified). Laboratory investigations showed that 70–90% of brucellosis cases were unknown to the health authorities; if 4900–9400 cases of unapparent or undiagnosed infection are added for 1965–1975, a total of 5900–10 900 brucellosis infections occurred, while only 120 were declared. This means that their number was 50–90 times higher than the number of notified cases. Only 3–5% of tuberculosis cases were notified by practitioners (7,8).

The national report for 1975 (part of the year only) registered 15 cases of leptospirosis, while the Pasteur Institute in Paris alone diagnosed 145 cases in the same period. In 1974 only 3500 cases of hepatitis were registered (9), while 100 000–150 000 were thought to have occurred (10).

Imported tropical diseases
Only seven countries report imported diseases other than malaria: Denmark, England & Wales, the Federal Republic of Germany, the Netherlands, Norway, Scotland and Sweden. It is impossible to obtain a clear picture of the number of tropical diseases imported into Europe and WHO is unable to answer the frequent questions about them, although at least for malaria the situation has improved and many countries have now included that disease in their notifications. Up to 1980 malaria was notified in France only if the transmission occurred locally (indigenous cases); introduced or induced malaria was not notified. Thus, from 1971 to 1977 only 101 cases, or about 15 per year, were officially notified. Replies to a questionnaire sent by the Ministry of Health and Social Security to the health authorities of the *départements* and regional hospitals showed 535 imported cases in 1978 alone. Even this is a vast underestimation; a survey among 319 physicians in Marseilles showed that treatment was given outside hospital in more than 90% of cases, which were not included in the official notification system. Since 1980 notification of all cases has been obligatory, whatever the origin.

Imported diseases are dealt with in Chapter 4.

A rational epidemiological service needs a base

A Communicable Diseases Surveillance Centre (CDSC) was established in 1977 in the United Kingdom to coordinate the investigation and control of communicable diseases in England & Wales. A similar centre had already been created in Scotland in 1964. These new centres have developed laboratory-based epidemiological functions with information centres at Colindale and Glasgow and specialist and community physicians located in different parts of the country. The association with laboratories has made possible the integration of surveillance programmes using both laboratory and clinical data (11). These are the first epidemiological units in Europe with services and responsibilities at a national level and come closest to the Centers for Disease Control (CDC) in Atlanta, USA. Although their function covers not only notification but also, more broadly, surveillance, investigation and control of communicable diseases and training of all levels of health and environmental personnel, it has led to the development of the weekly communicable diseases reports, compiled in their original form from laboratory reports, into wider-based information bulletins distributed not only to microbiologists but to all community physicians and senior environmental health officers. Through these national coordination centres the United Kingdom is in a position to take action in the event of a major communicable disease. Somewhat similar laboratory-based epidemiological centres exist in Bulgaria, Czechoslovakia, Norway and

Sweden, and are being developed in Italy and Spain. Excellent reports are received from Poland.

In 1975 a new notification system for infectious diseases was created on a nationwide scale in Norway, integrating notification, vaccination control, laboratory reports, seroepidemiological studies and surveillance of hospital infections. The system is as far as possible voluntary, but notification of specific diseases is compulsory and reporting in summary form with individual notification is included for certain cases.

Standardization or harmonization?

Because the notification of infectious diseases in European countries is not of recent origin but, in one form or another, based on a long tradition, it is very resilient and difficult to change. In view of the differences in the organization of health services and in socioeconomic development and traditions, and the geographical differences conditioning local pathology, no recommendations have been made by WHO for uniformity of reporting systems or for systematization of procedures for reporting infectious diseases, nor is it likely that countries would agree in the near future on a common system. The relative importance of any infectious disease varies with time and with the country, and a system applicable to one country might not suit another. The system must be flexible and able to adjust to changing situations. Comparison between countries is, however, all too often based on notifications and is useless if they do not accurately reflect the situation in the countries. However, there is a growing desire for harmonization of notification systems so as to make comparisons and a real assessment of trends possible. National authorities make periodic modifications in the reporting of diseases, omitting or adding diseases to the existing list. Thus, for example, several countries have recently added infections caused by *Yersinia enterocolitica*, *Campylobacter* and *Legionella* to their lists. The present hope is for at least agreement on the minimum common level of information needed.

International exchange of data

WHO collects, processes and disseminates internationally a certain amount of statistical material, including data on morbidity and mortality from notifiable infectious diseases. Another of its tasks is to compare the situation in different countries in a reliable way. In its effort to synthesize and consolidate health information from countries, WHO faces problems of relevance, timeliness, comparability and accuracy. It also receives many requests for up-to-date information, which it often does not possess. A special global notification scheme exists under the International Health Regulations (*12*) for diseases subject to the Regulations (cholera, plague and yellow fever; smallpox was deleted in 1981) with notification by telephone or telex within 24 hours of any outbreak and for the diseases under surveillance by WHO (louse-borne typhus, relapsing fever, paralytic poliomyelitis, viral influenza and malaria). Although smallpox has been eradicated, some countries still include it in their printed form. There are no statutory grounds for notifying other specific diseases that cause epidemics of national and international concern, such as cerebrospinal meningitis, dengue, viral haemorrhagic fevers, legionnaires' disease, foodborne epidemics, typhoid fever and dysentery. However, to promote the exchange of information on diseases not notifiable under the International Health Regulations or under international surveillance, the Thirtieth World Health Assembly requested Member States to endorse the opinion of the Committee on International Surveillance of Communicable Diseases that "prompt reporting of significant outbreaks of communicable diseases is the best foundation for their international control, irrespective of whether or not they are on any particular list".[a] This is intended to cover epidemics caused by agents that do not lend themselves to international specification. Moreover, virtually every outbreak has some aspect or aspects that cannot be envisaged in advance and covered by regulations. Opinions vary as to the value of negative (no case) reporting of "diseases under surveillance" and of "diseases on which routine information is necessary". While plague and yellow fever do not occur in Europe and only the latter has been imported in rare cases (e.g. two cases into France in 1980) the reporting of cholera, which does occur in several countries of the European Region, is different and presents problems.

Every Friday important information received during the week and intended for publication in the *Weekly epidemiological record* is summarized and fed into the automatic telex machine (see box). This enables national health administrations to obtain the information well before the *Weekly epidemiological record* reaches them.

The *Weekly epidemiological record* is published in English and French every Friday morning and a copy is sent to each national health administration by the fastest possible means. In addition, copies are dispatched by airmail to all subscribers.

The *Weekly epidemiological record* contains all the information the Organization is required to provide under the International Health Regulations, including the information already made available by telex. It also contains epidemiological notes and brief reviews of communicable diseases of international importance.

In certain countries, reporting has been suppressed by the authorities for "strategic" or prestige reasons. It is highly probable that diseases subject to the International Health Regulations are not reported from all places where they occur. Few people realize that the imperfect information WHO provides is intended merely to show trends. In all but one case of non-reporting, "WHO has been helpless" (13). In 1972 Dr Dorolle, Deputy Director-General of WHO, wrote: "We in the World Health Organization have been subjected to many criticisms on this score, and this is quite understandable on the part of the health administrations which want to be quickly informed. But we ourselves very often learn of epi-

---

[a] WHO Official Records, No. 240, 1977, p. 61.

demics in some parts of the world through the radio or the newspapers and we have to telephone or cable to the country concerned to obtain confirmation or rebuttal. Thus, one of the bases of the international system of surveillance and protection is weak, to say the least, because notification and diffusion of proper information have in most cases failed" (*14*). "The situation in the beginning of the present decade is at best unchanged. At least WHO should be able to make clear that the sign of underdeveloped health services is not the outbreak of a disease but the failure to report it, and that the rigid practices of the past century are a sign of weakness of the system rather than of its strength" (*13*).

The role of the Regional Office
The WHO Regional Office for Europe does not issue reports on infectious diseases. All other Regional Offices have one or more systems of reporting: monthly notes on communicable diseases, reports or leaflets on selected diseases preventable by immunization (under the global expanded programme on immunization) and/or immunizations carried out, specific surveillance reports, and annual bulletins on communicable diseases. The question has been raised by several countries of whether the Regional Office in Europe could give up-to-date information on infectious diseases. It is a matter of concern that the press is usually informed sooner of disease outbreaks and that diplomatic representatives have more complete data than WHO. The staffing situation and the low priority assigned to infectious diseases in the Region do not make it probable that this situation will be remedied in the near future. On special occasions the Regional Office takes action, for example to request information on imported malaria or poliomyelitis from European countries when they do not report it automatically. However, three specific notification schemes particular to Europe have been organized by WHO.

● European programme for the surveillance of foodborne infections and intoxications and early warning system at the FAO/WHO Collaborating Centre for Research and Training in Food Hygiene, Berlin (West). This programme has functioned since 1980 as the focal point in the European surveillance programme and collects, evaluates and disseminates data for the 13 countries participating. The early warning component of this programme is functioning well. A periodic newsletter is published.

- The Mediterranean zoonoses control project. Based at the Mediterranean Zoonoses Control Centre in Athens, this project collates the information and analyses of trends for Mediterranean countries (including non-European countries) on canine rabies, hydatidosis, brucellosis and Rift Valley fever. It is proposed to expand the coverage to other zoonoses. A monthly newsletter is published. This system has been in operation since 1980 only and cannot yet be evaluated though it is facing severe financial problems.

- European system for the surveillance of rabies. The WHO collaborating centre at the Federal Research Institute on Animal Viral Diseases, Tübingen, Federal Republic of Germany has for several years published a quarterly report on rabies in Europe, sponsored by WHO and the Office international des Epizooties (OIE). The report gives the numbers by animal species involved and by country, includes a map of the distribution, and comments on trends. This system functions very well.

- In January 1983 the European Centre for Health and Disease Surveillance was established in the Istituto Superiore di Sanità in Rome as a support to the Communicable Diseases unit and the Epidemiology and Information Support unit of the WHO Regional Office. This Centre will carry out analysis and make graphical presentations of data on communicable diseases provided by governments to the Regional Office, computerize them and produce yearly summaries. It will also supply countries with up-to-date information, on request.

Through the WHO collaborating centres for influenza and the national influenza centres, information is obtained about the types of virus isolated during the influenza season (Annex 2).

Other international information systems
Regular weekly, monthly and bimonthly reporting is carried out for animal diseases by the OIE in Paris. Although it reports for the world, European countries are particularly well represented. The reporting is according to the International Animal Health Code[a] (including such diseases as anthrax, rabies, glanders, tuberculosis, psittacosis and tularaemia) and has the advantage of giving not only up-to-date information but also the precise geographical localization and spread of the disease and the sanitary and veterinary control measures applied. While this system of surveillance of animal health also encounters some of the difficulties met with in the notification of human diseases (nomenclature, time limits, etc.) it has the advantage of providing information from countries that do not report to WHO.

FAO, in collaboration with WHO and OIE, publishes the *Animal*

---

[a] *International animal health code*. Paris, Office international des Epizooties, 1971.

health yearbook, in which the evaluation of animal diseases throughout the world can be followed year by year. This information is now being compiled by OIE.

Where the present system is faulty

The rapid decline in Europe of the classical acute infectious diseases that can be prevented by immunization, and of those reduced by the marked improvement in hygiene and living standards of the first five decades of this century, has given rise to the confident feeling that they will decline further. The reduction in mortality and the expanding armamentarium of effective drugs have eliminated the fear of or feeling of responsibility for controlling infectious diseases and, in part, the commitment to surveillance mechanisms such as notification. The classical infectious diseases have been equated with social and economic underdevelopment as opposed, for example, to cancer, accidents or chemical poisoning, which are seen to epitomize progress and development. Only the realization that the control of sexually transmitted diseases is a failure, the reappearance of malaria in Turkey, the increase in diseases attributable to modern mass food production, and the challenge created by the importation of infections by tourists and refugees have slowly brought about a gradual reawakening of interest in infections. Notification and epidemiological systems have not been prepared for respiratory syncytial virus, cytomegalovirus, the herpesvirus group, rotavirus, Norwalk agent, enteropathogenic *Escherichia coli*, *Chlamydia*, *Mycoplasma pneumoniae*, *Legionella*, *Yersinia*, *Campylobacter*, *Clostridium difficile*, hospital infections, and the unchecked spread of animal rabies.

With the emphasis on primary health services and the need for their evaluation, the problem of assessing priorities became urgent. The inadequacy of the notification system in general had already been noted in 1970 by Miller (*15*), who found that infectious and parasitic diseases and diseases of the respiratory system ranked first in inpatient days and outpatient visits but very low as the cause of death (although, if all infections are counted together, still in third place after accidents and diseases of the circulatory system). "If the administrator assigned priorities according to deaths, he would select accidents as the top priority. If he elected to use hospital data he would concentrate more on infections. If outpatient figures were selected, he would emphasize respiratory diseases. With few exceptions there is little agreement among traditional categories as to the rank order of diseases. Obviously, if priorities were assigned on the basis of mortality, they would conflict with the need reflected by the data in inpatients and outpatients" (*15*). In Europe health administrators pay special attention to data on deaths and not to needs that are manageable by the means available. The emphasis on primary health services requires a reversal of attention, a higher priority for diseases amenable to treatment or prevention. This is shown by a 48-hour survey carried out in France in March 1980. Out of 3216 diagnoses made by general practitioners in various parts of the country 998 (31%) were of infections, and in the age group 2–5 years they represented over 60%. In comparison, cardiovascular diseases accounted for only 13% (*16*). Only in 16% of cases was a laboratory or other diagnostic method sought and only exceptionally etiological clarification or confirmation. A specialist was consulted in 7% of cases and 1.5% of the 483 patients were sent to hospital. Sixty per cent of all patients were treated with antibiotics. In the United Kingdom, with a rather high standard of notification, a survey (*17*) showed that only about 50% of the cases of infectious hepatitis known to medical practitioners were reported during one year. Over and above those not notified are the atypical or anicteric hepatitis cases, which are likely to escape notification either because the patients do not seek medical help or the correct diagnosis is not made.

Notification as it now exists does not provide an adequate picture of the incidence or prevalence of infections, of their economic impact, of the workload on the services, or of other factors that concern the health authorities. Until it does the goals of primary health care will not be achieved. For example, even with incomplete reporting (at best 1 out of 50–100 cases is notified) cases of salmonellosis are increasing in Europe.

Clearly a fresh look is overdue, not only at the classical communicable diseases but also at all bacterial, viral and parasitic infections, including hospital infections with Gram-negative bacteria. New approaches are badly needed to collect better information on the whole spectrum of infections. It is reported, for example, that sales of pharmaceutical drugs are conservatively estimated for the year 2000 at US$560 000 million, the largest part being for antibiotics (*18*); this represents one of the largest non-salary outlays in hospital and primary health care. As antibiotics are used to prevent or combat infections, this raises the serious question of whether infections or the risk of infection are present or the whole preventive and therapeutic approach of the medical profession is wrong. In both cases the question requires thorough attention, there being a difference in theory and practice in the use of antibiotics. Whether routine notification in its present form could contribute at all is open to doubt. There were, for example, 125 000 pneumococcal infections in France in 1979 (not counted as infections according to the ICD). It is obviously difficult for physicians to renounce antibiotics in the prodromal stage of a febrile illness on the grounds that the majority of respiratory illnesses are caused by viruses.

Improving reporting

Possible methods of improving notification as at present practised are few and often inefficient, but there are areas where innovative cooperative effort might be attempted, such as through the periodic distribution of regulations, the continuous feedback of data, comments to suppliers of information on the updating of reports on particular diseases, instructions about the management of infections and immunization practices, and the supply of important scientific information in summary form. Written reminders that alert the medical profession to the arrival or risk of new diseases provide a national perspective and serve to educate. Meetings, talks (with case examples) at medical gatherings and seminars, and other contacts with practitioners may bring about a modification of notification practices, as shown in France in one *département* (4) where notifications were improved five times compared with the previous three years. Routine reporting could be reduced and a system of paid sentinel posts (including laboratories) instituted.

Education and training should start in schools of medicine. It is hard to believe, but unfortunately true, that epidemiology is not taught in all European faculties of medicine or that related courses such as hygiene, forensic medicine and clinical medicine do not always impart a full understanding of the value of reporting diseases. The physician needs to be clear what the purpose of reporting is and, if changes have frequently been made, what the current rules are.

The occasional distribution of pertinent information through the daily press, taking advantage of, for example, outbreaks of disease, and bringing the existence of the epidemiological services to the attention of the public and of health professionals has been of value. Postal surveillance on a sample basis has been tried occasionally to make underreporting visible. Among administrative measures that could help improve notification, other than feedbacks and simplification of procedures, are financial compensation for the notifying physician, telephone, telegraph and postal privileges, and special recognition by the health authority. The maximum exchange of information among the various sections of the institutions involved and the different institutions of the country, particularly at the primary health care level, would help and would also lay stress on the integration of the various sectors of the health system. Unfortunately it does not seem that record linkage schemes are sufficiently advanced in Europe to show the dynamic consequences of those infectious diseases (e.g. of the urogenital or locomotor organs) that are statistically recorded under chronic diseases. Changes in the system require complicated legislation and vast educational campaigns, which the health authorities are often unable to undertake.

The crucial aim is to establish a functioning system of day-to-day epidemiological evaluation in the health services and demonstrate that it is really used. Reporting officers should be offered assistance in epidemiological investigations. At present, however, the conclusion must be that options are limited and that undernotification is likely to continue.

Value of notification in epidemiological surveillance

"Surveillance means the continued watchfulness over the distribution and trends of incidence through the systematic collection, consolidation and evaluation of morbidity and mortality reports and other relevant data. Intrinsic in the concept is the regular dissemination of the basic data and interpretation" (19). Surveillance is thus more than just notification.

Notification and reporting systems have long-term documentary value, but without interpretation they are only a part of health statistics. Notification is just the first step in the system of epidemiological surveillance, which is a dynamic activity and includes an estimation of risks, further investigations, and recommendations for control measures. Notification is the most basic and least costly part of epidemiological surveillance, but it is the *sine qua non* for the setting of priorities, the formulation of policies, and the allocation of resources in any national health system. It is not limited to infectious diseases.

Miller[a] summarized the value of notification under three headings: clinical, epidemiological and administrative.

Clinical value
- It stimulates a more critical approach to diagnosis by alerting clinicians to currently prevalent agents and types of illness.

- Analysis of the correlation between the clinical features, personal characteristics of patients, and agents isolated may show combinations permitting better predictions of the etiology.[b]

- By sharpening the clinical assessment of the probable agents it assists decisions on treatment and management.

Epidemiological value
- The data can be used to show the relative significance of infections as a cause of sickness and death in the community and changes in incidence with time. They also enable the impact of control measures to be assessed. The prevalence of illness can be related to the prevalence of particular agents and their relative significance assessed. By analysing past experience and monitoring current incidence rates and the types of agents prevalent, it may be possible to predict future trends and the likelihood of epidemics (e.g. of influenza).

- The personal characteristics that predispose to illness and death can be studied to identify those groups in the population at highest risk. The risk of acquiring infection with particular agents and of developing particular types of illness in these groups can be estimated. The routes of spread of infection and the environmental and social conditions that favour infection and its transmission can be identified.

- The definition of risk groups directs attention to those sections of the population on which control action (e.g. vaccination) needs to be focused. The definition of risk factors that determine high incidence and fatality rates points to the type of control action that may be most

---

[a]**Miller, D.L.** *Acute respiratory diseases: methods of surveillance control.* Unpublished WHO report, Geneva, 1976.

[b]This may require comparison of the frequency of a particular attribute in a case population with that in the general population, or specific case-control studies.

relevant and effective. From knowledge of the agents currently prevalent in a community, the most appropriate treatment regimes or composition of vaccines can be decided.

Administrative value

- The information helps in assessing the need for health services and in planning the use of resources (accommodation, staff and finance).

- It permits measurement of the economic cost of infections to the individual and the community in terms of time lost from work and the utilization of medical care resources.

- It gives a warning about impending epidemics and the need for action by general practitioners in the organization of their work and by hospitals in relation to admission policy.

- In the interest of public relations the information must be readily available to the media and to politicians.

Future trends

Although there is at present (not only for political reasons) considerable pressure in favour of basing priorities on indicators other than morbidity — such as mortality, utilization of the health services, relationships within the structure of the health care system, or so-called "positive" indicators yet to be precisely formulated — the functioning of the health services is still best evaluated as a whole and within the perspective of a quantifiable reduction of morbidity. Morbidity assessment is based on notification, and this is incomplete. Mortality and morbidity indicators have been fully used in chronic diseases and cancer; morbidity from infection, on the other hand, not giving rise to any dramatic mortality because of the disappearance of large epidemics of the classical communicable diseases in Europe, has been largely disregarded. Mortality has lost its importance in the measurement of infectious diseases and can be used only rarely, for example as excess mortality in influenza or in particular situations as a measure of the effectiveness of the health services.

Other indicators are obviously needed, such as economic and social cost, use of drugs and laboratory services, and work absenteeism. However, here too there is a bias. Certified causes of absence from work are more likely to be weighted in favour of chronic diseases such as mental disorders, cardiovascular diseases or injuries rather than acute infections (with the exception of influenza) with their clear termination limits. The tendency therefore is to ignore unemployed women and the younger population groups who account for a large proportion of infections. The emphasis on mortality from so-called "big killers", undoubtedly more spectacular, usually disregards the age-specific rates at which death occurs but understandably captures the attention of the public, pressure groups and the authorities. Given the universal undernotification of infections and their classification elsewhere in the ICD, it is not surprising that health administrators no longer assess morbidity from infection appropriately.

The interest of health administrators has shifted towards the performance of the health care system, health care planning, and health problems not related to etiologically known and treatable diseases. Care and cure are not alternatives; both are needed. New and sophisticated techniques have been and are being developed to measure single and aggregate health outcome indicators, disease staging concepts, and classifications of impairments, disabilities and handicaps. They are undoubtedly useful, but could potentially be more useful if disease "can profitably be considered with reference to its cause, whether this is microbial, behavioural or genetic, environmental, or multifactorial".[a] All too often the classical etiology → pathology → manifestation → sequelae model is forgotten or no longer considered adequate by some administrators.

It is fashionable at present to be preoccupied not with disease but with health as though, in spite of the presence of bacteria, viruses, fungi and parasites, disease could be avoided by changing one's lifestyle. The constant deterioration in notification is in part due to this diminished attention to infectious diseases and to the neglect of epidemiology. Epidemiology and disease surveillance do not operate in a vacuum. Further reduction of infections is possible and probable in the future but, as Howie (1) warned: "There is less infection than there was; but there is still too much. Moreover, the control of what remains, let alone its elimination, calls for greater insight, more certainty of method, and burial of the illusion that it no longer matters".

*   *   *

Analysis of notifications of infectious diseases in countries of the WHO European Region shows wide differences, making comparison of reported frequencies and assessment of continental or regional trends difficult, if not impossible.

- Systems of notification, criteria for the use of diagnostic labels, and clinical appreciations vary widely and have not been standardized.

- Consistency in methods of compiling returns and adequate cooperation between the generators of data and the authorities are lacking in most European countries. Information systems themselves are often rudimentary and highly unreliable and the trend towards automation has so far not brought improvement in the quality of information, although it may have reduced the handling and made retrieval easier.

- With some exceptions, even countries with a good infrastructure and good supporting services are weak in epidemiological surveillance and in

---

[a]**Crew, F.A.E.** *Levels of living — the health component.* Document presented to the Study Group on the Measurement of Levels of Health, 1955 (WHO Technical Report Series No. 137, 1957).

managerial capacity to identify the magnitude of infections and their consequences. Often not even the visible part of the iceberg is shown.

- Health authorities are more interested in mortality than in morbidity, so that assessment of infectious diseases and the health status of the population is faulty. Yet the importance of assessing morbidity is greater since the drastic decline in infections preventable by immunization and the radical improvement in treatment.

- The notification systems are often anachronistic and slow in adapting to change. Statistical data rarely reflect the true incidence of infections. Undernotification of infectious diseases should accordingly be taken into account by the health authorities, especially as it is most marked at the primary health care level, where the need for continuous and correct information and assessment is greatest. On the other hand, the practitioner cannot be burdened with the administrative work involved in the notification of infections; the reporting can be assumed to be exact only from hospitals and laboratories, which give only minimum figures for the severe infections occurring.

- Assessment of infections has particularly suffered from the rigid application of the ICD, in which large numbers of diseases of bacterial and viral origin are included under different categories such as respiratory, neonatal, maternal, genitourinary and nervous system diseases. Irrespective of the classification, the basis of effective disease surveillance is identifying the cause of infection and doing something about it. Revision of the ICD will not take place until about 1990; until then the organ as opposed to the etiological classification will continue.

- There is lack of coordination between national agencies and international organizations on the subject of reporting requirements. WHO, the only body entrusted with the regional collection of data and trend assessment on a global scale, has yet to discuss with countries an eventual improvement of the situation. Assessment of regional trends, based on notifications as it now is, is only rarely possible except for some classical communicable diseases.

- Even with the best of all possible systems, the number of infections occurring in the community will remain approximate because of subclinical infection; only severe manifest diseases will stand a chance of being notified. Infections are always an iceberg phenomenon, the larger part consisting of unrecognized inapparent infections.

- While innovative approaches to the collection of better information over the whole spectrum of infections are badly needed, notification of all infections could easily lead to overloading of the system because of the avalanche of returns that could occur. Selective mechanisms might be needed based on sentinel cooperating posts of motivated physicians and laboratories, not as an alternative but as a complementary system. The use of modern electronic statistical and mathematical tools could help to assure carefully designed samples drawn from sentinel posts for better information on infections in each country, at less cost and with a smaller workload than at present.

● Even if notification is much improved, it will remain incomplete as a source of data on the frequency of infectious diseases in the population. The notification figures should be supplemented by information from other sources.

● The main argument for introducing notifications at the end of the last century was to keep the local health services informed so that they could take the necessary action: disinfection of dwellings, isolation of cases and possibly avoidance of contacts, etc. Statistics were a by-product. Nowadays, some sanitary measures are difficult to justify for many notifiable diseases even though they are still all too common (for example house disinfection for a disease caused by *Y. enterocolitica*). The same is true, in view of the present level of underreporting, for cost-effectiveness analysis based on the notification system for quite a number of diseases.

● The information a country has depends on an effective epidemiological service that not only collects, collates and analyses the information but also rapidly investigates and applies the appropriate control and preventive measures. Epidemiological services not only categorize diseases by their impact on morbidity, mortality, risk and cost but also influence and contribute to the development of the country's public health policy.

References

1. **Howie, J.W.** Infectious disease, does it still matter? *Public health*, **82**: 253–260 (1968).
2. **Barker, D.I.P. & Rose, G.** *Epidemiology in medical practice.* Edinburgh, Churchill-Livingstone, 1979, p. 22.
3. **Brès, P.** Les méthodes modernes de surveillance des maladies transmissibles: introduction générale. *Revue d'épidémiologie et de santé publique*, **25**: 351–359 (1977).
4. **Foulon, G. et al.** Enquête auprès des ménages sur les principales maladies transmissibles dans un département français: le Vaucluse. *Santé et sécurité sociale statistiques et commentaires*, No. 6A, pp. 75–83 (1980).
5. **Trifajova, I. et al.** Varicella morbidity in Czechoslovakia. *Journal of hygiene, epidemiology, microbiology and immunology*, **24**: 192–199 (1980).
6. **Haward, P.A.** Scale of under-notification of infectious diseases by general practitioners. *Lancet*, **1**: 873 (1973).
7. **Cabanel, G. & Stephan, J.C.** Pour une meilleure connaissance de l'état sanitaire des Français. *Concours médical*, **15**: 2497–2500 (1981).
8. **Bernard, E.** cited in **Boyer, J**. A propos de la déclaration obligatoire des maladies contagieuses. *Bulletin de l'Académie de Médecine*, **158**: 458–464 (1974).

9. **Mollaret, H.** Pour une approche nouvelle des maladies infectieuses. *In: Proceedings of the Annual Congress of the Societies of Social Medicine and Sanitary Engineering.* Paris, Ministry of Health, 1976, pp. 112–121.

10. **Charbonneau, P.**, cited in **Boyer, J.** A propos de la prévention de l'hépatite à virus type A. *Bulletin de l'Académie de Médecine*, **164**: 446–450 (1980).

11. **Galbraith, N.S. & Young, S.E.I.** Communicable disease control: the development of a laboratory associated national epidemiological service in England and Wales. *Community medicine*, **2**: 135–143 (1980).

12. *International health regulations.* Geneva, World Health Organization, 1981.

13. **Velimirovic, B.** Do we still need International Health Regulations? *Journal of infectious diseases*, **133**: 473–481 (1976).

14. **Dorolle, P.** International problems of communicable diseases control. *Lancet*, **2**: 525–527 (1972).

15. **Miller, I.E.** An indicator to aid management in assigning programme priorities. *Public health reports*, **85**: 725–731 (1970).

16. **Piccoli, S. et al.** Exposé des résultats de l'enquête 48 heures. *Médecine et maladies infectieuses*, **11**: 125–130 (1981).

17. **d'Alacron, R. & Lewis, M.** Failure in notification of infective jaundice. *Public health*, **85**: 223–238 (1971).

18. *World pharmaceutical news*, No. 509, 28 July 1980.

19. **Langmuir, A.** The surveillance of communicable diseases of national importance. *New England journal of medicine*, **268**: 182–192 (1963).

3

Figures and trends for selected infectious diseases in Europe, 1950–1980

B. Velimirovic, D. Greco,[a]
P. Piergentili[a] & A. Zampieri[a]

This chapter attempts to analyse the situation of certain diseases on the basis of official reports, notwithstanding their faults of undernotification, incomplete coverage and selectiveness. The diseases chosen are: five covered by the WHO Expanded Programme on Immunization (measles, diphtheria, pertussis, poliomyelitis and pulmonary tuberculosis), meningitis, brucellosis, parotitis, scarlet fever, varicella, typhoid and paratyphoid fevers, bacillary dysentery, hepatitis, influenza, and the two classical sexually transmitted diseases gonorrhoea and syphilis. It was felt that, while data from official notifications are incomplete, the bias may be consistent for each particular country, assuming that there is no change in the system or in readiness or lack of readiness to notify. Thus at least trends over time, if not incidence in its true perspective, can be determined. The diseases chosen were those likely to have come to the attention of the health services of the countries and thus be notified.

The data used are from the official reports of countries to WHO and have been published in *World health statistics annual*. Where those were not available, data were extracted from various national publications sent to the WHO Regional Office for Europe. Rates of incidence per 100 000 population per year for each disease were calculated using as denominator the census population figures for each country, adjusted for each year

[a]Istituto Superiore di Sanità, Rome, Italy.

according to the country's own estimates of population for the years between the census years. The graphs present the trends on a semilogarithmic scale. Where data were not available for a particular year, a space was preferred to any linking between the points. A BASIC language computer program was developed by the staff of the Istituto Superiore di Sanità in Rome, and the tracing was carried out by Textronix 4054 computer with 4368 plotter and printer. Note that the data available to WHO do not represent the total information available in countries, which in many instances is more complete than the official statistics distributed internationally. This also became evident when time trends were examined; it may appear that the diseases were notified only for the years shown in the graphs. This is not so, but the volume of work in compiling this information for earlier years proved to be beyond our capacity.

The data are presented on graphs, each for one disease in one country. Separate scale graphs were preferred to the net type of set-out, both for better visibility and for scale differences. The countries are arranged in alphabetical order. All data are presented in semilogarithmic graphs. Arithmetic graphs were also prepared but, not without hesitation, were omitted for reasons of space. A decline, where it occurs, is much more distinctly visible on an arithmetic presentation. The size of scale for each graph is a problem. For the semilogarithmic graph a single scale for each disease was chosen from the minimum–maximum range to include the whole country in the time period and all the possible fluctuations of rates. This dictates the use of quite large-range scales, with a certain flattening of the graphs as a consequence. For most countries the rates are in the central scale of 1–1000, but for a few they are squeezed onto a less fluctuating scale (the smaller the scale range the larger the fluctuation). Different scales could be chosen for each graph, but there is a danger that the reader might fail to notice the changes in scale and think that all the graphs have the same scale. It was therefore decided to have four scales for different diseases with the idea of presenting most diseases on the main scale graph, the other three scales being used for those that differed. A computer program allows for a more elaborate layout: mapping, linear trend analysis, histograms, etc. It was thought, however, that such a layout is unnecessary until a European agreement is reached on the definition of "case" and the first step is taken in approximating, if not standardizing, reporting and classification. Preliminary agreement is also needed on integration of laboratory notifications into national schemes. It is expected that this will be possible in the future and a system of regional analysis is being considered, based on a collaborating centre in the Istituto Superiore di Sanità in Rome.

Comparison among the various countries was not the objective. This would have been impossible, considering the variety of criteria for diagnosis and reporting and the different surveillance systems in countries. Moreover, diagnostic patterns and skills may have changed over the years studied and new techniques have been introduced. Nevertheless, those considerations are not expected to disturb significantly the trends in individual countries.

Table 9. Child population in Europe and the USSR
subject to immunization procedures in 1978 (millions)

Area	No. of births per year	Age group	
		0–4 years	5–14 years
Eastern Europe	1.9	9	16
Southern Europe	2.3	11	24
Northern Europe	1.1	6	13
Western Europe	1.8	11	25
USSR	4.7	22	45
Total	11.8	59	123

Source: WHO estimates, based on a variety of sources.

Immunization

Although the countries of the European Region, with the exception of
Algeria and Morocco, are not included in the WHO Expanded Programme
on Immunization, which aims at vaccinating *all* children by 1990, immunization procedures are carried out routinely in all countries. The child
population subject to primary or booster immunization is presented in
Table 9. There are about 12 million children born in the Region each year.
Some 59 million in the age group 0–4 years are subject to immunization
and about 123 million in the age group 5–14 years to some sort of revaccination. The immunization coverage for the six classical diseases is as
high as 85–95% in the countries in Europe where immunization is most
effective, although a trend towards a decline in acceptance has been noted.
Immunization is compulsory in 11 European countries, while in the rest of
Europe it is on the whole voluntary in six countries and compulsory only
for certain age groups, for example as a requirement for school entry or in
special situations (Table 10).

The vaccination schedules vary from country to country, and so many
recommendations have been made by national bodies and international
conferences that it is possible neither to quote them all nor to give a
meaningful synthesis of existing varieties. The available information is
summarized in Annex 3. The effectiveness of vaccination coverage is based
on surveillance of clinical cases and on interrogation of subjects (or
parents) about the clinical and immunization history. This assessment is
insufficient, and it seems that no government is satisfied with it; neither the
six target diseases of the WHO Expanded Programme on Immunization
nor the figures for the true coverage achieved through vaccination are
reported in all countries. In most cases vaccination in Europe is carried out
within the context of primary health care. In several countries, however,
mass campaigns are still used in specific situations for specific diseases.

71

The basic characteristic of immunization is that it must be undertaken each year *de novo* if the results are to be maintained. In order to reverse the declining trend of immunization observed in a number of countries in recent years, intensive educational and motivational action is needed to make people aware of the importance of routine vaccination. While efforts to extend the benefits of immunization must be permanent, this does not mean that vaccination must permanently be undertaken against specific diseases; the epidemiological situation, the need for the approximately 25 individual vaccines currently used in Europe, and immunization techniques

Table 10. Summary of immunization practices
in the WHO European Region, 1982

Country	Vaccine						
	BCG	Diphtheria	Pertussis	Tetanus	DPT	Poliomyelitis	Measles
Albania	C	C	C	C	C	C	C
Austria	V	V	V	V	V	V	V
Belgium	S	V	V	V	V	C	V
Bulgaria	C	C	C	C	C	C	C
Czechoslovakia	C	C	C	C	C	C	C
Denmark	V	V	V	V	V	V	V
Finland	V	V	V	V	V	V	V
France	C	C	V	C	V	C	V
German Democratic Republic	C	C	C	C	C	C	C
Germany, Federal Republic of	S	V	V	V	V	V	V
Greece	V	C	C	C	C	C	V
Hungary	C	C	C	C	C	C	C
Ireland	S						
Italy	S	C	V	C	—	C	V
Luxembourg	V	V	V	V	V	V	V
Malta	V	C	V	C	V	C	V
Morocco	C	V	V	V	V	V	V
Netherlands	S	V	V	V	V	V	V
Norway	C	V	V	V	V	V	V
Poland	C	C	C	C	C	C	C
Portugal	V	C	C	C	C	C	C
Romania	C	C	C	C	C	C	C
Spain	V	V	V	V	V	V	V
Sweden	S	V	—	V	V	V	V
Switzerland	V	Cᵃ	V	V	V	V	V
Turkey	V	V	V	V	V	V	V
USSR	V	C	C	C	C	C	C
United Kingdom	V	V	V	V	V	V	V
Yugoslavia	C	C	C	C	C	C	C

C – compulsory; V – voluntary; S – compulsory for certain age groups or in special situations only.

[a] In the French and Italian speaking regions only.

must always be evaluated anew and decisions taken accordingly. It should be remembered that the success of an immunization programme is not measured by the number of persons employed, the number of vaccinations, or the geographical areas or populations involved, but by what actually happens to the incidence of the disease concerned. The sad fact is that, at the minimum, and disregarding the fact that many countries did not provide reports, over 1.3 million cases of disease preventable by basic immunization occurred in Europe in 1980.

Europe is self-sufficient with respect to vaccines. It is expected that by 1986 all countries will use vaccines known to conform to WHO requirements and establish systems for monitoring the quality and potency of vaccines at the time of use. Consequently, no outbreaks of measles, poliomyelitis or pertussis should theoretically occur in fully immunized children.

Periodic serological surveys to check the immunity profiles of the child population and better determine the target age are carried out routinely in five countries on stratified random samples.[a] Typhoid vaccine is given in five countries in endemic areas or to selected groups. Several countries offer vaccines against rubella (the slow acceptance of this vaccine is surprising in view of the fact that neonatal rubella syndrome can be completely eliminated) and parotitis, routinely combined with measles and rubella in two countries. In geographically selected areas specific vaccines are given seasonally against influenza and tick-borne encephalitis. Currently safe polyvalent (23-type) pneumococcal polysaccharide vaccines, containing purified capsular material of *Streptococcus pneumoniae* extracted separately and combined in the final vaccine, have become available. They are effective against 90% of types responsible for bacteraemic disease. They have been given experimentally in field trials in Finland and the Netherlands, while in Belgium, Norway and Sweden they are given to certain high-risk individuals. Theoretically, to be effective it is important to have vaccines representing those types of pneumococci responsible for most cases of pneumonia and otitis media. Some 18 types are responsible for more than 85% of infection and 7 types have been found to account for 70% of pneumococcal otitis media. Children under one year of age, however, respond poorly to polysaccharides. WHO has initiated a collaborative typing study on the long-term changes in circulating serotypes. However, except for those countries mentioned previously where information is available, only a few European countries have joined so far, even though there is no lack of competent laboratories and although the reference laboratory at the Statens Seruminstitut in Copenhagen willingly offers training and group antisera. This shows how difficult it is to obtain joint cooperative action between laboratory workers and clinicians, perhaps because some authorities believe that there is little evidence so far that the vaccine is effective for the chronically ill or elderly (1). There is evidence that its efficacy is diminished in those with chronic bronchitis. Older people

---

[a] Except for pertussis, for which there is no ready serological test to evaluate the protective effect of the vaccine.

have high levels of circulating antibody, but not necessarily to all types; vaccination is thought to be able to fill the antigenic gaps, and may be useful during influenza pandemics. It is vitally indicated in splenectomized patients. Various types of meningococcal vaccine have so far been used in selected groups in several European countries.

Every vaccine presents some problems; thus there is room for improvement in their efficacy and safety. Still lacking in most of Europe is adequate record linkage for surveillance of the complications of vaccination (it began in the United Kingdom in 1963), a step that is particularly important in view of the increasing opposition of certain consumer groups to systematic vaccinations. In the USSR a special paediatric department is responsible for surveillance and investigation of complications within the Scientific Research Institute for the Standardization and Control of Medical Biological Preparations. Most estimates of side-effects and complications are based on published observations from certain geographical and socioeconomic areas; so osteitis after BCG was observed in 1974–1976 mainly in Finland and Sweden, and persistent screaming and shock after pertussis vaccine mainly in the United Kingdom. Some of the side-effects observed may have been caused by a specific brand of vaccine and have disappeared when it was changed.

The occurrence of complications must be separated from chance events. For example, in 1976 in the United States over 40 million people were vaccinated against swine influenza, and some 2–3 weeks after vaccination they were 5–6 times more likely than the rest of the population to develop Guillain-Barré syndrome (2,3). This seems to have been due to a special feature of this particular vaccine, for the vaccine used in a smaller influenza vaccination programme in 1978–1979 did not increase the likelihood of developing the syndrome (4). However, without a surveillance programme the occurrence of this complication would not have been assessed. The risk of brain damage after pertussis vaccination was estimated by the National Childhood Encephalopathy Study at from 1 in 100 000 to 1 in 30 000 after a full course of pertussis vaccine; there were 1300 claims for compensation in the United Kingdom, of which 300 were admitted. The seriousness of such events, rare as they might be, calls for systematic surveillance. This was highlighted in July 1978 in Naples by an unexplained illness in children under two years of age vaccinated with diphtheria–tetanus toxoid in the 24 hours before admission to hospital. Five of the children died, and 59 additional deaths occurred between October 1978 and February 1979. In spite of all the efforts of the Italian authorities and a team of international experts this outbreak, eventually suspected to have been caused by vaccination associated with simultaneous respiratory syncytial virus infection, remained unexplained.

The six diseases subject to routine immunization procedures under the WHO Expanded Programme on Immunization are measles, diphtheria, pertussis, tetanus, poliomyelitis and tuberculosis. There is a constant decline in the incidence of these diseases except for measles, where a relatively high number of cases still occurs in some countries. Table 11 indicates the latest situation (1981) available to WHO.

74

Table 11. Reported annual incidence of the six target diseases of the WHO Expanded Programme on Immunization, 1976–1981

Country	1977 population (millions)	1976 D	1976 M	1976 Per	1976 Polio	1976 T	1976 TB	1977 D	1977 M	1977 Per	1977 Polio	1977 T	1977 TB
Albania	2.55												
Algeria	17.91	282	15 646	2 862	78	78	2 506	169	12 025	666	40	79	2 311
Austria	7.52	5		311	0	9	5 118	9		313	1	5	6 531
Belgium	9.83	5			1	28		3			0	29	3 475
Bulgaria	8.80	0	16 877	141	0	10		0	806	1 393	0		
Czechoslovakia	15.03	1	28 153	141	1	14	17 846	1	5 335	130	0	12	7 469
Denmark	5.09	0	57 756	16 385	0		400	0	52 308	11 453	0	8	375
Finland	4.74	0	8 706	105			3 095	0	2 837	99	0		3 027
France	53.08	26	2 607	353	9	288	19 660	20	2 186	184	9	268	20 917
German Democratic Republic	16.76		3 694	171	9	27	5 742	0	1 067	598	0	6	4 988
Germany, Federal Republic of	61.40	88			40	38	32 857	26			25	34	31 617
Greece	9.28	9	7 905	7 781	7	114	8 101	8	15 690	2 238	3	99	7 981
Hungary	10.64	17	243	55	3	56	5 790	2	130	27	3	48	968
Iceland	0.22	0	36	91	0	0		0	2 994	58	0	0	3
Ireland	3.27		1 651	308	0		1 061		1 501	1 149	3		
Italy	56.46	202	53 618	18 354	12	263	4 782	173	42 112	8 076	10	256	4 516
Luxembourg	0.36	0	41	28	0	2	226	0	424	56	0	1	107
Malta	0.33	0	38	150	0	0	37	0	472	15	0		28
Monaco	0.03												
Morocco	18.36		87 011	33 636	264	44	26 547		156 598	25 970	269		25 889
Netherlands	13.85	0	2 512	4	0	4	2 081	2	1 812	25	1	7	1 974
Norway	4.04	1	3 204	1 094	1		466		13 487	1 053	0	3	427
Poland	34.70		125 168	512	14	112	24 741	0	44 949	1 068	10	115	26 419
Portugal	9.73	3		150	2	97	6 002			32	0	91	7 498
Romania	21.66	672	113 907	15 602	15	53	17 893	296	124 227	13 471	24	46	15 893
San Marino	0.02												
Spain	36.35	10	133 060	1 190	41	6	3 335	4	129 375	6 464	39	5	3 685
Sweden	8.26	1	8 774	5	0		1 307	0	10 313	19	3		1 105
Switzerland	6.33	3			0	2	1 823	5			0	1	1 648
Turkey	42.08	170	21 740	2 440	500	1 076		142	16 123	1 739	328	1 109	
USSR	259.03	200	320 800	33 000	110	430		240	315 300	22 600	264	420	
United Kingdom	55.85	2	67 934	4 278	15	15	11 581	6	190 505	18 717	18	16	9 520
Yugoslavia	21.78	9	31 487	6 706	6	167	19 358	4	27 918	5 829	141	169	19 188
Total	815.34	1 706	1 112 568	145 853	1 120	2 933	222 360	1 110	1 170 494	123 442	1 191	2 827	207 559

D – Diphtheria; M – Measles; Per – Pertussis; Polio – Poliomyelitis; T – Tetanus; TB – Tuberculosis

continued

Table 11. (contd)

Country	1979 population (millions)	1978 D	1978 M	1978 Per	1978 Polio	1978 T	1978 TB	1979 D	1979 M	1979 Per	1979 Polio	1979 T	1979 TB
Albania	2.79												
Algeria	18.90	108	10 690	283	106	83	2 240	73	14 942	482	40	81	2 362
Austria	7.35	1		376	1		2 546	1		425	2		2 200
Belgium	10.18	3	423		1	7		1	249	145	2	3	2 819
Bulgaria	8.86		3 135	909	0	19	3 575		6 561	108		21	3 396
Czechoslovakia	15.24	3	18 593	50	0	18	7 012	0	66 493	3 510	0	11	5 528
Denmark	5.10		2 325	4 056	0	8	303	2	2 396	97	0	4	343
Finland	4.79		2 026	84	1		2 757				1		2 508
France	53.24	14	941	163	26	268					11		
German Democratic Republic	16.29	0		197	0	13	4 798	0	2 128	149	10	26	4 189
Germany, Federal Republic of	59.67	20			13	27	29 536	13				24	27 845
Greece	9.45	4	2 169	2 437	1	72	8 160	1	7 762	6 368	9		
Hungary	10.79	3	334	67	0	54	5 509	2	216	46	1	57	
Iceland	0.22	0	240	234	0	0	2	0	32	566	0	0	5
Ireland	3.25		1 585	831					1 668	588			
Italy	57.55	91	67 860	12 680	8	218	4 316	46	23 270	17 741	2	166	4 105
Luxembourg	0.36		263		0	2	87		121	50	0		128
Malta	0.30	0	3 348	83	0	8	24		30	34	0	5	42
Monaco	0.02							0					
Morocco	19.48		94 094	15 942	151		27 916	59	113 486	13 408	207	107	24 795
Netherlands	14.10	1	133	1	110	2	1 911	1	56	26		2	1 765
Norway	4.09	0	15 942	1 812	2	2	352	0	2 724	2 059	0	2	378
Poland	35.40	1	84 073	633	6	105	26 408	0	30 653	508	1	104	26 605
Portugal	9.84	249		66	1	68	7 651	154		95	1	87	6 635
Romania	22.03	9	118 124	5 614	22	48	13 101	5	66 371	12 734	0	34	12 628
San Marino	0.02												
Spain	37.05	8	129 712	8 609	82	6	3 642	17	93 476	4 105	11		4 165
Sweden	8.32	2	6 908	13	0		1 127	4	8 667	7	1	3	991
Switzerland	6.16	6	12 517	2 267	1		1 575	6		3 094		0	
Turkey	43.87	93	545 400	17 000	253	1 981	100 808	107	11 747		223	749	1 447
USSR	261.31	270	124 754	67 008	152	360	9 899		93 390	33 197	214	20	10 490
United Kingdom	55.76				4	15	18 817	0			6	124	17 701
Yugoslavia	22.15	0	27 667	6 187	20	127		8	18 596	6 369	5		
Total	823.93	886	1 273 256	147 602	958	3 511	284 072	500	565 034	105 911	747	1 630	163 070

D – Diphtheria; M – Measles; Per – Pertussis; Polio – Poliomyelitis; T – Tetanus; TB – Tuberculosis

Table 11. (contd)

Country	1981 population (millions)	1980 D	1980 M	1980 Per	1980 Polio	1980 T	1980 TB	1981 D	1981 M	1981 Per	1981 Polio	1981 TNN	1981 Total T	1981 TB
Albania	2.85	3	0	137	1	5	2 702							2 061
Algeria	19.52	28	14 665	737	116	86	2 191							2 479
Austria	7.34	0		186	1		2 623	1		264	0			5 975
Belgium	9.86	1			1	4		1			0		3	
Bulgaria	8.90	2	10 763	154	15	18	3 280	0	9 239	391	0		18	329
Czechoslovakia	15.32	2	3 533	84		11	6 674	0	8 800	46	0		2	1 378
Denmark	5.11	0	27 533	4 733	0	0	6	0	35 651	4 365	1	0	4	
Finland	4.80	1	2 147	187	0	0	2 247							
France	53.45	51	1 244	100	8	208	17 199				9		8	3 725
German Democratic Republic	16.80	19	28 745	258	0	6	4 067	0	5 290	209	0		8	
Germany, Federal Republic of	60.33		13 456		7	15	25 924	7			8		14	
Greece	9.50	6	1 198	3 082	2	24	7 051							4 565
Hungary	10.83	0		22	1	48		0					0	9
Iceland	0.22		13	41	0	0			24	26				
Ireland	3.28		1 090	547		0								
Italy	57.78	30	23 827	13 605	1	176		34	64 884[a]	6 646	1		197	24
Luxembourg	0.36	0	63	46	0	0	90							
Malta	0.30	0	14	2	0	8	31	0	1 530	144	0			
Monaco	0.02													
Morocco	20.36	43	79 547	14 873	52	81	24 878	38	77 107	7 248	0		1	28 637
Netherlands	14.17	0	178	30	0	8	1 701	0	77	50	57	3	94	1 763
Norway	4.10	0	1 322	2 003	2	3	403	0	4 586	2 017	1		2	358
Poland	35.75	90		223	0	89	25 807			281	1		0	24 087
Portugal	9.95	13	22	71		59	6 873	18		69	0		91	7 249
Romania	22.05		10 476	11 441	40	33	12 093	4	35 283		0		61	5 552
San Marino	0.02													
Spain	37.42	7	144 153	5 221	17	500	4 847	4	147 575		14	0		
Sweden	8.32	4	1 786		0	4	926			2 256	0		5	875
Switzerland	6.18	1			0	2	1 397	2	3 540		0	0	2	1 389
Turkey	45.55	86	8 618	1 520	182	683								
USSR	263.40	850	352 990	139 000	170	290								
United Kingdom	55.90	5	147 053	21 131	2	18	10 578	3	60 815	21 261	3		15	9 215
Yugoslavia	22.35	2	37 441	6 710	4	99	16 645	0	20 878	4 593	0	15	112	16 714
Total	832.09	1 244	911 877	226 144	621	2 478	180 233	111	475 279	49 866	96	18	629	116 384

D – Diphtheria; M – Measles; Per – Pertussis; Polio – Poliomyelitis; T – Tetanus; TB – Tuberculosis; TNN – Tetanus neonatorum.

[a] Data from four regions missing.

continued

Fig. 4. Reported cases of diphtheria
in some European countries, 1960-1981

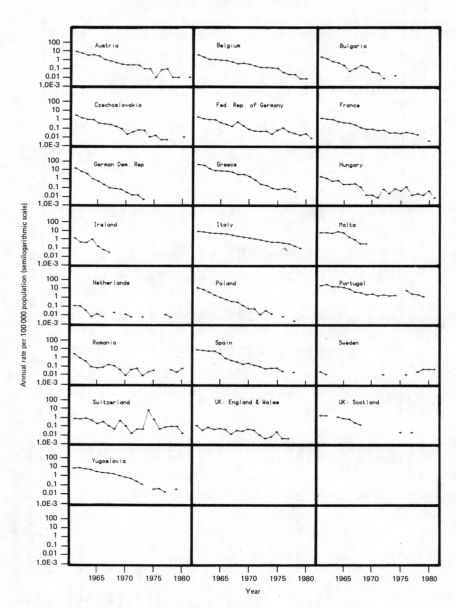

Annual rate per 100 000 population (semilogarithmic scale)

Year

Diphtheria (Fig. 4)

The prevalence of disease caused by toxigenic strains of *Corynebacterium diphtheriae* has so declined in all countries that it is no longer regarded as a public health problem. In 1980, the last year for which data are complete, there were only 1244 cases of diphtheria in the European Region[a] — most occurred in Algeria (28 cases), the German Democratic Republic (51), the Federal Republic of Germany (19), Italy (30), Morocco (43), Portugal (90), Romania (13), Turkey (86), and the USSR (850). Other countries had fewer than 10 cases, and 10 countries had none at all. Only 111 cases have so far been reported for 1981 for the whole European Region.

Tetanus

This disease still occurs sporadically. Some 2480 cases were reported in 1980 in the whole Region.[b] No cases occurred in Denmark, Finland, Iceland or Luxembourg. In all other countries of the Region there were fewer than 100 cases in the year, with the exception of France (208), Italy (176), Spain (500), Turkey (683) and the USSR (290). The immunization boosters at school age and for males in military services provide sufficient protection against the disease. In Europe tetanus is now predominantly seen in older, unvaccinated people.

Measles (Fig. 5)

Although the incidence of measles was declining even before vaccine became available, analysis of its annual incidence suggests that the drop in its level reflects immunization policy. The effects of measles immunization began to be evident in France in 1963, in Poland in 1973, in Norway and notably in Hungary in 1975, and in Bulgaria in 1976. The overall incidence declined from over 1000 per 100 000 population to 10 per 100 000 in those countries where vaccination was carried out extensively; in Czechoslovakia in 1982 the incidence was 0.09 per 100 000. There seems to be little change and even an increase in the rates in Algeria, Denmark, Greece, Italy, Luxembourg, Romania, Spain, Turkey, the USSR and Yugoslavia. In some countries there has been hesitation in introducing the vaccine for reasons of cost, fear of a shift in the pattern of infection towards older children or adults, or doubt whether immunization coverage (more than 95%) could be maintained. Another reason perhaps is lack of data on the incidence of complications, which are estimated as: otitis media 25–89 per 1000, pneumonia 38–73 per 1000, and particularly encephalitis, which seems to occur in 1 per 1000 of all naturally acquired infections. About 25% of children with measles encephalitis die and one third of the survivors have severe brain damage requiring institutionalization (5). The risk

---

[a] Ireland and Monaco did not submit reports.

[b] Austria, Ireland and Switzerland did not submit reports.

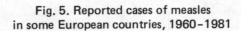

Fig. 5. Reported cases of measles
in some European countries, 1960–1981

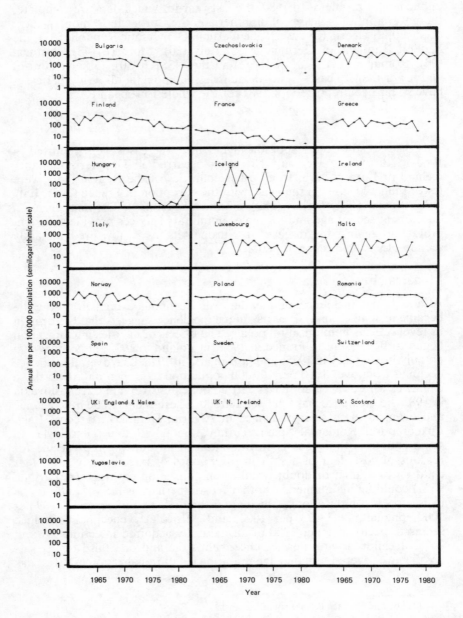

80

of severe complications in vaccination, on the other hand, appears to be lower than 1 per million. Vaccination might, it is hoped, also eliminate the risk of subacute sclerosing panencephalitis in countries where mass vaccination against measles has been successful; it appears that its incidence is markedly lower some seven years after vaccination and persistence of the virus in the brain occurs far less frequently, if at all, after vaccination than after natural infection.

The semilogarithmic presentation eliminates the cycle of epidemics every 2–4 years (before the immunization programmes the cycle was annual) and the seasonal peaks. There are strong fluctuations, however, in some countries, notably Bulgaria and Hungary, which are possibly due to notification artifacts. Note when looking at the graph that probably only 10% of cases are registered in some areas where measles are notifiable, as epidemiological studies in Italy have demonstrated (so that the incidence there is about 400 000 cases yearly) (6). This is particularly so for the rural population. A serious limitation to assessment is that, in some countries, such as the Federal Republic of Germany, only fatal cases or institutional mass outbreaks are notifiable, not sporadic cases occurring at home. There were 912 877 cases of measles reported in 1980 in Europe.[a] Vaccination coverage for 1980 was: Albania 90%, Austria 90% (estimated), Czechoslovakia 95%, Greece 98.7%, Iceland 63% (1979 data), Malta 75% (estimated), Netherlands 91% (estimated), Poland 65% (1979 data) and Yugoslavia 50%.

An interesting measles epidemic occurred in 1980 in the German Democratic Republic, reaching a rate of 171.7 per 100 000 population (28 745 cases). This increase by 12.5 times over 1979 brought the levels to only slightly below those existing before the introduction of compulsory measles vaccination in 1970. The reappearance of measles in epidemic form after ten years of successful immunization is explained by the cumulative effect of an increase in the susceptible population and the absence of natural endemicity; after 1972 the morbidity was around 1% of the level before the introduction of immunization. The herd immunity gap in about 20% of the children, who were not immunized or not successfully immunized, was not closed, generating appropriate conditions for epidemics. This was evident in the age structure of the children affected. Whereas before the introduction of immunization 50% of cases occurred before the fourth year of life, in 1980 children 10 years old or more accounted for 50% of cases. This epidemic illustrates the importance of periodic serological checking of the immunity status of the susceptible population and of meticulous attention to the cold chain and vaccine quality.

It is believed that measles, despite its high infectivity, can be eliminated from Europe if vaccination coverage of at least 96% of children of one year of age can be achieved and cumulation in the immunity gap prevented. The failure of the earlier killed measles vaccines has been attributed, at least in

---

[a]No reports were received from Austria, Belgium, the Federal Republic of Germany, Monaco, Portugal, San Marino or Switzerland.

81

part, to a lack of antibody response to the fusion protein. Live attenuated measles vaccine is produced and sold in Europe under different brand names and this often causes problems in deciding which one to use. The vaccines used in Western Europe and Yugoslavia all derive from the original Edmonston B strain isolated by Enders in 1954, and differ only in the number of passages (Schwarz 85, Beckenham 20–71, Moraten 64, and Milovanović 94 passages). No egg culture vaccines are produced at all today; all are tissue culture vaccines. In Eastern Europe the vaccine used is derived from a strain isolated by Smorodintsev in the USSR in 1959; he developed, also in chick embryo tissue culture, a different parent seed known as Leningrad 16. Vaccines from strains isolated in Japan are not used in Europe. All the vaccines mentioned are effective in inducing active immunity in about 95% of susceptible children and show only minor differences in tolerance. Several countries (Czechoslovakia, the USSR, Sweden) currently administer a second dose of measles vaccine as a routine.

Pertussis (Fig. 6)

The rates of pertussis show great variation. While there appears to be an increase in Algeria, Iceland, Ireland, Luxembourg, Sweden, the USSR and the United Kingdom some countries, such as Czechoslovakia, France, Finland, the German Democratic Republic, Hungary and Portugal, have an incidence of around 1 per 100 000 below the European average. In the late 1970s there was an increase in Bulgaria and Denmark. Over 226 000 cases of pertussis were reported in Europe in 1980.[a] In a number of countries the incidence is about 10 per 100 000 population and in some, such as Denmark, Greece, Ireland, Romania, the United Kingdom and Yugoslavia, it is 100 per 100 000 or more. Vaccination coverage rates reported for 1980 were: Albania 94%, Austria 90%, Czechoslovakia 95%, Denmark 85%, Greece 31%, Hungary 99.8%, Ireland 33%, Malta 75%, Morocco 61%, the Netherlands 95%, Poland 95%, Turkey 64% and Yugoslavia 35%. Prediction models indicate that 96% of children have to be vaccinated before their fourth birthday if effective control is to be achieved.

Acceptance of pertussis vaccination has met with difficulties because of questions regarding the degree of protection it confers[b] and uncertainty about the level of risk of more serious side-effects from the toxic effects of the pertussigen component of *Bordetella pertussis* in the vaccine (con-

---

[a]Belgium, the Federal Republic of Germany, Monaco, San Marino, Spain and Switzerland did not report. In Spain in 1982, however, there were over 50 000 cases.

[b]The current vaccine is made of whole cells containing lipopolysaccharide endoxin. Separation of the protective components of the cells is difficult to achieve as protection requires three surface components (agglutinogens 1, 2 and 3) and the lack of any one renders the vaccine inadequate.

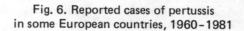

Fig. 6. Reported cases of pertussis
in some European countries, 1960-1981

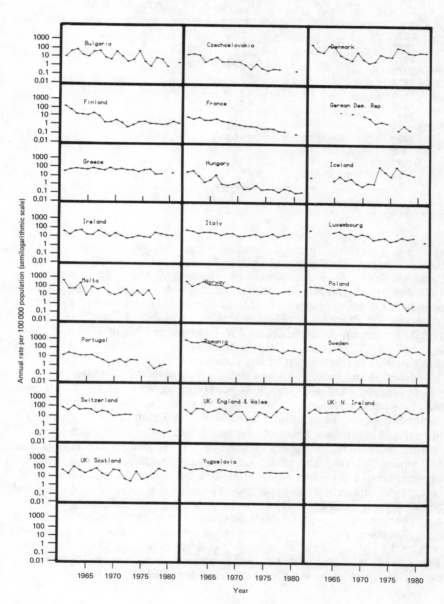

83

Table 12. Pertussis in England and Wales, 1970–1982

Year	Cases notified	Percentage vaccinated	
		England	Wales
1970	16 597	79	
1971	16 846	79	
1972	2 069	79	
1973	2 441	79	
1974	16 230	72	
1975	8 910	60	44
1976	4 278	39	23
1977	18 717	41	24
1978	67 008	31	16
1979	33 197	34	10
1980	21 131	—	23
1981	21 261	—	—
1982 (first 9 months)	47 508	50	—

Source: Community Disease Surveillance Centre.

vulsions, hypotonic episodes, permanent neurological sequelae).[a] After the acceptance rate dropped to about 8% in Scotland in 1974, the largest epidemic since 1967 was experienced. The same seems to have occurred in 1977–1980 in England & Wales, the vaccination acceptance rate (children completing a primary course of three doses of pertussis vaccine by the age of two years) dropping to 41% in England and 23% in Wales (8) (Table 12). The acceptance rate increased in England in 1981 to 45% and in the first half of 1982 to 50%. The incidence (over 3000 cases a week) in the third quarter exceeded that of any quarter since 1957.

Although the current intense debate on whole-cell pertussis vaccine is not yet closed, and although it is generally recognized that it can have adverse effects and needs improvement (a safer,less reactogenic vaccine or a subcellular one such as that being tested in Japan at present), there is little doubt about the value of systematic vaccination of children of 3–18 months in reducing mortality and the severity of complications in infants and young children. The effects on morbidity are as yet not too clear; the experience of later years shows that 35% of reported cases were in fully vaccinated children; in an epidemic in Malmö, Sweden, 78% of cases had been fully vaccinated (9). Sweden stopped using pertussis vaccine in 1979. In general, pertussis among those immunized occurs more often in children aged four years or more. However, good immunization coverage will reduce the risk in all groups including children less than three months old. Typing of *B. pertussis* and comparison with the types used in vaccines may perhaps help in assessing the situation. Some European countries regard

---

[a] A careful three-year study in the United Kingdom put the risk at 1:300 000 injections (7).

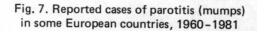

Fig. 7. Reported cases of parotitis (mumps)
in some European countries, 1960–1981

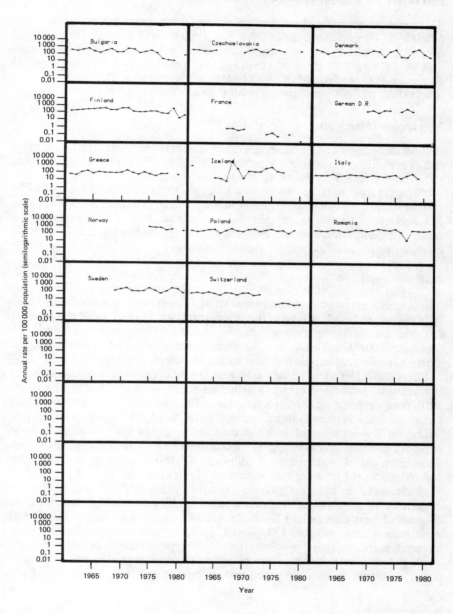

antibiotic treatment of asymptomatic family contacts as an alternative or addition to immunization.

Parotitis (mumps) (Fig. 7)

The trends essentially show persistence in all countries for which data are available. Routine immunization has begun in Finland, Iceland and Sweden. Immunization is carried out between 12 and 15 months of age, and at unknown degrees of coverage, in Austria, Bulgaria, the Federal Republic of Germany, Malta, the Netherlands, Norway, Portugal, Switzerland (also at 12–14 years of age) and the USSR.

Varicella (chickenpox) (Fig. 8)

A clear decline has been observed only in Scotland; in all other countries it has remained stationary. Vaccines are being developed in Japan (Oka strain) and tested in immunocompromised people. They are safe and immunogenic in normal children and adults. Recent trials in 1981–1982 in Belgium have shown excellent tolerance. The importance of this vaccine has become clear since evidence has grown that Reye's syndrome occurs more often after chickenpox. None is yet in general use but this is likely to change in the near future.

Poliomyelitis (Fig. 9)

The effects of large-scale immunization of the whole susceptible child population are clearly visible in the trend from 1960 to 1978. In all countries of Europe the decline is remarkable, the incidence being even less than 0.01 cases per 100 000 population. The decline is most marked in countries that started immunization earlier and in those where the coverage was satisfactory; the difference in rate of decline in other countries reflects delays in application, lack of vaccine, which had to be imported, or perhaps insufficient primary health care services. In a number of countries cases occurred only in small ethnic groups such as gypsies (as in England & Wales in 1976–1977 and in France in 1978) or specific religious groups refusing vaccination (as in the Netherlands in 1978 in an outbreak involving 110 cases, 80 of which were paralytic). All those cases were caused by poliovirus type 1 or were imported cases in immigrant children.

Poliomyelitis has not yet disappeared entirely from the European Region. There were 622 reported cases in 1980,[a] of which 116 were in Algeria, 182 in Turkey and 170 in the USSR. An outbreak occurred in 1980 in Romania that involved 15 children aged between five months and three years in a small area; six children died. A type 2 virus was isolated from these patients, who had received either no vaccine or only monovalent type 1 oral vaccine. Nine cases occurred in France in 1981. A survey of the

---

[a]Ireland, Monaco and San Marino did not report.

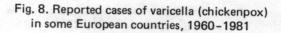

Fig. 8. Reported cases of varicella (chickenpox) in some European countries, 1960-1981

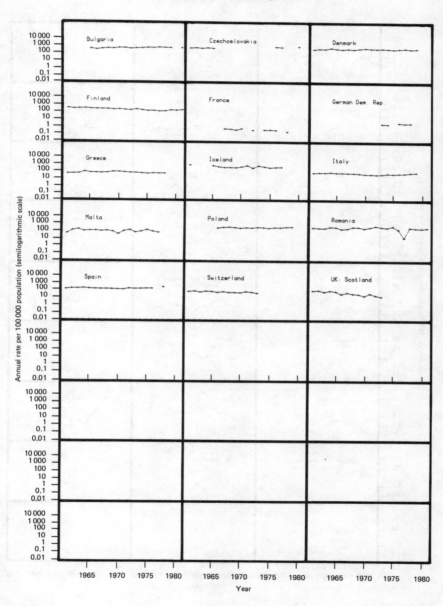

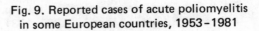

Fig. 9. Reported cases of acute poliomyelitis in some European countries, 1953–1981

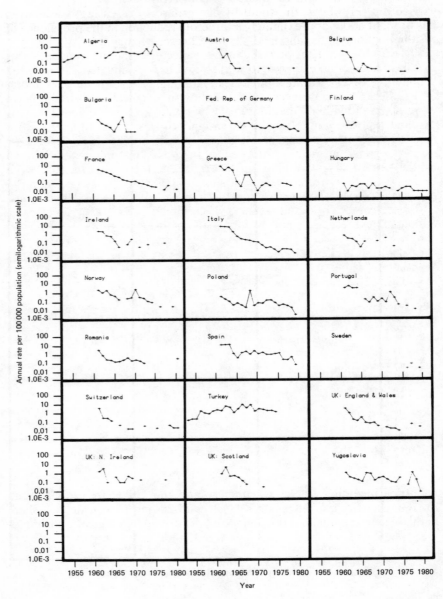

prevalence of residual paralytic poliomyelitis in Casablanca[a] estimated that the average annual incidence rate between 1976 and 1980 was 0.4 cases per 1000 children, enough to produce approximately 150 new cases of residual poliomyelitis per year. The overall prevalence rate in Casablanca is the second highest of any area in the world where similar surveys have been carried out. However, the trend by age group is decreasing; vaccination has brought about approximately a threefold reduction in the prevalence of residual poliomyelitis, and in 1980 only 52 cases occurred.

The problem in Europe is the maintenance of immunity in populations that have little or no exposure to wild poliovirus to stimulate constantly the production of circulating antibodies. Although it has been found that under these circumstances serum poliovirus neutralizing antibody in immunized individuals may diminish over time to titres below 1:4, it is possible that challenge by wild or vaccine viruses would rapidly restore protective levels. Further investigation of this condition is needed. A rather more serious matter is the decline in interest in immunization shown by the community after long periods of freedom from the disease. It is known that wild virus can and will spread and cause disease in unimmunized sections of a population under European environmental conditions, and there can be little doubt that, unless immunization coverage is maintained at high levels, some countries in the Region will experience an increase in the incidence of poliomyelitis (10).

All but four European countries use the live oral trivalent vaccine based on the Sabin strain. Finland, the Netherlands and Sweden use inactivated vaccine, and in Finland and Sweden circulation of wild virus no longer occurs. Norway used live vaccine exclusively up to 1978 and shifted to inactivated vaccine in 1979. Denmark uses both the inactivated vaccine (the first three doses) and follows it up with the live vaccine. Both vaccines are effective. The question of the choice of vaccine re-emerged in some affluent countries in the late 1970s when the production of highly purified inactivated vaccine became cheaper and easier and clinical studies showed that two doses reliably stimulate neutralizing antibody in infants. Advocates of inactivated vaccine pointed to the possibility of paralysis with live oral vaccine (1 case per 3 million doses), vaccine-associated poliomyelitis in parents (mostly with type 3 virus) (11), and the inadequate effectiveness of immunization in tropical and subtropical countries. However, all this cannot offset the advantages of live oral vaccine: low cost and easy application.

A polio-like disease caused by enterovirus 71 occurred in several countries including Bulgaria, Hungary and the USSR in 1975. Certain other enteroviruses (enterovirus 11, 16 and 20 and Coxsackie B5) share antigenic determinants with poliovirus. The epidemiological and immunological significance of these shared antigenic determinants in different

---

[a]**Bernier, R. et al.** *Prevalence of residual paralytic polio in Casablanca.* Paper presented at the IX Scientific Meeting of the International Epidemiological Association, Edinburgh, 23–28 August 1981.

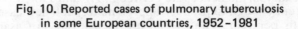

Fig. 10. Reported cases of pulmonary tuberculosis
in some European countries, 1952–1981

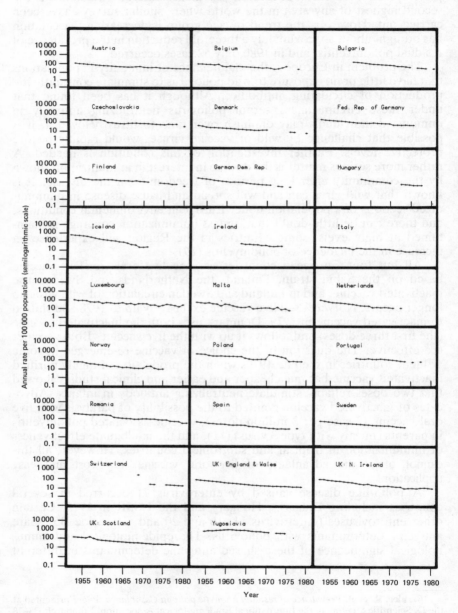

human enteroviruses requires further elucidation. Enterovirus 71 was also isolated during an epidemic of aseptic meningitis in Sweden.

Pulmonary tuberculosis (Fig. 10)

Although the reporting of tuberculosis is obligatory in almost all countries, has a long tradition, and is of universally recognized importance, caution is needed in interpreting and comparing data between countries and even within one country, because of the different criteria used for reporting (bacillary and nonbacillary cases, extrapulmonary tuberculosis), different coverage, different diagnoses (clinical without bacteriological confirmation, smear-positive, culture-positive) and different methods of case finding and the completeness with which this is carried out (Tables 13–16). A warning has been given about placing too much trust in statistical reports, although in Europe they are more reliable than in the developing world.

Notifications of pulmonary tuberculosis show a uniform, constant and linear decline over the last 25 years for all European countries (thus continuing the trend over the last century). Some Mediterranean countries (Italy and Spain) have relatively lower rates than the rest of Europe, which casts doubt on the completeness of their reporting; however, they are in harmony with the linear trend in decline over time. Countries in Eastern Europe have higher rates than countries in Western Europe. The incidence in 1979, as reported by 24 countries, was 169 364 cases, a rate of 49.3 per 100 000. There were over 180 000 new cases notified by 22 countries in Europe in 1980 (Table 17).

With the cheap treatment available, adequate coverage by the health services, and statutory notification in all European countries, it is thought that tuberculosis has ceased to be a major public health problem in most countries of Europe; in some countries it is definitely a disappearing disease. Nevertheless, when tuberculosis becomes rare underdiagnosis occurs. "Indeed an increasing percentage of patients is not being diagnosed until autopsy. As for mortality data, they really lost their significance when chemotherapy was introduced, and with tuberculosis occurring more and more at old age, they become less accurate, many patients dying *with* tuberculosis being notified as dying *of* tuberculosis" (*12*). In the developed countries, owing to the greatly reduced risk of infection, less than 10% of cases reported were in children under 15 years of age. The decline is notable in nonrespiratory tuberculosis, and tuberculosis meningitis has almost completely disappeared. The decline slowed down in the late 1970s and in some countries there has been no decline in the number of new infectious cases. Tuberculosis is a controllable disease generally and particularly so in Europe, where there is a 4–5% natural decline in the absence of any specific measures. In spite of the continuous decline, notably in younger generations, it is estimated that there may be up to about 200 000 new tuberculosis cases discovered annually in Europe by the year 2000, assuming that detection will be more complete, particularly in the older age groups, and that migrations continue at the present level.

Table 13. Reported "incidence" of tuberculosis (all forms) in Europe,
according to the World Health Statistics Annual, 1979

Population (in millions)	Reporting countries or areas		Reported cases		Countries or areas not reporting		Total population (× 1000)
	No.	Population (× 1000)	No.	Rate/100 000	No.	Population (× 1000)	
<1	4	847	148	17.5	8	426 (33%)	1 273
1–10	11	71 232	33 707	47.3	4	18 209 (20%)	89 441
11–20	3	42 444	19 504	46.0	1	13 856 (25%)	56 300
21–30	2	43 433	33 727	77.7	—		43 433
31–50	2	71 370	29 761	41.7	1	49 120 (41%)	120 490
51–75	2	114 490	52 517	45.9	1	56 461 (33%)	170 951
Total	24	343 816	169 364	49.3	15	138 072 (29%)	481 888
USSR	—				1	258 932 (100%)	258 932

Source: **Styblo, K. & Rouillon, A.** Bulletin of the International Union Against Tuberculosis. **56** (3/4): 129–138 (1981).

Table 14. Proportion of bacteriologically confirmed tuberculosis cases, 1980

Country	Proportion bacteriologically confirmed	Country	Proportion bacteriologically confirmed
Algeria	64%	Luxembourg	not available
Belgium	50%	Netherlands	63.4%
Bulgaria	not available as a percentage	Norway	62.5% males, 56.1% females (1979)
Czechoslovakia	56–58% (1979)	Poland	68%
Denmark	85% (1978)	Spain	67–74%
Finland	65% (1979)	Sweden	approx. 80%
Germany, Federal Republic of	30–33%	Turkey	unknown
Greece	unknown	USSR	50%
Hungary	44.8%	Yugoslavia	96%
Ireland	37% (1976)		

Table 15. Reported incidence of respiratory tuberculosis in Europe, 1976–1977[a] (rates per 100 000)

≤ 10	Denmark, Italy, Malta, Northern Ireland, Norway, Spain
11–25	England & Wales, German Democratic Republic, Netherlands, Sweden, Switzerland
26–50	Austria, Bulgaria, Finland, France, Federal Republic of Germany, Hungary, Ireland,[b] Luxembourg
51–75	Belgium, Czechoslovakia, Poland, Portugal, Romania, Yugoslavia
76–100	Greece

Source: **Bulla, A.** *Bulletin of the International Union Against Tuberculosis*, **56** (3/4): 122–128 (1981).

[a] 1976 or 1977 or latest available results.

[b] All forms of tuberculosis.

Table 16. Reported mortality in Europe from respiratory tuberculosis, 1974–1977[a] (rates per 100 000)

< 2	Denmark, England & Wales, Iceland, Luxembourg,[b] Northern Ireland, Malta, Netherlands, Norway, Scotland, Sweden
2–5	Austria, Belgium, Bulgaria, Czechoslovakia, Finland, France, German Democratic Republic, Federal Republic of Germany, Greece, Ireland, Italy, Romania, Switzerland
6–10	Hungary, Portugal, Spain, Yugoslavia
11–20	Poland

Source: **Bulla, A.** *Bulletin of the International Union Against Tuberculosis*, **56** (3/4): 122–128 (1981).

[a] Latest available results.

[b] All forms of tuberculosis.

Table 17. Newly registered tuberculosis cases (all forms) in Europe, 1976–1981

Year	Number of reporting countries	Population in thousands	Newly registered cases
1976	26	388 056	201 131
1977	24	430 737	181 667
1978	24	493 526	284 070
1979	23	481 888	163 065
1980	22		180 586
1981	17		110 441

Table 18. BCG vaccination policies in Europe

Country	Main policies	Coverage in children under 5 years of age
Algeria	Compulsory in newborn and at 5 and 7 years of age	85% at 5 years
Belgium	Not compulsory	—
Bulgaria	Compulsory in newborn and at 7, 14 and 18 years of age	99.7%
Czechoslovakia	Compulsory in newborn and at 7, 14 and 18 years of age	98.7%
Finland	Compulsory in newborn	close to 100%
Germany, Federal Republic of	Different policies in the *Länder*; most stopped vaccinating in 1975–1977	10–90%
Greece	In contact children	—
Hungary	Compulsory in newborn and at 7, 13, 17 and 20 years of age	99.3%
Ireland	Policy left to local public health officers	47 159 children vaccinated (1975)
Luxembourg	Risk groups only	not available
Netherlands	Restricted to high-risk individuals	—
Norway	School-leaving age	—
Poland	Compulsory in newborn and at 2, 6, 10, 14 and 18 years of age	94–96%
Spain	Not compulsory (replaced by chemoprophylaxis)	—
Turkey	Compulsory in children 0–6 years, and at 7 and 12 years of age	74.1% (4–6 years) 93.8% (7–14 years)
USSR	Compulsory in newborn and at 7, 12, 17 and up to 30 years of age	96%
Yugoslavia	Compulsory in newborn and at 7, 14 and 19 years of age	90%

In the European Region tuberculosis control in most countries is in the hands of specialists, but tuberculosis units are incorporated administratively into the network of general health services, and BCG vaccination and ambulatory treatment are in the process of being integrated into primary health care. A vertical control system is maintained in some countries, for example Algeria, Finland,[a] Norway, Poland and Turkey.

The proportion of newly detected cases given inpatient treatment varies from 40% in Spain and 50% in Finland to 90% in Poland and 98% in Czechoslovakia. In the majority of countries the drugs are free of charge or at least partially free, and the short-course regimen now predominates. Treatment failures are reported to amount to as much as 5–10%, the lowest failure rate (1%) being reported from Denmark. Primary drug resistance seems not to exceed 7–10%. Patient non-compliance remains a

[a] Information provided to Joint IUAT/WHO Study Group on Tuberculosis Control held in Geneva, 14–18 September 1981.

problem even with short-course regimens. The situation of BCG vaccination in European countries is shown in Table 18.

Although it is as yet unclear why BCG vaccine provides varying degrees of protection, it remains in the WHO Expanded Programme on Immunization and is recommended for continuation by WHO. After BCG vaccination of newborn infants in Sweden was stopped in 1975, an increasing number of patients suffering from atypical cervical lymph-node mycobacteriosis were seen. In a report from Lund, 15 cases were described (13). Similar cases requiring surgery were seen in Czechoslovakia, Denmark and other countries. The Society of Social Paediatrics in the Federal Republic of Germany strongly recommends that BCG vaccination of all newborn infants should be started again. Since the time that it was suspended (June 1975) to August 1977, 1198 children contracted tuberculosis and there were 53 cases of meningitis with 11 deaths (14). In those aged 1–5 years tuberculosis has increased in all of the federal states, and also particularly in Berlin (West).

Rubella

No attempt has been made to assess graphically the extent of rubella, a widespread disease in Europe; it is notifiable in only 16 countries. The clinical diagnosis is not easy if based only on rash and lymphadenopathy, which can occur in a number of other diseases, and there are about two asymptomatic infections to every symptomatic one. Vaccination has started in several countries during the past decade, but there are still countries where it is not considered indicated because the natural infection is mild and the number of complications small. However infection during early pregnancy can have a devastating effect on the fetus, causing fetal death or severe malformations in a high proportion of those infected. The incidence of prenatal rubella infection becomes progressively greater as the natural transmission rate grows *less*, with the result that a higher proportion of pregnant women are susceptible to the disease. Congenital rubella syndrome imposes a severe and continuing load on the family and on the social and educational services, as well as incurring tremendous life-long financial costs. A systematic annual assessment of susceptibility to rubella by examining serum-specific haemagglutination-inhibiting (HAI) antibodies began recently in a number of countries. A simple card test (latex agglutination) for assessing immunity status by qualitative detection of rubella antibodies has now become available but still needs to be evaluated. Serological testing prior to vaccination is unnecessary for children.

There is as yet no unanimity about the effectiveness (estimated at 90–95%) of the three types of relatively costly vaccine available in Europe (HPV 77 derived, Cendehill and RA 27/3), the choice of age and sex for vaccination, the way of administering the vaccines (intranasal or subcutaneous), the teratogenic potential of the vaccines, or the duration of vaccine-induced immunity, but observations now extending for up to 16 years indicate that vaccine-induced immunity is long lasting. Further studies will be needed to demonstrate whether immunity is life-long; this is an important issue since the vaccine is typically given several years before the individual is at risk of having a rubella-damaged pregnancy. In several countries that have started immunization, such as Sweden, the recommendation is for vaccination at the age of 15 months with trivalent vaccine (measles, mumps and rubella) of all children, male and female, to stop epidemics. The general opinion appears to be that no revaccination is needed. The preference in Europe at present seems to be to vaccinate girls aged 9–10 years only, since after 14–15 years about 82–85% of females appear to be seropositive, but acceptance of this vaccination by the population in some countries has so far been unenthusiastic. Rubella epidemics occur in Europe without clear periodicity and can be prevented by vaccination in the youngest preschool age groups; rubella might continue, however, in the older age groups. An increase in rubella was observed in the Federal Republic of Germany in 1982 and in the United Kingdom in 1982 and 1983.

In the third edition of *Health services in Europe* (*15*) only Ireland, the Netherlands, Norway, Sweden and the United Kingdom specifically mention carrying out rubella vaccination (France began in 1983 in combination with measles vaccination). Finland and the United Kingdom vaccinate mothers after delivery, if they are seronegative. Routine screening of sera from pregnant women started in Iceland in 1975 and was followed in 1976 by the screening of 12-year-old schoolgirls. Vaccination began in 1977. A severe epidemic occurred in December 1978–January 1979 with 6568 cases. A nationwide screening and vaccination programme was carried out from June 1979 to June 1981. The consequences of this last epidemic have not yet been evaluated, but there were 104 therapeutic abortions. The previous epidemic in 1963–1964 left 33 deaf children, even though 91 abortions were then carried out following the clinical diagnosis of rubella.[a] Vaccination is carried out on request in some countries but the number of requests and the vaccination cover achieved are unknown.

The effectiveness of rubella vaccination programmes in practice depends on the acceptance rate and on the choice of strategy. The minimal acceptance requirements differ according to the choice of strategy and, conversely, the choice of strategy must depend on the likelihood of these minimal acceptance requirements being met. There are two main strategic options.

— A programme of protecting women from the effects of exposure without (necessarily) influencing the transmission rate of rubella itself; a reduction in the transmission rate can be counterproductive among women who are not vaccinated. This strategy is attained through vaccinating schoolgirls and women of childbearing age.

---

[a]**Antonsdottir, S.** *Rubella epidemic in Iceland 1978–79.* Document presented at the Eighteenth Symposium of the European Association against Viral Diseases, Stirling, 31 August–3 September 1981.

— A programme of protecting pregnant women from being exposed in the first place by very considerably reducing the transmission rate to levels far below those observed in nature. This strategy is attained through vaccinating young children of both sexes.

The choice of strategies or combinations of strategies is necessarily influenced by considerations of feasibility, especially those concerning the current accessibility of the respective populations and the possibility of attaching a rubella vaccination programme to an existing programme. Programmes based on vaccination of preschool children of both sexes have the advantage of a more rapid response, and can be expected to produce their full response within about 10 years of initiation. However, the response is not linear with input. In particular, uptakes less than about 70% may produce long-term results significantly worse than the schoolgirl vaccination system, whereas responses greater than 70% should produce better results. Moreover, uptake rates of less than 70% could produce oscillations such that intermediate term results were worse than if no vaccination programme had been started at all.

It therefore follows that a choice for the preschool child vaccination strategy must be preceded by firm reassurance that high levels of compliance (voluntary or imposed) can be achieved. In addition, the possibility of decay of vaccine immunity seriously influences the choice. For the schoolgirl vaccination system, the effect of decay is simply to reduce effectiveness in a linear manner. For the preschool vaccination system, by contrast, the potential effect is to delay the age at infection from childhood to adult life and to set off a severe "rebound" phenomenon which, in the worst projected calculations, could be disastrous.

While the passage of time has so far failed to demonstrate decay rates on a scale that would cause serious concern, it may yet be a few years before countries that have already adopted a schoolgirl programme, and which are only just beginning to reap its benefits, might find it appropriate to adopt a strategy of vaccinating preschool children of both sexes or a combination of vaccination approaches.

In the mean time it is essential that, within individual countries, and possible within Europe itself, a compatibility of policy should be sought such that one district or country does not find itself in the position of trying to reduce transmission rates while another neighbouring district or country is trying to maintain them. Countries or districts that opt for interrupting transmission will face the subsequent task of protecting their populace from reintroduction of rubella and of maintaining high uptake rates for the indefinite future. For many countries it is doubtful whether this can be achieved without the introduction of compulsory vaccination, e.g. at school entry.

Whichever approach or combination of approaches is taken, prenatal rubella infection can and should be eliminated from Europe before the end of this century. Achievement of this objective will require attainment of immunization levels in excess of 90% in designated target populations.

There are no consolidated data in Europe on the amount of congenital

Fig. 11. Reported cases of influenza
in some European countries, 1953-1981

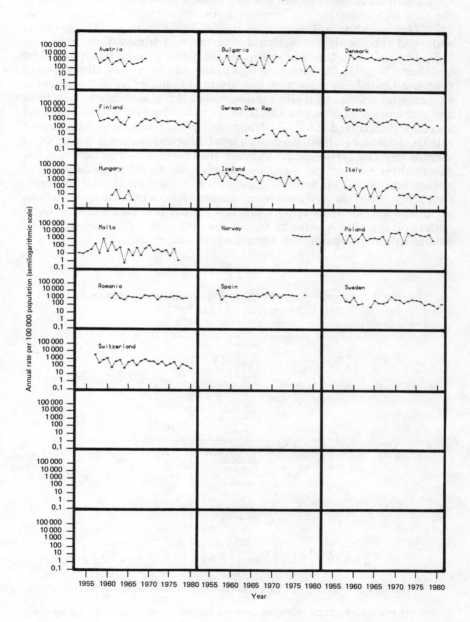

Annual rate per 100 000 population (semilogarithmic scale)

Year

defects from rubella, variously estimated as ranging from 1 per 1000 to 1 per 6000 births, or on the risk of placental or fetal infection of women vaccinated in the first trimester of pregnancy. The risk of congenital malformations in children of pregnant women known to be susceptible at the time of vaccination has been theoretically estimated to be as high as 3.3% (*16*), which is far less than the overall 20% or greater risk associated with wild rubella virus infection during the first trimester of pregnancy (*17*). The risk to fetuses of mothers of unknown immune status would be less than 1% (*18*). The largest body of information on this subject comes from the United States, where data are now available on 174 susceptible women who received rubella vaccine within three months of conception and who carried their pregnancies to term (94 received HPV 77 or Cendehill vaccines, 80 received RA 27/3). None gave birth to infants with congenital rubella syndrome, although a few infants had serological evidence of intra-uterine infection. These data indicate that rubella vaccines have a low potential for teratogenicity and that vaccination during pregnancy should not be considered an automatic indication for termination of the pregnancy. All in all, the available information indicates that the potential risk of rubella vaccine is extremely low and should not interfere with vaccination of susceptible women of childbearing age, although in general women known to be pregnant should not be vaccinated (*19*).

Fig. 12. Epidemiological monitoring of respiratory infections in Berlin (West),1981–1983[a]

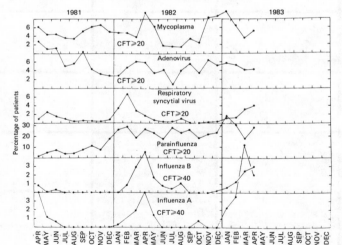

[a] Based on examination of 60 000 patients using the complement fixation test (CFT).

Source: **Habermehl, K.O.** Deutsche Vereinigung zur Bekämpfung der Viruskrankheiten, Munich.

Fig. 13. The surveillance of acute respiratory diseases in Czechoslovakia

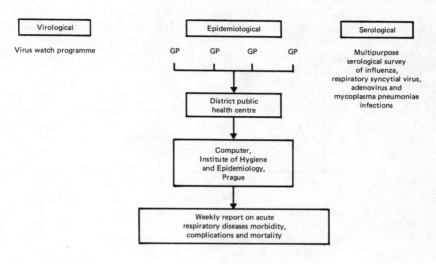

Source: Syruček, L. (20).

Influenza (Fig. 11)

In many countries influenza (or acute respiratory infection, often called influenza or influenza-like disease) is not systematically notified because of its volume, which is thought likely to overburden the notification process at the peripheral and central levels, and also in some countries because it is not included among infections in the ICD. But a WHO network of about 110 national collaborating centres keeps a watch on circulating influenza strains and subtypes in order to detect the appearance of any new variant that may be of importance in decisions about the production of vaccine and about vaccination policy.

While this system functions satisfactorily, the magnitude of influenza remains under-assessed and good incidence data are available only from a few countries. Examples of the surveillance system and the morbidity curve by weeks of acute respiratory infections from Berlin (West), Czechoslovakia (20) and the United Kingdom are given in Fig. 12–15. It is esti-mated that about 20 million persons among the employed population suffer from influenza every year in the USSR. The variation even within a country in the degree of assessment of the incidence of influenza is clearly seen in the graphs presented, ranging from less than 100 per 100 000 population to 10 000 per 100 000 and often representing the degree of efficiency of health service systems rather than the real difference. Exact assessment of the incidence of influenza seems impossible at present.

101

Fig. 14. Reported morbidity from acute respiratory diseases in Czechoslovakia, 1979-1980

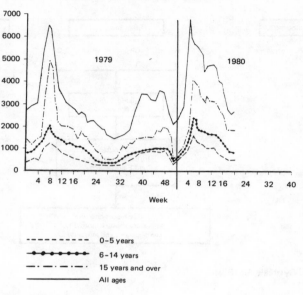

Source: Syruček, L. (20).

Various alternative systems have been proposed or introduced for assessment: sentinel areas, sample surveys, excess mortality, and absenteeism from work and schools in countries where no better evaluation on the basis of notification is possible. The rates in our graphs are in general high, with large natural year-to-year fluctuations. They were below the European average in Italy and Malta. The information from the German Democratic Republic, which is among the best in Europe, was unfortunately available for only four years in the 13-year period. However, in 1980 there were about 6 million cases of acute respiratory disease, involving 35.3% of the total population, in that country. Obviously it is not possible to clarify virologically all acute respiratory infections, which include parainfluenza, adenoviruses, respiratory syncytial virus and, particularly, *Mycoplasma pneumoniae* infections, these last-mentioned being on the increase in all European countries. Various types and subtypes of influenza have occurred over the years and it is thus not possible to comment on them in detail; see the reports for the respective years in the special issues on the influenza situation in the *Weekly epidemiological record*. In general influenza has been clinically mild since the early 1970s. Systematic surveillance, at present among the top priorities for infections in Europe, is carried out by WHO to detect the continuous influenza antigenic shifts (changes of haemagglutinins) and drifts (changes in amino acids at one antigenic site) as a prerequisite to preventive immunoprophylactic control measures

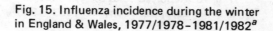

Fig. 15. Influenza incidence during the winter
in England & Wales, 1977/1978-1981/1982[a]

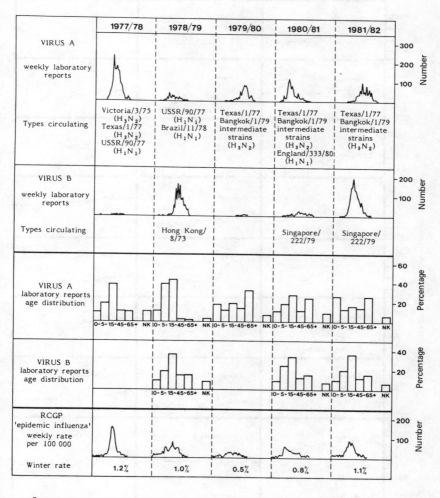

[a] NK = not known.

Source: Communicable Disease Surveillance Centre. London, Department of Health and
Social Security, 1982 (CDR 82/40).

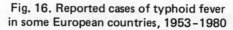

Fig. 16. Reported cases of typhoid fever in some European countries, 1953-1980

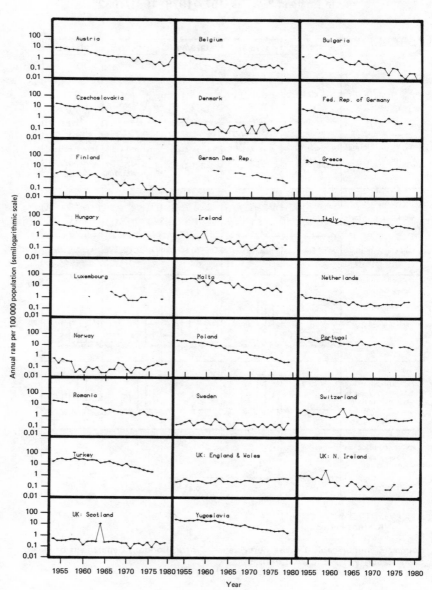

and/or specific therapy; its importance will increase even further if a clinically serious type appears and effective immunoprophylactic and chemoprophylactic antiviral drugs become available. Amantadine, the antiviral drug most used at present, protects against influenza A but not against influenza B infection.

Typhoid fever (Fig. 16)

All countries of Northern and some of Central Europe show a definite decrease in typhoid fever. Ireland and the United Kingdom have the lowest incidence since the post-war years (except for a peak in Scotland owing to the epidemics in Aberdeen). Countries of Eastern Europe, which started in the 1950s with incidence rates ten times higher than those in Northern Europe, have arrived in the 1970s at the same low levels. On the other hand, rates in countries of the Mediterranean area (the highest in Europe are Greece, Italy, Portugal, Spain and Turkey) are still considerable, although there was also a substantial decline in the 1970s.

A large outbreak of typhoid fever involving over 1000 suspected cases and 12 deaths, of which 695 cases were confirmed in the laboratory as typhoid fever, occurred in November–December 1981 in Ankara among people using well water on the outskirts of the city. Smaller outbreaks occurred in 1980 in the German Democratic Republic, such as that in Jena involving 50 cases, and in Potenza, Italy involving 35 cases (water-associated). Morocco in 1980 reported 14 478 clinical and 2873 laboratory confirmed cases of typhoid fever. There were 4667 cases in Spain in 1981.

In the United Kingdom typhoid fever has been declining by about 50% every 10 years. Such a decline, attributable to improved sanitation and standards of living and the control measures instituted, brought typhoid fever close to eradication, but this did not happen because of infection imported either by tourists or by immigrants. This same situation is met with in several other countries, such as Denmark, Finland and Sweden. Typhoid fever will continue to decline in all countries of Europe once it has been reduced to a certain critical level.[a]

Typhoid fever in Northern and Western Europe is mainly imported from outside Europe and from Mediterranean countries. In the United Kingdom 90% of cases (about 250 per year), and 90% of paratyphoid fever cases (100 per year) are contracted abroad or originate from unrecognized typhoid carriers among immigrants.

Paratyphoid fever (Fig. 17)

It is not possible to comment with any degree of reliability on trends in paratyphoid fever, which are more sensitive to variation since in some

---

[a]For details of the process of decline see **Cvjetanovic, B. et al.** *Bulletin of the World Health Organization*, **56** (Suppl.): 45–65 (1978).

Fig. 17. Reported cases of paratyphoid fever in some European countries, 1953–1979

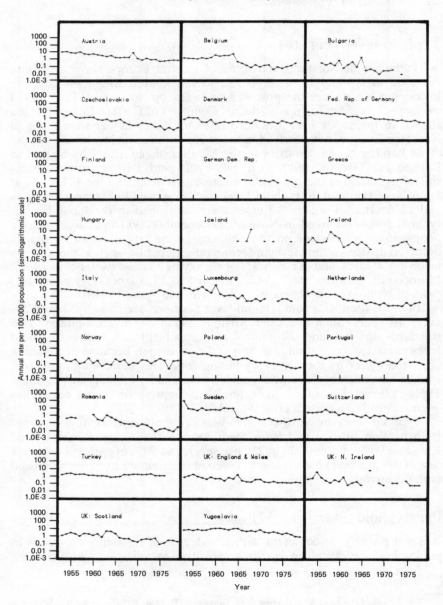

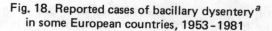

Fig. 18. Reported cases of bacillary dysentery[a] in some European countries, 1953–1981

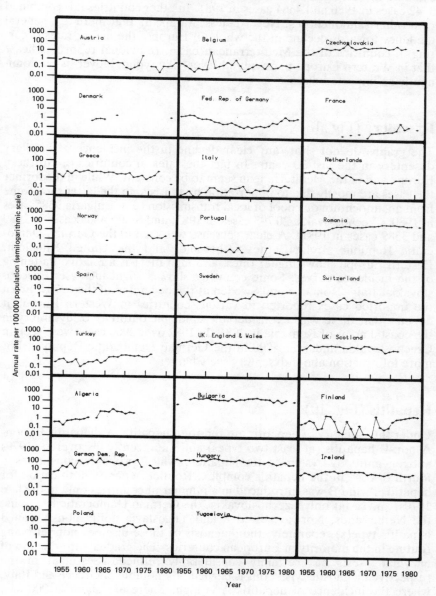

[a] The numbers of cases reported in England & Wales and Scotland include amoebiasis as well as bacillary dysentery, while those reported in Algeria, Bulgaria, Finland, German Democratic Republic, Hungary, Ireland, Poland and Yugoslavia include all forms of dysentery.

countries notification of cases is combined with that of typhoid fever; for example in the USSR, 169 000 cases were reported in 1980, and in Spain 3742 cases in 1980 and 4664 cases in 1981. In other countries it is combined with other salmonelloses. Nevertheless, it appears that there is a general tendency towards decline in the whole of Europe, the higher rates occurring in countries of the Mediterranean basin. Individual reports indicate that in Western Europe paratyphoid fever, like typhoid fever, is predominantly an imported disease.

Dysentery (Fig. 18)

The graphs do not show any clear decline in the incidence of bacillary dysentery in the last 30 years. In fact the rates in countries of Northern Europe and of the Mediterranean seem to be constant. While in the former the cases are mostly due to importation by tourists, in the latter they come from an autochthonous pool of local transmission (e.g. Bulgaria 9385 cases in 1980; Czechoslovakia 20 793 cases in 1982; and Spain 4805 cases in 1980 and 3589 cases in 1981). A clear decrease was seen in the German Democratic Republic, Ireland, the Netherlands and the United Kingdom. Eastern Europe shows higher rates, although there is a relative flattening of the incidence curves. Some countries show a slight increase: Czechoslovakia, Italy, Romania and Sweden at the beginning of the 1970s. From the imported cases reported in various countries in Western Europe it appears that there was a considerable epidemic outbreak of dysentery in the coastal areas of Romania in 1981. In 1982 over 2900 cases were seen in Czechoslovakia and over 4000 in the German Democratic Republic. For more information about dysentery see Chapter 5.

Hepatitis (Fig. 19)

Under the category of hepatitis are reported hepatitis A, hepatitis B, non-A non-B hepatitis (at least two types) and the recently discovered (1979) antigen–antibody system delta hepatitis, which probably constitutes a fourth disease in the hepatitis complex. Routine separate notification for hepatitis A and B was introduced in a number of countries only in the late 1970s, and so far only Czechoslovakia, the German Democratic Republic, the Netherlands, Norway, Sweden and Yugoslavia notify non-A non-B hepatitis type(s) separately, the diagnosis of those diseases not yet being routine in the majority of European countries. The gradual introduction of enzymatic tests has certainly considerably refined assessment of the respective diagnostic types; this is particularly notable in Greece and Italy, where the incidence of hepatitis A is high. There are about 20 000 new cases (about 32.9 per 100 000 population) yearly in the Federal Republic of Germany. The incidence of anicteric cases seems to be around 16%, as is reported for example from the German Democratic Republic. The graphs (referring most unfortunately to *all* infectious hepatitis and therefore of

Fig. 19. Reported cases of viral hepatitis in some European countries, 1953–1981

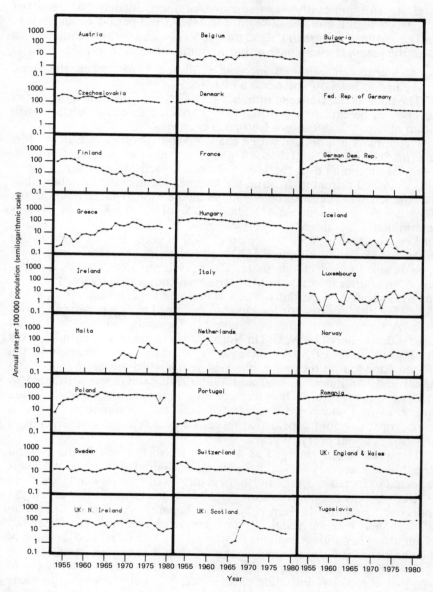

Annual rate per 100 000 population (semilogarithmic scale)

Year

rather limited value) indicate that it is possible to divide Europe into three areas.

— Central and North-West, with actual ratios of 10 cases per 100 000 population and a clear decrease in the last 20 years.

— East, with constantly elevated ratios of approximately 100 cases per 100 000 population and a slight decrease in the period under review. The distinct increase in Poland probably coincides with the introduction of the serum transaminase test as a routine procedure in 1955–1960.

— Mediterranean, with an increase until the 1970s, when the trend seemed to level off and reach a plateau.

The notable difference in rates between Eastern Europe and the rest of Europe can be explained by the much more complete and stricter notification of hepatitis in Eastern European countries.

Hepatitis A is a disease with a changing epidemiology in Europe. It is rare in Scandinavia and becoming less common in several European countries, declining over the last 15–20 years, particularly in urban areas, with a marked retreat in Austria, the German Democratic Republic, Italy and Switzerland. The situation is static in the Federal Republic of Germany. Hepatitis A is responsible for about 50% of cases where the type is determined. The disease is still common in Greece, Portugal, Spain, Turkey and the Maghreb, where up to 90% of adult persons demonstrate antibodies as measured by anti-HAV solid-phase radioimmunoassay, but it appears also to be declining there. The prevalence of antibodies to hepatitis A virus after infection in Mediterranean countries (Greece, Portugal, Spain) is about 90% in adults, whereas in Scandinavia it varies from 9% to 35%. Hepatitis A does not lead to chronic infection or a persistent carrier state. A slight increase has been noted in Denmark, where 1 in 3 of all cases is due to hepatitis A, and in Norway, where the incidence in 1980 was the highest since 1975. An increase in hepatitis A notifications in the United Kingdom in the age group 5–14 years, which began in 1979 (3203 cases) and continued in 1980 and 1981 (9740 cases), was attributed to foodborne outbreaks, such as through the consumption of shellfish. Three outbreaks in London were associated with the consumption of frozen raspberries. It would appear that there is a cyclic epidemic resurgence of hepatitis A about every 10 years.

Hepatitis A has emerged as a major risk to tourists. In the Federal Republic of Germany 64% of hepatitis A is acquired abroad and the risk is expected to increase. In the northern countries of Europe adults are more at risk, whereas in Southern Europe children are the main risk group. As collective immunity in Europe declines hepatitis A, a mild disease in children, may become a clinically more severe disease in adults. The policy of admitting hepatitis A patients to hospital needs to be revised, because of the absence of infectivity some eight days after the onset of jaundice.

Hepatitis B is more important clinically. It has a high frequency (up to 10%) of chronicity, including chronic active hepatitis, leading in some cases to cirrhosis of the liver and other chronic conditions. In about 10% of cases it is followed by a persistent carrier state, sometimes for life (80% of carriers are HBeAg positive). There is a strong association between hepatitis B virus and liver cancer. It is estimated that there is a large reservoir of carriers (about 200 million people) in the world, though there are relatively fewer in Europe than in Africa and Asia. It appears that the prevalence of carriers, particularly among blood donors, is about 0.1% in Northern Europe, and 5% in Central and Eastern Europe. There is a higher frequency in Southern Europe and countries bordering the Mediterranean. The overall prevalence rate of HBsAg in Italian men aged 18–26 years was found to be 3.9%; among poorly educated men with large families in southern Italy, however, it was 14.6%, the highest carrier rate reported for a general population in Europe (21). The high-risk groups include persons requiring multiple transfusions of blood or plasma or injections of blood derivatives (there are about 100 000 haemophiliacs in Europe), those receiving prolonged treatment or frequent injections into the tissues or veins, patients with natural or acquired immune deficiency, patients with malignant diseases, and people undergoing acupuncture, tattooing or ear-piercing. Sexual and vertical transmission occurs and in tropical environments insects now seem probably to play a role. Particularly high rates of infection have been reported in drug addicts, prostitutes and homosexual men. In a review in the Federal Republic of Germany in 1982 (22) the carrier rate of HBsAg was found to be 40 per 100 000 population in the general population, but 240 per 100 000 in physicians and 529 per 100 000 in dentists.[a] The risk increases with the length of work in medicine or dentistry so that, for example, after 5 years of work it is around 15%, after 25 years around 55% and after 49 years around 70% (22). This again clearly demonstrates the already well documented professional risk, usually associated with carriers, for dentists and medical and laboratory personnel in practice and in institutions.

While there are no laboratory tests as yet available for identifying the agent(s) of non-A non-B hepatitis, the diagnosis can be made by exclusion of hepatitis A and hepatitis B. The highest rate of transition to the chronic state occurs with this form of hepatitis. It can also be transmitted at birth and possibly also orally; it seems to be responsible for about 80%

---

[a]The specific prevalence rates of hepatitis B virus markers depend on the age of the group examined. A WHO collaborative study (**Sobeslavsky, O. et al.** *Bulletin of the World Health Organization*, **58**: 621–628 (1980)) found 1.3% of positive HBsAg in the general population of Berlin but 21.9% in haemodialysis staff and patients, 35.6% in psychiatric patients, 13% in patients with sexually transmitted diseases, and 3.6% in hospital and laboratory staff. In all European countries age-specific anti-HBs prevalence increases with age. The study found, for example, 35.7% in Athens, 4.6% in Munich and 43.7% in Moscow for the general population, but a much higher percentage in people over 50 years of age — 49.8%, 13.8% and 64%, respectively. The conclusion was that, in Southern and Eastern European countries, the HBsAg prevalence rates were generally higher, some of them being comparable with the prevalence rates in Asian and African countries. A high prevalence of antigen can frequently be detected in preschool children; this suggests early contact with infection, possibly as a consequence of intrafamilial spread or genetic transmission from mothers to children in countries with high carrier rates, or both. The risk of prenatal hepatitis B infection in countries with high carrier rates of HBsAg may reach 40–50%.

Table 19. Use of hepatitis B vaccine in Europe as of March 1983

Country[a]	Vaccine				Written instructions	Trial use
	H.B. Vax		Hevac B			
	Licensed	Date of licensing	Licensed	Date of licensing		
Austria	yes	Jan. 1983	yes	Jan. 1983	no	
Belgium	yes	Nov. 1983	yes	Oct. 1981	yes	
Czechoslovakia	yes	1983				yes
Denmark	in process		no		in process	
Finland[b]	no		no		yes	
France			yes	Jun. 1982		
Germany, Federal Republic of	yes	Jun. 1982	yes	Jun. 1982		
Hungary						yes (1982)
Iceland	yes	Dec. 1982			yes	
Ireland	yes	Sep. 1982				
Italy	yes	Jan. 1983	yes	Jan. 1983	yes	
Luxembourg			yes			
Monaco	no		no		no	no
Netherlands[c]	yes	May 1982			yes	
Norway	yes	1982			in process	yes
Poland[c]	in process		in process			
Spain[b]	no		no			yes
Sweden	yes	Oct. 1982	no			
Switzerland	yes	1981	yes	1982	yes	
Turkey	no		no		no	
USSR	no		no		no	
United Kingdom						
England & Wales	yes	Oct. 1982	no		yes	
Northern Ireland	yes	1982				
Scotland	yes		no		yes	
Yugoslavia[d]	no		no			yes

[a] No information received from Albania, Algeria, Bulgaria, Greece, Malta, Morocco, Portugal, Romania or San Marino.

[b] Licensing expected in 1983.

[c] Preparation of own vaccine under consideration.

[d] A certain quantity imported.

of post-transfusion hepatitis and for about 20% of hepatitis in drug addicts. Although exact assessment of trends of hepatitis B and the non-A non-B type(s) is not yet possible (they accounted for about 50% and 16.9%, respectively, of examined cases in the Federal Republic of Germany in 1980) it is generally recognized that they are among the most serious problems of infectious diseases in Europe today.

A new antigen–antibody system associated with the delta agent has recently been identified in Italy in the liver and blood of HBsAg carriers. The delta agent appears to be partly responsible for the aggressivity, sudden onset, fulminant course and chronicity of hepatitis B. It has been seen in epidemic form, for example recently in Dublin, particularly in drug addicts and in patients with haemophilia who have frequent transfusions, but the parenteral route seems not to be the only mode of transmission. It appears to be a defective virus requiring synthesis of hepatitis B virus for its own replication. Sensitive assays have been developed for detecting delta agent infections.

Hepatitis in all its forms is a heavy financial burden on the health services owing to high hospital costs — the length of and criteria for hospitalization varying considerably in different countries — and appears to be in the range of US $20 000 to $75 000 per 100 000 population in countries that participated in a WHO study (23). Prophylactic measures by inactivated vaccine against hepatitis B for high-risk persons are today exceedingly costly, about US $100 per person for three doses (24). Passive prevention by hepatitis B hyperimmunoglobulin costs about US $450 per dose, and the dose has to be repeated several times in cases of a clear maternal–fetal transmission risk. Two subunit vaccines have now been licensed (Table 19) but they can be produced only from the pooled plasma of chronic carriers with a high titre of HBsAg by costly and lengthy extraction of HBsAg and strict safety testing and removal of possible extraneous adventitious substances. They are safe, immunogenic and effective, except for clearance of the carrier state.[a] Research on the development of a second-generation hepatitis B polypeptide of synthetic hepatitis B peptide vaccines is being carried out, and it is hoped that it may become available in the not too distant future. Although hepatitis A virus has not yet been cultivated in vitro, the problem of both inactivated and live attenuated hepatitis A vaccine has been solved theoretically and clinical trials have been initiated, but the vaccine has yet to be produced commercially.

Brucellosis (Fig. 20)

The incidence of brucellosis demonstrates a notable difference between Northern and Southern Europe. Whereas the countries of Northern Europe show a considerable decline in brucellosis over the last 30 years, in Mediterranean countries (Greece, Spain) the situation is either stationary or there is a slight increase. In Eastern Europe there has been no notable decrease, although the rates are lower than in the Mediterranean countries. Of particular interest are two trends: an increase in Ireland and a sharp decline in Bulgaria (no cases since 1970) and Yugoslavia, where a control programme put into effect in the 1950s seems to have had a substantial effect.

Brucellosis is a typical and very widespread occupational zoonosis and its occurrence coincides with infection in sheep, goats, bovines, dogs, pigs and camels. In general, the incidence is low where control measures have

---

[a]For a short but excellent review of hepatitis B vaccine see **Krugman, S.** Journal of the American Medical Association, **247**: 2012–2015 (1982).

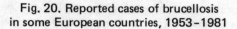

Fig. 20. Reported cases of brucellosis in some European countries, 1953–1981

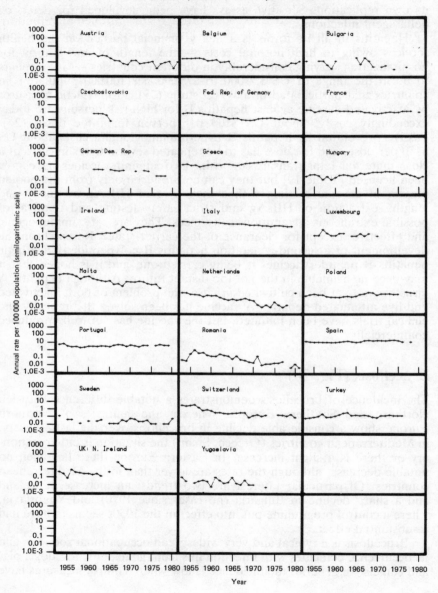

114

been carried out, although sporadic cases occur in most European countries. Brucellosis is a typical Mediterranean disease of the rural milieu in persons involved with animal husbandry and dairy and meat processing, and represents about 75% of the occupational pathology of salaried agricultural workers; it also affects tourists consuming fresh cheese and unpasteurized milk sold through uncontrolled distribution channels. It is particularly prevalent in France (about 500 cases a year), Greece (about 1750 a year), Italy (about 3000 a year), Portugal (about 300 a year), Spain (about 5400 in 1980 and 7400 in 1981), Algeria, Morocco and Turkey. However, because of the frequency of mild cases it is not adequately diagnosed; in France it is prevalent in all but ten *départements* and the rate exceeds 6 per 100 000 population. It also occurs in Ireland and Poland and sporadically in other countries. The United Kingdom was declared brucellosis-free in 1982. In the USSR infections are mostly confined to the Asian parts of the country. The decline is due to vaccination of sheep flocks, from which about 87% of cases appear to have been derived. At present 40% of sheep flocks are brucellosis-free (25).

Three main groups of *Brucella* (*abortus*, *melitensis* and *suis*) are represented among animals but it seems, curiously enough, that host specificity is disappearing.

Meningitis (Fig. 21)

The graphs show that in some European countries there has been a substantial decline in meningitis in the last 20 years, while in others there was an increase in the 1970s (France, Greece, Norway, United Kingdom), an increase between 1965 and 1975 in Austria, Italy, the Netherlands, Spain and Yugoslavia, and an increase in Finland in 1974. The rates vary from a minimum of about 0.7 per 100 000 population to a maximum of about 26 per 100 000. Although there are little differences in the diagnosis and in clinical definitions of the illness, it is impossible to define the trends clearly as some countries notify only "purulent meningitis" (often called epidemic meningitis in reports), others only "meningococcal meningitis" (e.g. Austria), some meningitis of any etiology, and some only those cases where meningococci or other bacterial agents and viruses are isolated in the laboratory (e.g. Switzerland). Norway has five separate etiologically differentiated classes. A constant trend has been noted in some countries, for example in the Federal Republic of Germany in the last 15 years, where there was an average of 6300 cases and about 233 deaths each year, or 9.9 per 100 000 population; however, meningococcal meningitis accounted for only one fifth of the cases. Although only 12 856 cases of meningococcal meningitis were reported in 1980, on average about 20 000 cases occur annually in Europe (excluding Albania and the USSR).

Epidemic outbreaks of meningococcal meningitis (Table 20) were seen in Belgium in 1972–1973, in Finland in 1973–1975, and in Norway in 1974–1975, and regularly in different cities in Algeria in 1968, 1970 and

Fig. 21. Reported cases of meningococcal infection in some European countries, 1961–1981

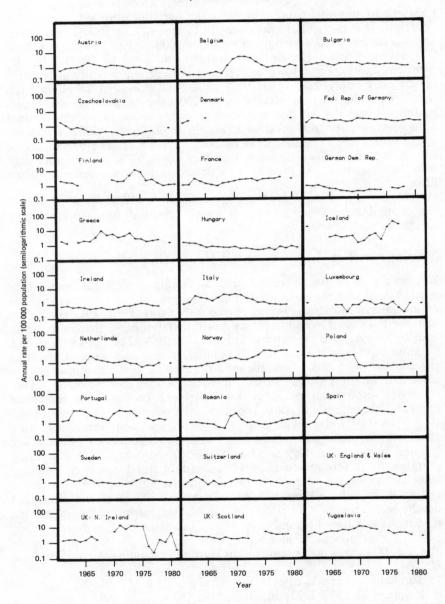

Table 20. Cases of meningococcal meningitis in Europe, 1973–1981

Country	1973	1974	1975	1976	1977	1978	1979	1980	1981
Albania				no information					
Algeria					847				
Austria	80	90	76	66	61	73	72	69	58
Belgium	418	228	136	94	114	127	99	158	
Bulgaria	128	117	134	136	128		106	107	64
Czechoslovakia	51	57	57	79	94	94	116	136	143
Denmark	165	223	206	190	99	149	147	177	163
Finland	255	646	456	120	147	84	55	64	66
France	1560	1109	1505	1591	1596	2016	2036	1661	1374
German Democratic Republic	82	78	95	107	95	128	118	156	186
Germany, Federal Republic of	1400	1474	1366	1135	1066	1208	1400	1145	1153
Greece	765	313	306	268	271	286	244	188	151
Hungary	65	63	60	75	55	95	74	103	82
Iceland	13	5	35	83	55	20	25	14	18
Ireland	29	40	47	41	55	30	7		114
Italy	1250	790	848				597		
Luxembourg	6	4	3	5	2	1	4		4
Malta	0	1	0	0	0	1	1	0	
Monaco				no information					
Morocco[a]	732	976	580	507	295	278	309	292	319
Netherlands	171	162	95	129	117	186	154	143	179
Norway	112	167	327	376	271	327	328	227	260
Poland	233	228	212	241	248	272	305	326	
Portugal	733	348	273	249	183	249	209	193	251
Romania	279	212	191	216	261	355	417	496	503
San Marino				no information					
Spain	2244	2089	1932	1834	2549	4419	6620	4806	5171
Sweden	100	160	233	205	142	139	116	110	89
Switzerland	107	113	86	92	77	68	87	80	98
Turkey		3923	2051					906	1027
United Kingdom									
England & Wales	1067	1296	864	718	500	501	525	509	
Northern Ireland	268	286	249	246	11	4	30	20	
Scotland	122	216	324	242	200	207	216	232	214
Yugoslavia	1593	1119	1322	847	1011	986	712	542	617

Source: National reports.

[a] Bacteriologically confirmed cases. Additional clinically or epidemiologically implicated cases ranged from 115 (in 1976) to 396 (1981).

1974–1979, particularly in the north of the country, with a rising yearly incidence. About 1000 cases are reported on average every year in Algeria, with a rate between 5 and 12.5 per 100 000 population, but the figures are based mostly on hospital admissions and do not include fatal cases before diagnosis or hospitalization. The last epidemic, in Blida in 1979, involved more than 670 cases (serogroup A). On this occasion polysaccharide meningococcal vaccine A + C was used for the first time in children at risk in Algeria to limit the spread of the infection (26).

117

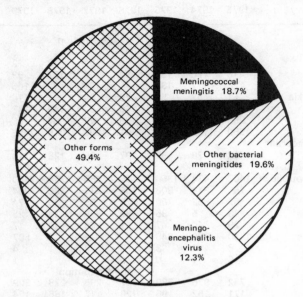

Fig. 22. Etiological classification of meningitis
in the Federal Republic of Germany in 1980 (6071 cases)

Meningococcal
meningitis 18.7%

Other forms
49.4%

Other bacterial
meningitides 19.6%

Meningo-
encephalitis
virus
12.3%

Source: **Weise, H.J.** *Bundesgesundheitsblatt,* **25**: 81 –87 (1982).

In Spain, on the other hand, serogroup B is dominant (about 89% in 1980), the distribution being group A 7.9%, group C 2.8–12%, all the other groups together not exceeding 20%. The rising trend started intermittently in 1962 and continued to 1981, with peaks about every five years. In 1980 there were about 4800 cases, a rate of 12.8 per 100 000 population, and in the first half of 1981 there were 3262 cases. In a number of countries the increase has been particularly notable in infants. There seems to be a shift from group A to group B predominance. Serogroup B is also dominant in Belgium (80%), France, Hungary (76% in 1980) and the Netherlands (69.2%). Group B accounted for about 57% in Austria in 1979–1981, 70.4% in the Federal Republic of Germany in 1981; and 75% in Norway in 1981. In the United Kingdom a very slight increase seems to have been observed since 1977 (after a peak in 1973–1974), but the numbers were relatively small, only about 500 cases per year. Of cases in which the serogroup was recorded, 61% were due to group B. In Italy a peak was observed between 1969 and 1970 with several local epidemic foci. From 1976 onwards the number of sporadic cases remained around 600–850 per year, with a clear increase of serogroup B. An outbreak involving 8 cases caused by serogroup C occurred in Sweden in 1982.

Although the clinical diagnosis of purulent bacterial meningitis is reliable even without laboratory examination, the etiological agent remains undetermined. In most countries only a very low percentage of isolates come to reference laboratories for bacterial classification and serological grouping (nine serogroups if the agent is meningococcus). Typing is necessary to enable the health authorities to decide on general or special preventive action, as so far only serotype A and C meningococcal vaccines, single or combined, are available.[a] However, a trial group B meningococcal vaccine is being tested in Norway. The usefulness and general applicability of A+C vaccines have been confirmed. Control policy inclines towards vaccination at 2–5 years of age for the control of both epidemic and endemic meningitis. Vaccination against meningitis might be undertaken in special situations when the group distribution is well known, as it can prevent at least 50% of cases. The problem remains of children less than a year old; they are the largest age group affected and also have the highest mortality rate (about 15–17%, while in older children it is 6.9–9%).

Meningococci are, however, not the only cause of suppurative bacterial meningitis in Europe; other bacterial meningitides are up to seven times more frequent. *Pneumococcus*, for which a safe and effective polyvalent vaccine is now available for preventing blood-borne disease, plays a very prominent role; so to a lesser extent do *Haemophilus influenzae*, *Escherichia coli* (particularly in neonatal meningitis), staphylococci and streptococci, *Pseudomonas* and Klebsidiae (*Klebsiella pneumoniae*, *Enterobacter*, *Serratia marcescens*). A promising new vaccine for *H. influenzae* type B, active in children under two years of age, is being tested. A rare disease in Europe recently reported is meningitis due to group R streptococci, as an occupational disease in persons handling pigs or meat products. In all countries viral meningitis (often reported simply as "other forms" of meningitis) is more frequent than bacterial, as can be seen for the Federal Republic of Germany in Fig. 22 and Table 21. In Poland in 1979 some 6836 cases were registered as meningitis and encephalitis, the meningitis cases consisting of:

meningococcal meningitis	305
other pyogenic meningitis	2122
enteroviral meningitis	3995

Acute viral encephalitis accounted for 172 cases, arboviral meningoencephalitis for 35 cases, and other infectious encephalitis for 207 cases. Among viral encephalitides, enteroviruses or mumps account for more than 75% of all cases; infections by lymphocytic choriomeningitis virus are next in importance. Between August and October 1982, over 11 500 cases of viral meningitis occurred in Poland, caused by echo 4 and Coxsackie A9, B3 and C4 viruses. There are no statistics available in Europe on mycotic meningitides or primary amoebic meningoencephalitis.

---

[a]Information on the prevention of meningococcal disease by immunization with meningococcal polysaccharide vaccines is to be found in unpublished WHO document EPI/GEN/81/7, Geneva, 1981.

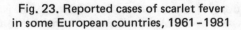

Fig. 23. Reported cases of scarlet fever
in some European countries, 1961–1981

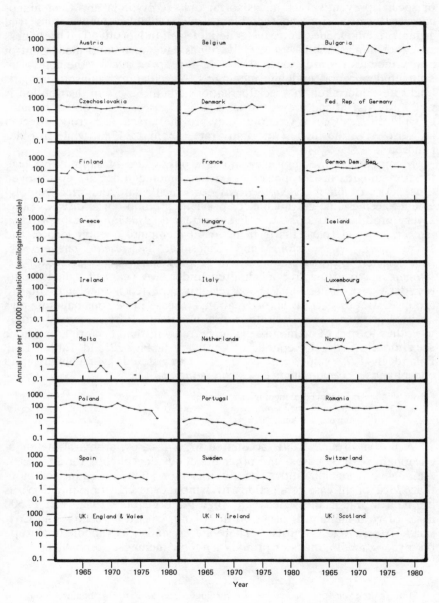

Scarlet fever (Fig. 23)

The figures for scarlet fever are incomplete and for most countries are available only to 1976–1977. Thus they do not reflect the increase in scarlet fever observed in the last five years. Nevertheless, an increase is seen in Bulgaria, Finland, the German Democratic Republic, Hungary, Iceland, Ireland, Northern Ireland, Norway and Scotland. The newer data indicate an increase or at least persistence in most countries of Europe, but their collation is still in progress and it was not possible to include them here in graphic form.

Gonorrhoea (Fig. 24)

The trend in gonorrhoea shows a steady increase, being more pronounced in Austria, England & Wales, Finland, the German Democratic Republic, the Netherlands, Northern Ireland, Norway and Sweden, all (except Austria) countries with high standards of notification. The decline shown in a few countries may be apparent only; it is admitted that in general undernotification and self-treatment are common for this disease. Gonorrhoea is probably the disease with the largest number of cases unaccounted for (up to 10% of cases in males and 50% in females can be asymptomatic) and the lowest standard of reliability of statistical assessment. A good example of this is France: out of 18 389 cases of gonorrhoea reported in 1980, some 17 447 were notified by the public health services and only 742 (4%) by practitioners (27). On the assumption that 35 503 practising physicians did not treat any case of gonorrhoea, which is highly unlikely, and that only dermatovenereologists treated cases, then each of those

Table 21. Reported incidence of non-meningococcal, non-bacterial meningitis in the Federal Republic of Germany, 1970–1979

Year	Morbidity		Mortality[a]	
	No.	Rate per 100 000	No.	Rate per 100 000
1970	5016	8.3	164	0.27
1971	4648	7.6	166	0.27
1972	4980	8.1	170	0.28
1973	5003	8.1	134	0.22
1974	6262	10.1	126	0.20
1975	5135	8.3	141	0.23
1976	5398	8.8	114	0.19
1977	4200	6.8	110	0.18
1978	4614	7.5	104	0.17
1979	4917	8.0	138	0.23

Source: Weise, H.J. Bundesgesundheitsblatt, 25: 81–87 (1982).

[a] Note that the mortality is higher than the combined mortality from typhoid and paratyphoid fevers, dysentery and infectious enteritis.

121

Fig. 24. Reported cases of gonorrhoea in some European countries, 1952–1981

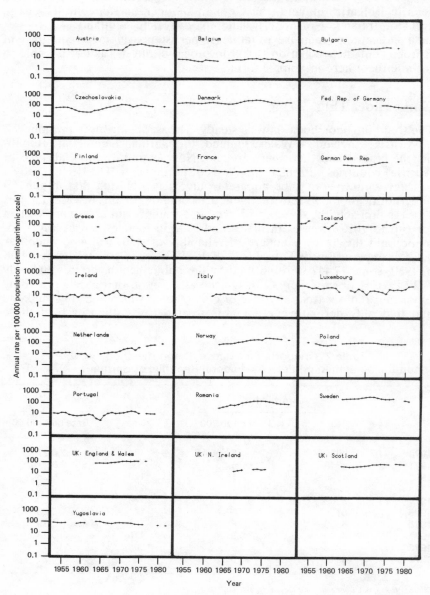

1086 specialists reported only 0.6 cases in that year. From the few countries where the information can be considered reliable, the trend towards an increase continues, as it did in the years following those presented in the graphs. In the German Democratic Republic in 1980 morbidity, at 303.9 per 100 000 population and with 50 835 registered cases, reached the level of 1947. The highest incidence was in males of the age group 18–25 years. There seems to have been an increase of cases in a number of countries in females and, particularly, in homosexuals. There is also an increase in pharyngeal localization, which may be asymptomatic.

A few countries experienced a decline in gonorrhoea rates, for example the United Kingdom with 60 824 cases in 1980, but this was offset by an increase in other second generation sexually transmitted diseases. For the first time attendance at clinics in the United Kingdom in 1980 exceeded half a million, a more than five-fold increase since the 1950s. There was also an increase in the United Kingdom in laboratory reports of β-lactamase (penicillinase)-producing strains of *Neisseria gonorrhoeae*, from 104 in 1979 to 211 in 1980, 255 in 1981, and 420 for the first half of 1982.

The incidence of gonorrhoea rose in Denmark (where it had been on the decline since the early 1970s), reaching over 11 000 cases in 1980. As in other countries, there was also an increase in pharyngeal gonorrhoea-positive cultures: 18% of 1218 females examined and 12% of 2291 males. The prevalence of gonorrhoea in Greenland is still about 100 times that registered in Denmark (about 8000 cases per year in a total population of about 45 000).

Penicillinase-producing strains largely acquired from abroad have appeared in Denmark and the Netherlands as well as in other Nordic countries, particularly Norway and Sweden, and in the United Kingdom. Plasmid-mediated resistance of gonoccocal strains is also on the increase in other parts of Europe, this presenting therapeutic problems that are expected to become more complex in future — extended infectivity and increase in complications, especially in females. β-lactamase-producing *N. gonorrhoeae* strains were also identified in 1981 in Austria, Belgium, Finland, France, the Federal Republic of Germany, Ireland, Italy, Morocco, the Netherlands, Poland, Portugal, Spain, Switzerland and, judging from reports on imported cases, also in the USSR. In 1982 they were also observed in the German Democratic Republic. This development has been preceded by years of diminishing susceptibility of the gonococci to penicillin as a consequence of chromosomal mutations, making "one-shot" therapy less and less effective or requiring a radical increase in dosage. From the late 1970s onwards, the strains that emerged were totally resistant to penicillin because of their ability to produce a penicillin-destroying enzyme (penicillinase). This resistance spread through interbacterial transfer of extrachromosomal plasmids. At least two such plasmids exist, originating in West Africa and South-East Asia, the latter displaying a much lower spontaneous rate of loss of resistance and also carrying a special transfer factor. In the Netherlands, where β-lactamase-producing strains constituted about 15% of all gonococcal isolates, strains were recently discovered that carry both the African and the South-East Asian resistance factor. In 1981 there were 1180 cases of gonorrhoea caused by β-lactamase-producing strains in 11 West European countries. This is a matter of serious concern and calls for systematic monitoring of the development of resistance in Europe. The percentage of cases imported has declined relatively, whereas since the end of 1981 the number of infections contracted locally has increased.

Syphilis (Fig. 25)

In most European countries the incidence rates of primary syphilis are increasing. In some countries (Bulgaria, Finland, Hungary) there was a sharp decline in the curve towards the end of the 1950s, with a corresponding epidemic peak at the beginning of the 1960s. The relatively small numbers contribute to natural variations of the trends on the graphs. The increase is particularly notable in urban areas, and specifically among homosexual males.

Notifications of secondary and tertiary syphilis and its sequelae show a constant trend in the majority of European countries from the beginning of the 1960s, but data are available from 1962 to 1978 only. While the rates are homogeneous for the whole of Europe, in some countries (Austria, Bulgaria) there has been a notable increase since the beginning of the 1970s. Only those countries that had rates higher than 10 per 100 000 population in the 1960s recorded an appreciable decrease in the 1970s, thus arriving at the rates common in the rest of Europe. However, it should be remembered that notification of syphilis is optional in some countries. In 1981 in Portugal 735 cases were notified.

The rates of congenital syphilis in European countries are generally very low, below 1 per 100 000 population and in most countries negligible. This indicates that the system of preventive prenatal examination has been successful.

Rabies 1977–1982[a]

In 1980 rabies was reported in animals from 18 countries participating in the European Rabies Surveillance System. Finland, Malta, Sweden and the United Kingdom continued to be rabies-free, and no cases were reported from Bulgaria, Greece, the Netherlands or Portugal. Norway reported rabies for the first time on the island of Svalbard; of the 17 cases, 13 were in the arctic fox *Alopex lagopus*.

A total of 18 606 rabies cases were reported in 1980. There were 4348 cases (23.4% of the total) in domestic animals, 14 255 (76.6%) in wild

---

[a]Data, graphs and maps are taken from *Rabies bulletin Europe*, issued by the WHO Collaborating Centre for Rabies Surveillance and Research.

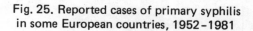

Fig. 25. Reported cases of primary syphilis
in some European countries, 1952–1981

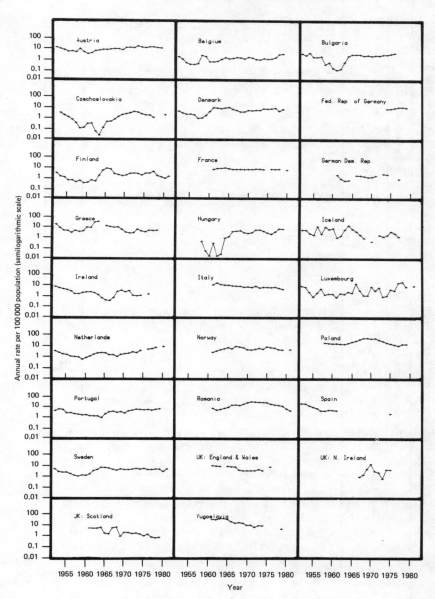

Table 22. Cases of rabies in domestic and wild animals and man in Europe, 1980

Country	Domestic animals							Wild animals						Man	Total
	Dogs	Cats	Cattle	Horses	Sheep and goats	Others	All domestic animals	Foxes	Badgers	Other mustelids	Deer	Others	All wild animals		
Austria	3	21	16	—	3	—	43	652	58	19	42	2	773	—	816
Belgium	—	2	8	1	—	—	11	35	1	—	—	—	36	—	47
Bulgaria							0						0		0
Czechoslovakia	27	45	2	—	5	2	81	1 079	4	22	20	6	1 131		1 212
Denmark	—	—	3	—	4	—	7	29	—	1	—	—	30		37
Finland							0						0		0
France	47	53	111	26	69	—	306	1 261	19	5	13	15	1 313	1	1 620
German Democratic Republic	81	137	77	10	65	2	372	1 523	11	58	83	9	1 684		2 056
Germany, Federal Republic of	117	203	423	44	130	5	922	4 895	104	283	353	46	5 681		6 603
Greece							0						0		0
Hungary	13	28	9	—	—	—	50	864	—	—	3	1	868		918
Italy								10	2	—	—	—	12		12
Luxembourg			6	—	—	—	6	17	—	—	—	—	17		23
Netherlands							0						0		0
Norway[a]							0	—				17	17		17
Poland	53	97	55	5	2	3	215	649	12	21	22	25	729		944
Romania	11	10	14	1	6	—	42	39	3	1	—	2	45		87
Spain[b]	1	—	—	—	—	—	1	—	—	—	—	—	0		1
Switzerland	12	84	40	5	48	1	190	832	81	33	48	6	1 000		1 190
Turkey	1 289	142	482	10	97	43	2 063	2	1	2	—	20	25		2 088
Yugoslavia	16	12	4	—	—	7	39	862	—	—	—	32	894	2	935
Total	1 670	834	1 250	102	429	63	4 348	12 749	296	445	584	181	14 255	3	18 606
Percentage	9.0	4.5	6.7	0.5	2.3	0.3	23.4	68.5	1.6	2.4	3.1	1.0	76.6	0.0	100.0

[a] Island of Svalbard.

[b] Contracted in North Africa.

126

Table 23. Incidence of rabies in domestic and wild animals and man for the ten European countries with the highest incidence in 1980

Country	Domestic animals							Wild animals						Man	Total
	Dogs	Cats	Cattle	Horses	Sheep and goats	Others	All domestic animals	Foxes	Badgers	Other mustelids	Deer	Others	All wild animals		
Germany, Federal Republic of	7.0	24.3	33.8	43.1	30.3	7.9	21.2	38.4	35.1	63.6	60.4	25.4	39.9		35.5
Turkey	77.2	17.0	38.6	9.8	22.6	68.3	47.4	0.0	0.3	0.4	—	11.0	0.2		11.2
German Democratic Republic	4.9	16.4	6.2	9.8	15.2	3.2	8.6	11.9	3.7	13.0	14.2	5.0	11.8		11.1
France	2.8	6.4	8.9	25.5	16.1	—	7.0	9.9	6.4	1.1	2.2	8.3	9.2	33.3	8.7
Czechoslovakia	1.6	5.4	0.2	—	1.2	3.2	1.9	8.5	1.4	4.9	3.4	3.3	7.9		6.5
Switzerland	0.7	10.1	3.2	4.9	11.2	1.6	4.4	6.5	27.4	7.4	8.2	3.3	7.0		6.4
Poland	3.2	11.6	4.4	4.9	0.5	4.8	5.0	5.1	4.1	4.7	3.8	13.8	5.1		5.1
Yugoslavia	1.0	1.4	0.3	—	—	11.1	0.9	6.8	—	—	—	17.7	6.3	66.7	5.0
Hungary	0.8	3.4	0.7	—	—	—	1.1	6.8	—	—	0.5	0.6	6.1		4.9
Austria	0.2	2.5	1.3	—	0.7	—	1.0	5.1	19.6	4.3	7.2	1.1	5.4		4.4

animals, and 3 in man. The animals most frequently recorded with rabies were foxes (68.5%), cattle (6.7%), and mustelids (4%). Dog rabies accounts for 9% of the total when Turkish data are included, but for only 2% of cases in the rest of Europe. Rabies cases by species and rabies rates are presented in Tables 22 and 23.

Fig. 26–30 show the rabies cases recorded in Europe. Data from some countries (Romania, Turkey, the USSR and Yugoslavia) are incomplete. Information on human rabies is also incomplete; 3 cases were recorded in continental Europe. In Yugoslavia there were 49 cases in the period 1971–1980 (at present about 2 cases yearly). In Morocco, 46 cases of human rabies were reported in 1981. One case occurred in the German Democratic Republic, one (imported) in the United Kingdom, and two in France.

All participating countries with rabies are included in Fig. 26, except those where rabies has occurred only in single cases and sporadically, as in Greece, the Netherlands and Norway or by importation, as in Spain. The figures indicate some of the changes that have taken place in the incidence of rabies. In Austria the first wave of fox rabies reached a peak in 1978 and has since dropped steadily. In Denmark and Italy the incidence has also markedly fallen since 1978, but rabies again invaded Vintschgau in Italy over the passes from Austria and Switzerland and

Fig. 26. Incidence of animal rabies in Europe, 1977–1980

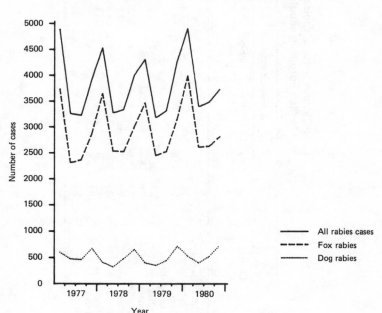

128

cases are now found 140 km south and in areas open to the Po Valley. In Czechoslovakia, rabies increased mainly in the north and west of the country near the borders with the German Democratic Republic and the Federal Republic of Germany, and in Yugoslavia it increased markedly during 1980 by spread into the north-west from Austria. In France an extension took place in the north-west of the country towards the English Channel. In general there is a spread south and south-west of about 30 km a year. A total of 4832 persons have been treated in France because of bites by animals suspected of being rabid.

The extent to which the fox is involved also varies greatly. In Czechoslovakia, Hungary and Yugoslavia, foxes account for more than 85% of recorded cases. Austria, France, the German Democratic Republic, the Federal Republic of Germany, Poland and Switzerland usually record a 60–80% fox involvement, rarely higher or lower. In Turkey fox rabies and wildlife rabies account for almost no cases; the involvement of dogs is between 55% and 70% (Fig. 29). The closest and most active cooperation is urgently needed between the health and the veterinary departments in the effort to contain this disease and reduce the reservoir of the virus; so far it has met with little success.

Listeriosis

An example of a rare disease on which comprehensive statistical and epidemiological information is lacking in Europe is listeriosis, an infectious disease of animals and man and a sapronosis–geonosis. Up to 1950 the total number of cases of human listeriosis in the world was no more than 70 (28); during the 1950s an increasing number were observed in many countries. In Europe the increase was marked in Czechoslovakia and the Federal Republic of Germany in the 1960s (1964, 1966, 1968), but smaller and larger epidemics occurred (up to 300 cases) in the German Democratic Republic and the Federal Republic of Germany, and the disease increased in France and in the 1960s, and particularly in 1970, in Sweden. Between 1950 and 1970 over 2000 human cases were identified bacteriologically in the Federal Republic of Germany and even greater numbers serologically.[a] The yearly average of known cases in Europe seems to be about 400. The scarce data available come mostly from Czechoslovakia, Denmark, France, the German Democratic Republic, the Federal Republic of Germany, Hungary, the Netherlands, Poland, Sweden, the USSR and the United Kingdom and rarely from other countries (a reflection, perhaps, of better developed laboratory diagnosis in those countries). The best information seems to come from the German Democratic Republic, where the disease has been notifiable since 1955. A big outbreak in 1966 in the Halle district of septic listeriosis in the newborn accounted for 279 cases and 83 deaths. In the years 1967

---

[a]**Gyorgy, B.** *Data on the epidemiology of Listeria infections.* Paper presented at the VIII Listeriosis Symposium, Madrid, September 1981.

Fig. 27. Rabies incidence in 16 countries of the WHO European Region, 1977-1981 (quarterly totals)

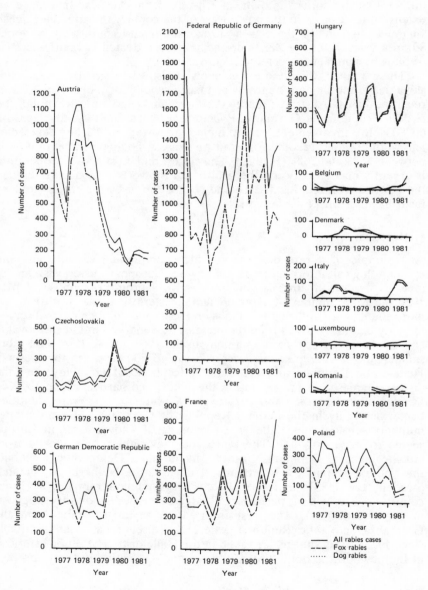

Fig. 27 (contd)

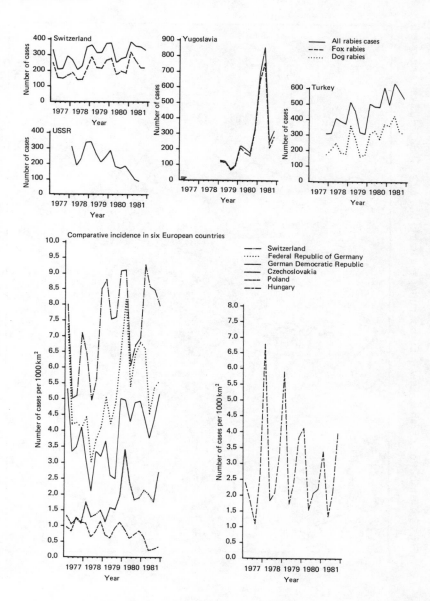

Fig. 28. Distribution of rabies cases in Europe during the fourth quarter of 1982 (6132 cases reported)

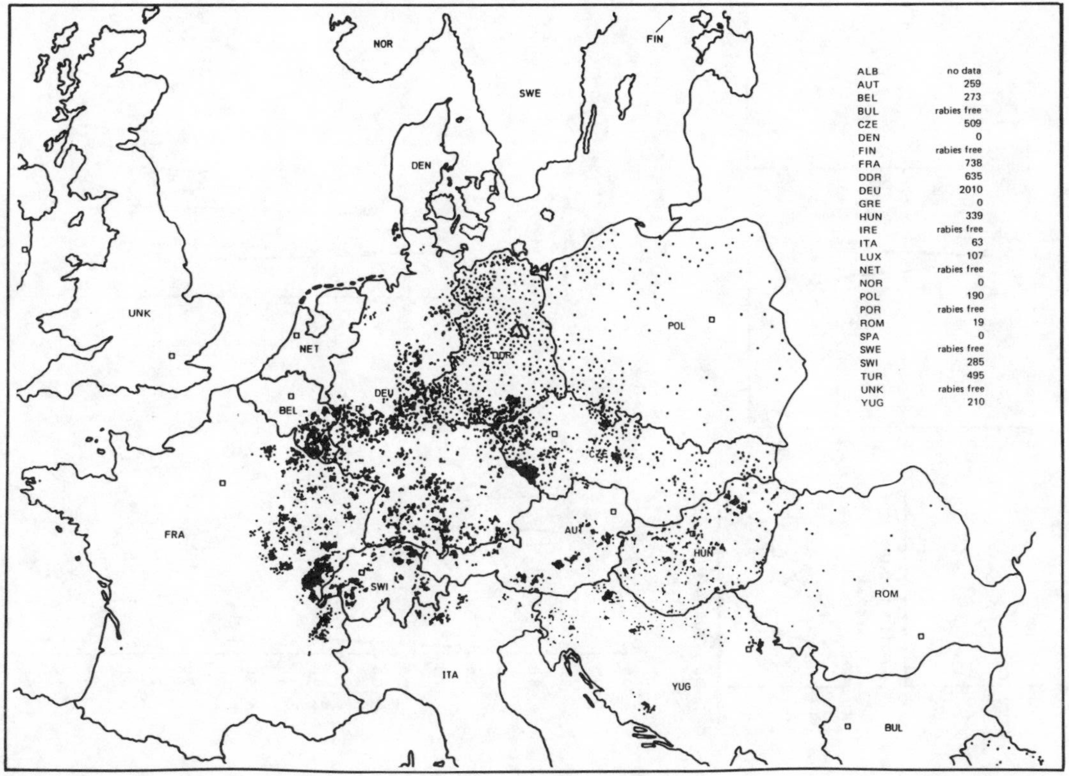

ALB	no data
AUT	259
BEL	273
BUL	rabies free
CZE	509
DEN	0
FIN	rabies free
FRA	738
DDR	635
DEU	2010
GRE	0
HUN	339
IRE	rabies free
ITA	63
LUX	107
NET	rabies free
NOR	0
POL	190
POR	rabies free
ROM	19
SPA	0
SWE	rabies free
SWI	285
TUR	495
UNK	rabies free
YUG	210

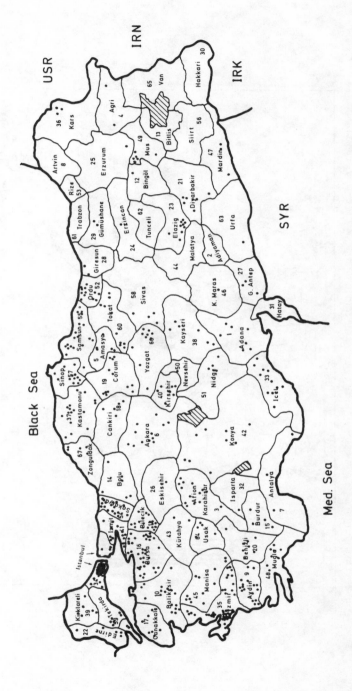

Fig. 29. Distribution of rabies cases in Turkey during the fourth quarter of 1982 (495 cases reported)

133

Fig. 30. National incidence and distribution of rabies cases in Europe, 1977–1982

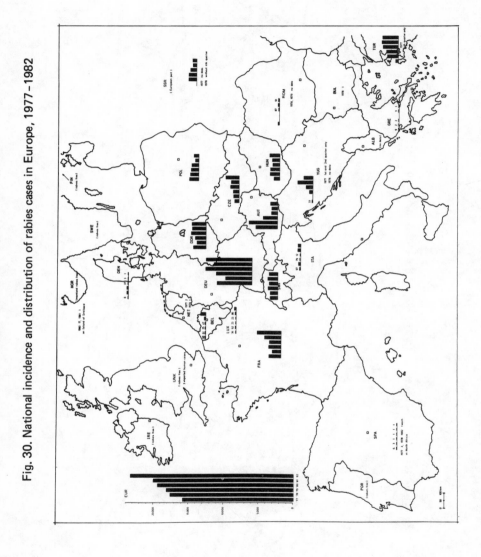

(118 cases) and 1968 (189 cases) the disease was predominant in the newborn (90%) and about 40% of all cases came from the same district of Halle; the morbidity was four times higher in the city than in the rural areas of the district (29) and was not milk-borne. Apart from the German Democratic Republic, only in Czechoslovakia, the Federal Republic of Germany and Sweden is listeriosis a notifiable disease. Voluntary notification depends on the degree of collaboration of microbiological laboratories and pathological institutes with the epidemiological services. The clinical diagnosis is non-specific, particularly in light infections (meningitis, encephalitis, septicaemic form with pharyngitis, cutaneous form, etc.).

Listeriosis is, however, a most important bacterial cause of abortion, premature birth and neonatal infection. The lethality rates in identified clinical cases are high and range in newborn and premature infants from 33.4% to 61.5% and in other patients from 28% to 43.7%, in France and Hungary respectively (28). The amount of fetal wastage from abortion is unknown.

Listeria monocytogenes has been isolated from about 60 different species of animals. Animal listeriosis (sheep, cattle) is on the increase in Bulgaria, the German Democratic Republic and Hungary (28), and its relationship to human disease is not parallel. The organism has also been found in soil and in patients in whom an animal source could not be established (28). Neither the epidemiology of single cases nor that of outbreaks is clear, except in veterinarians attending aborting cows and in premature infants owing to maternal infection. Only in a few cases has infection been traced to the consumption of raw milk from infected cattle and goats or of eggs or meat. Association with the consumption of raw cabbage as salad was observed during an epidemic in Canada in 1981. The recognition that listeriosis affects primarily newborn and immunodepressed persons, and that it has been implicated in AIDS, has brought renewed interest in the disease.

The isolation of *L. monocytogenes* from the stool samples of the healthy population showed an average of 5% excretors of various serotypes and variants (1 and 2a, about 40.4%, and 4a, about 33.5%) the lowest being in slaughterhouse workers (3.5%) and the highest in pregnant women (24.2%) and laboratory personnel (91.6%) (29). Shift of serovars does occur, the reasons for it being unknown (28). *Listeria* may form part of the normal faecal flora with potential pathogenic properties, an hypothesis that would help to explain the widespread prevalence of *Listeria* antibodies in the human population in the absence of clinical disease (28).

References

1. **Hirshmann, I. et al.** Pneumococcal vaccine in the United States. *Journal of the American Medical Association*, **246**: 1428–1432 (1981).
2. **Schonberger, K.B. et al.** Guillain-Barré syndrome following vaccination in the National Influenza Immunization Program, United States, 1976–77. *American journal of epidemiology*, **110**: 105-123 (1979).
3. **Marks, J.S. & Halpin, T.J.** Guillain-Barré syndrome in recipients of A/New Jersey influenza vaccine. *Journal of the American Medical Association*, **243**: 2490–2494 (1980).
4. **Hurwitz, E.S. et al.** Guillain-Barré syndrome and the 1978–1979 influenza vaccine. *New England journal of medicine*, **304**: 1557–1561 (1981).
5. **Halsey, N.** The epidemiology of measles and complications associated with measles in the United States. *Igiene moderna*, **2**: 139 (1978).
6. **Santoro, R. & Zampieri, A.** Il programa nazionale di sorveglianza epidemiologica del morbillo e delle sue complicanze. *Igiene moderna*, **2**: 175–193 (1978).
7. **Miller, D. et al.** Pertussis immunisation and serious acute neurological illness in children. *British medical journal*, **282**: 1595–1599 (1981).
8. **Stewart, G.** Whooping cough in relation to other childhood infections in 1977–79 in the United Kingdom. *Journal of epidemiology and community health*, **35**: 139–145 (1981).
9. **Bank, G. et al.** Whooping cough – an epidemic in Malmö. *Läkartidningen*, **77**: 1293–1295 (1980).
10. *Weekly epidemiological record*, **54**: 361–368 (1979); **56**: 329–332, 337–341 (1981).
11. **WHO Consultative Group**. The relation between acute persisting spinal paralysis and poliomyelitis vaccine — results of a ten-year enquiry. *Bulletin of the World Health Organization*, **60**: 231–242 (1982).
12. *Weekly epidemiological record*, **56**: 313–400 (1981).
13. **Afezetius, L.E. et al.** Mycobacteriosis in the cervical lymph glands – an unforeseen consequence of the cessation of BCG vaccination of new-born infants? *Läkartidningen*, **78**: 121–122 (1981).
14. Entschliessung zur BCG Impfung. *Sozialpädiatrie*, **3**: 28 (1981).
15. *Health services in Europe*, 3rd ed. Copenhagen, WHO Regional Office for Europe, 1981, Vol. 2.
16. *Congenital malformation surveillance*. Atlanta, Centers for Disease Control, 1980 (Publication No. 640).
17. **Dugeon, J.** Congenital rubella, pathogenesis and immunology. *American journal of diseases of children*, **118**: 35–44 (1969).
18. **Preblud, S. et al.** Fetal risk association with rubella vaccine. *Journal of the American Medical Association*, **246**: 1413–1417 (1981).
19. Rubella prevention recommendation of the Immunization Practices Advisory Committee. *Morbidity and mortality weekly report*, **30**: 37–42, 47 (1981).

20. **Syruček, L.** Surveillance of acute respiratory diseases in the Czechoslovak Socialist Republic (CSSR). *Czechoslovak medicine*, **4**: 185–188 (1981).

21. **Pasquini, P. et al.** Prevalence of hepatitis B markers in Italy. *American journal of epidemiology* (in press).

22. **Kuwert, E. et al.** Hepatitis: Berufskrankheit des Zahnarztes. *Zeitschrift für arztliche Fortbildung*, **1**: 39–41 (1982).

23. *Economic aspects of communicable diseases:* report on a WHO Working Group. Copenhagen, WHO Regional Office for Europe, 1982 (EURO Reports and Studies No. 68).

24. **Mulley, A. et al.** Indications for use of hepatitis B vaccine, based on cost-effectiveness analysis. *New England journal of medicine*, **307**: 644–652 (1982).

25. **Abdussalam, M. & Fein, D.A.** Brucellosis as a world problem. *Developments in biological standardization*, **31**: 9–23 (1976).

26. **Ait Khaled, A. et al.** La méningite cérébrospinale en Algérie. *Médecine et maladies infectieuses*, **11**: 484–490 (1981).

27. **Martin Bouyer, G. et al.** Maladies sexuellement transmissibles: données statistiques sur les cas déclarés en France métropolitaine. *Santé et sécurité sociale*, **6**: 45–56 (1981).

28. **Seeliger, H. & Finger, H.** Listeriosis. *In:* Remington, J. & Kline, J., ed. *Infectious diseases of the fetus and newborn infant.* Philadelphia, Saunders, 1976, pp. 333–365.

29. **Ortel, S.** Listeriose und Listerienausscheider in der DDR. *In: Proceedings of the Second International Colloquium on Natural Foci of Infectious Diseases in Central Europe, Graz, 25–28 February 1976*, pp. 261–271.

4

The challenge of tropical, imported, unusual and "new" diseases in Europe

B. Velimirovic

Strictly speaking, Europe has no tropical areas but only, at best, in the Mediterranean region something akin to subtropical areas. There are no true tropical diseases in Europe, i.e., diseases in which the ecology of the agents, hosts or vectors is linked with the specific climatic conditions found roughly between latitude 30° north and 30° south. True tropical diseases are thus of interest to the medical profession in Europe almost entirely as imported clinical problems. It is quite wrong to speak of, for example, tuberculosis, hepatitis, salmonellosis, tetanus or poliomyelitis as "facultative" tropical diseases, simply because they occur more frequently in tropical countries at present. (Classifying such diseases as "tropical" can make a great deal of difference when it comes to compensation or sickness benefits.) On the other hand, from the geographical standpoint of, say, Central or Northern Europe, diseases such as malaria, leishmaniasis and leprosy might be called "exotic" or "tropical", even though they may occur (mostly in small ecologically suitable focal areas) in parts of Europe. In general, therefore, tropical diseases *sensu stricto* do not occur in Europe but can be imported.[a] While importation of infectious diseases from warm climates is a serious clinical problem that merits every attention, a distinction should be made between true tropical diseases and diseases foreign to a particular country.

In this review only infectious diseases are dealt with. Noninfectious genetic diseases frequently considered tropical diseases, such as thalassaemia (Cooley's or Mediterranean anaemia), favism (acute haemolytic anaemia caused by a genetic enzyme deficiency) and a few other rarer haemoglobinopathies are disregarded here.

---

[a]The question of what are tropical diseases has been adequately discussed by Macdonald (*1*) and Maegraith (*2*).

Diseases commonly considered tropical but existing in Europe

Malaria

Malaria has been eradicated in most countries or territories of the European continent where it occurred in the past, but the African and Eastern Mediterranean Regions immediately bordering on the European Region have countries where malaria transmission continues, thus creating a situation fraught with potential danger. The geographical distribution of mosquitos that transmit malaria is frequently continuous; several border countries may constitute one large eco-epidemiological area, as do Iraq, Syria and Turkey. Malaria transmission continues in certain parts of Algeria, Morocco and Turkey. The following formerly malarious countries have been officially registered as having achieved eradication of the disease: Bulgaria, Greece, Hungary, Italy, the Netherlands, Poland, Portugal, Romania, Spain and Yugoslavia.[a]

Infection with *Plasmodium malariae* and occasionally other species occurs from time to time in relation to blood transfusion, particularly, as a special problem of importation, from donors originating from endemic countries. There is, however, a persistent reservoir of *P. malariae* in Romania that has caused three relapses and 19 post-transfusional cases, reported during 1968–1979.

In Europe, receptivity to malaria is generally nil from November to May, as the mean temperatures are too low to allow completion of the sporogenic cycle. It is well known that no malaria at all occurs in areas on the colder side of the 15.6° isotherm of the hottest month, and no falciparum malaria on the colder side of the 20° isotherm (*3*).

The spread of malaria in Turkey in the 1970s is of particular interest as it illustrates the build-up of an epidemic. In 1968 Turkey was engaged in its national eradication campaign and the areas that had been most malarious were in the consolidation phase; the annual parasite index had fallen from a 1960 level of 10.3 to 0.002 per 1000 inhabitants, and falciparum malaria was no longer found in the area. The eastern provinces, however, were still in the attack phase. In 1970 a recrudescence of *P. vivax* transmission was detected in the south–central part of the country (the Çukurova area), 149 cases being seen, of which 82 were autochthonous and scattered through some 50 villages. From 1970 to 1977 the parasite index rose dramatically in the three provinces of the region (Adana, İçel, Hatay), as shown in Table 24. By 1977 a true epidemic situation had developed, with the total number of cases in the whole country reaching 115 512.

"The situation in this region is aggravated by the recent extension of agriculture through the construction of a dam on the Seyhan river and the introduction of industries with attendant rapid and uncontrolled urbanization. While the resident population of the region is about 2.8 million (1.16

---

[a] Readers interested in the history of malaria in Europe can consult: **Bruce-Chwatt, L.J. & de Zulueta, J.** *The rise and fall of malaria in Europe.* Oxford, Oxford University Press, 1980.

Table 24. The build up of the malaria epidemic in Turkey:
number of malaria-positive localities and cases,
Çukurova/Hatay region only, 1968–1976 (a total of 1691 localities)

| Year | Localities positive | | Total cases | Parasite index |
	No.	Percentage		
1968	5	0.29	37	0.002
1969	10	0.59	49	0.004
1970	51	3.01	149	0.02
1971	167	9.87	978	0.35
1972	312	18.4	1 341	0.50
1973	386	22.8	1 293	0.47
1974	391	23.1	1 825	0.70
1975	709	41.9	5 665	1.20
1976	1 014	59.9	28 849	10.30

urban, 0.36 suburban, 1.31 rural) there is also a large 'floating' population of seasonal workers numbering some 560 000 and mostly occupying temporary accommodation such as tented encampments in grain, cotton and rice fields in harvest seasons" (3). These labourers carrying malaria migrate especially from the south-eastern part of the country, with the consequence that the malaria epidemic in the Çukurova area became the source of nationwide dissemination of the disease, with cases brought to 43 out of 67 provinces and re-establishment of transmission in 13 provinces. Malaria has also been found in Turkish migrant workers in other countries. The vast majority of autochthonous cases in Turkey are caused by *P. vivax*, with a few isolated cases caused by *P. falciparum* among people living near the borders with Iran and Iraq.

"The situation in Turkey has been recognized there and in the outside world as a major emergency, and funds and supplies have been made available together with international staff to assist the authorities to contain the epidemic. The position is made more difficult by virtue of the broad spectrum of insecticide resistance exhibited by the local vector, *Anopheles sacharovi*, which is present in abundance. This resistance is largely attributable to the uncontrolled use of many insecticides [for pest control in agriculture], 32 different compounds having been applied in recent years. *A. sacharovi* is now sensitive only to malathion in the Çukurova area, although DDT can still be used further east. A multiple attack is being made to control transmission, based on the use of malathion against adult anophelines and Abate against larvae, fogging in urban areas, treatment of cases and follow-up of migrant workers" (3). Those measures brought the infection down. In 1979 there were 29 324 cases, but in 1980 the numbers rose again to 34 154, in 1981 to over 54 000 cases, and in 1982 to over 62 000 (see Fig. 31).

In Greece the last cases occurred in 1974. However, five indigenous cases occurred in 1975 and 1976, in villages on the west bank of the river

Fig. 31. Malaria in Turkey, in mid-1978 (top) and at the end of 1982

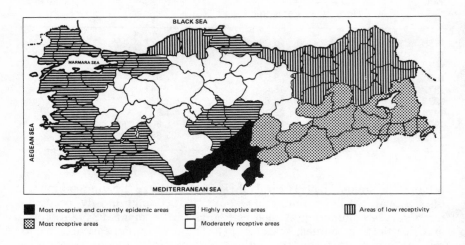

■ Most receptive and currently epidemic areas	▤ Highly receptive areas	▥ Areas of low receptivity
▦ Most receptive areas	□ Moderately receptive areas	

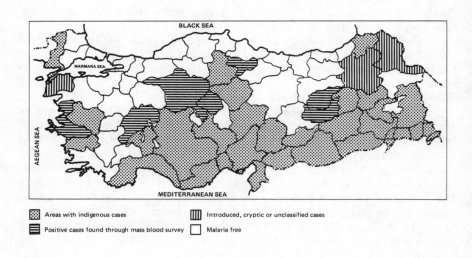

▦ Areas with indigenous cases	▥ Introduced, cryptic or unclassified cases
▤ Positive cases found through mass blood survey	□ Malaria free

142

Table 25. Malaria cases in Algeria, 1977–1981

Year	Total population at risk (thousands)	No. of blood slides examined	No. of positive slides	Plasmodium species				Type of case		
				vivax	falciparum[a]	ovale	malariae	Indigenous	Relapse	Imported
1977	10 728	710 502	58	58				48	10	
1978	11 117	965 103	30	20	9	1		13	4	13
1979	11 366	1 072 136	74	60	11	1	1	51	7	13
1980	9 732		36	7	25		4	7		27
1981	9 732		67	56	5			52	—	9

Source: Oddo, F. Unpublished WHO document.

[a] All imported from abroad (African countries).

Table 26. Malaria cases in Morocco, 1977–1981

Year	Total population at risk (thousands)	No. of blood slides examined	No. of positive slides	Plasmodium species					Type of case				
				vivax	falciparum	ovale	malariae	mixed	Indigenous	Relapse	Imported	Non-classified or unknown	Cryptic
1977	3 631	249 753	159	155	4[a]				103	36	11	3	6
1978	1 493	112 969	64	59	3[a]	1	1		31	16	4		3
1979	1 668	184 867	397	389	8[a]				313	58	9	8	9
1980	5 908	437 153	367	361	6		—		187	126	26	10	13
1981		172 359	98	91	6[a]			1	25	27	39	6	—

Source: Periodic reports from the Government of Morocco to the WHO Regional Office for Europe.

[a] All imported from abroad.

143

Evros on the Greek–Turkish border. Malaria also occurs in Algeria (Table 25) and Morocco (Table 26). In Algeria, where malaria has been limited in the past to a few cases, a local reactivation of transmission occurred in 1981 in a valley at the foothills of the coast (El Hamiz, Blida area) with 67 cases. In 1980 in Morocco 21 provinces were affected, compared with 15 in 1979. However, 80% of cases occurred in a single province, Khemisset, where transmission was reactivated in 1979. The government report stated that the outbreak was proof of the disastrous consequences that follow a slackening of surveillance in areas that formerly represented important foci of transmission. In both countries the number of imported cases is increasing.

In Corsica importation led to the renewal of transmission in 1970–1971, with 50 autochthonous cases. The focus has been efficiently dealt with, but surveillance and vector control were still being carried out in 1982.

Leishmaniasis
Leishmaniasis, the most important "tropical" disease in Europe, is a complex of diseases of zoonotic origin caused by various parasites of the genus *Leishmania*. Current taxonomic studies indicate that a number of distinctive species and subspecies are involved in the etiology of the cutaneous form (oriental sore) and the visceral form of the disease (kala-azar) in the European Region and elsewhere. In spite of a large number of publications, the exact prevalence and epidemiology of the leishmaniases in Europe are unknown, the information available being fragmentary and incomplete. "The diseases [are] grouped in the classical manner as follows:

(1) infantile kala-azar caused by *L. infantum*: a zoonosis with domestic and wild Canidae as the major reservoirs;

(2) urban cutaneous leishmaniasis caused by *L. tropica* (*L. tropica minor*): possibly an anthroponosis, although a dog reservoir may occur;

(3) rural cutaneous leishmaniasis (typical OS [oriental sore]) caused by *L. major*: a typical zoonosis with a wide variety of wild rodents as reservoirs" (*3*).

Taxonomic identification of European leishmaniasis will be clarified when a specific diagnostic test using monoclonal antibodies is developed, both for direct diagnosis and for distinguishing between species causing a determined type of disease.

The leishmaniases are transmitted in the European Region by a number of sandflies of the genus *Phlebotomus*. Kala-azar and urban cutaneous disease are transmitted mainly by endophilic species, many of which have decreased or disappeared in areas where insecticidal campaigns have been carried out against malaria vector anophelines. Conversely, some species are returning where spraying operations have been halted.

There is evidence that the different species of *Leishmania* may not be as strictly limited in their trophism as previously believed; for example, *L. infantum* may cause cutaneous disease in some individuals and this may account for the rare cases reported, as in Portugal and Spain (*3*).

144

Adult kala-azar and infantile kala-azar (1–10 years of age) are typically seen in small foci in practically all the countries around the Mediterranean basin. However, they are not seen in the south of France. In the USSR they occur sporadically in large areas of Transcaucasia and Central Asia, the northernmost foci being in the Syr-Darya Valley at latitude 46° north. In the focal areas it has been estimated that 40–50% of persons 50 years of age or more have been infected at one time or another.

The difficulty in assessing the importance of leishmaniasis is compounded by the long time elapsing between the sandfly bite and the appearance of the lesion: 3–6 months, but extending to as much as 3 years for *L. tropica*. It is also suspected that many asymptomatic or chronic infections occur. What information exists is mostly derived from occasional published reports. Leishmaniasis is not a notifiable disease in all countries where it regularly occurs. Although human cases do not give an adequate evaluation of the importance of leishmaniasis, notifying them would enable epidemiological investigation to be carried out at the place of infection. The major emphasis must continue to be on epidemiological research.

The situation has been subject to change since the Second World War, owing not only to residual spraying for malaria but also to economic changes and extension of urban types of habitat to the countryside; pre-war statistics and those of the first two decades after are not applicable at present. Local transmission occurs in Algeria, France, Greece, Italy, Malta, Morocco, Portugal, Spain, Turkey, the USSR and, now rarely, in Yugoslavia. Sporadic cases also occurred formerly in Albania, Bulgaria (the last case in 1972), Hungary and Romania, but there have been no reports to WHO in the last two decades from those countries. While the endemicity levels are considerably lower than 20 years ago, the increasing numbers of reports on importation from Mediterranean to other countries in recent years indicate that the disease may have a larger transmission potential than is generally thought, and may require more detailed up-to-date epidemiological studies. In France, Greece and some places in Italy, for example, cases of visceral leishmaniasis in adults have become more frequent, while cutaneous leishmaniasis has increased in Algeria and Morocco. In Algeria, several thousand cases were declared in 1982 in four provinces in the High Plateaux, while the disease is endemic in only two provinces of the Lower Plateaux — Bechar and Ardar. The number of infected dogs in the Marseilles area, where 12 cases of visceral leishmaniasis were detected in 1981, is on the increase. The main active focus in France of the cutaneous form is the Cévennes-Languedoc area, while there are foci of the visceral form in the *départements* of Ardèche, Gard, Hérault, Pyrénées-Orientales, Bouches-du-Rhône, Vaucluse, Var, Basses-Alpes and Corsica. In Spain an increase has been observed since the 1960s and the cutaneous form now clearly dominates the clinical picture. In Portugal there was an increase in 1979 and between 40 and 80 cases are recorded yearly, predominantly in infants; most cases come from the Alto Douro region, Vila Real, Viseu and Bragança. In Italy, in the outbreaks of Emilia-Romagna in 1971–1972 there were 13 fatalities (21.7%) among 60 cases of visceral leishmaniasis. Sporadic cases occur in Tuscany, where

Fig. 32. Distribution of visceral and cutaneous leishmaniasis in the Mediterranean and Middle Asian regions

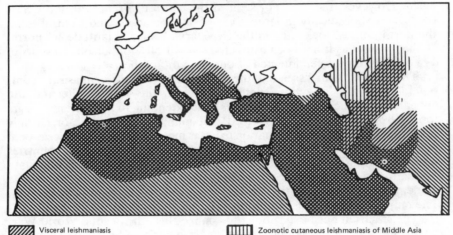

//// Visceral leishmaniasis	||||| Zoonotic cutaneous leishmaniasis of Middle Asia

\\\\ Cutaneous leishmaniasis

Source: **Lysenko, A.J. & Belaev, A.E.** Some problems of primary importance concerning the epidemiology of leishmaniasis in the Mediterranean — Middle Asian region. *In: Ecologie des Leishmanioses, Colloques Internationaux du CNRS, Montpellier 18-20 août 1974* (No. 231, p. 249-251).

29% of dogs were found to be infected in 1979–1980, and in Sicily all over the central and southern areas, where 37% of dogs were found to be infected in 1981. In Yugoslavia visceral leishmaniasis cases formerly occurred in Serbia, Macedonia, Montenegro and Dalmatia, but have now become rare. There was an increase in Greece (island of Zante) in both the cutaneous and the visceral forms, and also in the Peloponnese and Attica in strictly limited foci. In Turkey half or more of the 161 cases occurring in 1974–1975 were detected in areas where antimalarial spraying has been discontinued, particularly in central Anatolia, the western provinces and the southern parts of the country, but there has been a resurgence of the disease and in 1981 some 500–600 cases were seen. In Morocco the disease was considered rare until 1975, when large foci were discovered in the south.

The distribution of visceral and cutaneous leishmaniasis is illustrated in Table 27 and Fig. 32. In all these countries dogs, and in some cases wild Canidae and rodents (the fox, *Vulpes vulpes*, and the rat, *Rattus rattus*) have been incriminated as reservoirs of *L. infantum* (*4*). In Turkey and the USSR various species of rodent have been incriminated as major reservoirs.

In outbreaks a preponderance of infantile cases is not usually seen, presumably because the immune status of the population is uniformly low, as was shown, for example, in the outbreaks of 1971–1972 in Emilia-Romagna, Italy (*5,6*). The frequency of infantile cases is thought to be still relatively high in Sicily (*7*).

146

Table 27. Latest available information on leishmaniasis in Europe

Country	Year	No. of cases		Author and notes
		Visceral	Cutaneous	
France	1970–1977	25	15	Rioux (1977)(*8*),[a] south-east of the Rhône
	1975–1978	71	3	Rouque et al. (1975, 1977)(*9*)
	1981	23		Quilici et al. (1979)(*10*)
				van Damme.[b] About 50 cases treated yearly, 25 east of the Rhône, of which 11 in the vicinity of Nice. No compulsory notification
Greece	1970–1975	228	47	Léger et al. (1979) (*11*)
	1971–1977	442		In a recrudescence in 1966–1970 half of the cases were detected in Athens
	1979	48	2	Marcelon Kinti [b]
				More than half in Attica/Athens
	1980	48	2	No compulsory notification
	1981	57	11	
Italy	1970	10	21	Biocca et al. (1977) (*12*)
	1971	11	29	Sicily, eastern Italy, south of the
	1972	57	28	Po valley
	1973	24	33	
(Emilia-Romagna, Tuscany)	1971–1973	60		Pampiglione et al. (1974, 1975) (*5,6*) Emilia-Romagna, along the Adriatic
	1974	20	37	Bettini et al. (1977, 1981) (*4*)
	1975	32	39	22.9% of 1285 persons tested intra-
	1976	40	51	dermally positive in Grosseto Province
Malta	1970–1971	13		Busuttil (1974) (*13*)
	1977–1980	10 (yrly. ave.)		Gradual decline from 1948 (213 cases)
Portugal	1960–1976	1 134		Lecour et al. (1978) (*14*) Ministry of Health statistical returns
	1977	78	1	Amarachande (1982) [b]
	1978	42	—	Only state, not university hospital reports
	1979	42	—	Mostly caused by zoophilic
	1980	55	2	*P. perniciosus*
	1981	46	10	

continued

[a] **Rioux, J.A.** *Les leishmanioses en Europe méditerranéenne.* Unpublished WHO document TDR/MPD/SWG-LEISH(1)/77.18. Geneva, 1977.

[b] Unpublished paper presented at a WHO meeting in Mahón, Spain, 1982.

Table 27. (contd)

Country	Year	No. of cases		Author and notes
		Visceral	Cutaneous	
Spain	1951–1972	1 064		Hörder et al. (1978) (15)
	1970		52	
	1971		51	
	1972		76	Gil Collado (1972) (16) Granada, Jaén, Lérida
	1973		39	
	1977		2	Urbano Jiménez (1977) (17)
	1976–1981	17	256	Luengo [b] Increase since 1960s owing to rise in canine population and spread of urbanization in the countryside. Dogs infected 1.7–7.8%, foxes 4.7%. Made notifiable in 1982. Most cases detected in Murcia and Alicante provinces
Turkey		65 yearly		Osmen et al. (1977)[c] Izmir, Diarbakir, Mardin, Urta, Gaziantep
			500–600	Unsal.[b] Eastern and south-eastern part of the country
USSR	1966–1976	385		Genis (1978) (18) Kyzil-Orda Ashacabad
	1965		711	Sofyanova (1977)[d]
Yugoslavia	1970–1978	1–4 yearly		Official notifications
	1976–1980	11		Ristic[b]
Algeria	1965–1975	497		Addadi & Dedet (1976) (19) Abadla oasis
			497	Bobin et al. (1978) (20)
Morocco	1925–1974	9	16	Meyruey et al. (1974) (21) Benallégué & Tabbakh (1977) (22)
	1975	?	1 000	Benmansour (1982) Since 1975 in the focus of Alnif, Province of Errachidia, Fafslalet, 1230 cases, Ouarzazate, 800 cases. Semi arid areas north of High Atlas, Tangier, Fez, Meknès, Kenitra, Nador, Zara, Oujda
	1977	1	726	
	1978		564	
	1979	5	?	
	1980	7	?	
	1981	?	3 456	

[b] Unpublished paper presented at a WHO meeting in Mahón, Spain, 1982.

[c] Osmen, K. et al. *The early diagnosis of kala-azar and the characteristics of kala-azar cases encountered in the vicinity of Izmir, Turkey. In:* Summaries of the First Mediterranean Conference on Parasitology, 5–10 October 1977.

[d] Sofyanova, V.M. *Leishmaniasis in the USSR, 1977.* Unpublished WHO document WHO/TDR/MPD/SWG-LEISH 77.17, Geneva, 1977.

Both forms can be found (Fig. 32) not only in the coastal areas of the Mediterranean but also in the rural areas of the interior up to a height of 700 m above sea level, within the limits of about the 10°C isotherm. One autochthonous case has been reported from Switzerland in the region of Lausanne *(23)*. Autochthonous leishmaniasis in Europe is almost exclusively a rural disease, and the large accumulation of cases in Athens seems exceptional.

A number of sandfly species have been found to be possible vectors of *L. infantum*, either by the identification of infected sandflies or on epidemiological grounds,[a] but the situation regarding vectors in the Mediterranean countries is not entirely clear.[b] The species are:

P. papatasi	Greece, Italy, Spain
P. perniciosus	Algeria, France (in Provence up to 600 m above sea level), Italy, Portugal, Spain, Turkey, Yugoslavia
P. longicuspis	Algeria
P. major	Bulgaria, Greece, Italy, Spain, Turkey, USSR, Yugoslavia
P. perfiliewi	Italy, Turkey, Yugoslavia
P. sergenti	Greece, Italy, Spain, Turkey
P. ariasi	France (three focal areas up to 1400 m above sea level), Italy, Spain

Dengue

Common in the past in the Mediterranean basin, particularly in Greece, dengue fever has vanished with the disappearance of *Aedes aegypti* from that area.

Cholera

Cholera is now established in the Mediterranean basin and has occasionally been reported in Algeria, Italy, Malta, Morocco, Spain and Turkey. There were about 8000 cases in Algeria in 1982. Although Europe is not generally receptive and no large epidemics are likely to develop, smaller outbreaks can occur (in Spain in 1979 there were over 260 cases and in 1980 four cases, and in Sardinia in 1979 there were ten cases). No quarantine measures will prevent the cholera vibrio from entering a country, a fact that should be accepted if the challenge is to be adequately met. Because of its emotional overtones its notification is incomplete (see below and Chapter 5).

Leprosy

Leprosy is today considered an eminently tropical disease. There are, however, indigenous cases in 13 countries of the European Region: Algeria, Bulgaria, France, Greece, Italy, Malta, Morocco, Portugal,

---

[a]**Zahar, A.R.** *Studies on leishmaniasis vector reservoirs and their control in the Old World.* Unpublished WHO document WHO/VBC/79, Geneva, 1979.

[b]Other diseases transmitted by the bites of phlebotomines infected with the sandfly fever group of viruses — sandfly fever, Pappataci fever, and Naples and Sicilian fevers — are at present not seen around the Mediterranean, except rarely in Italy and possibly in other countries, but definitive virological confirmation there is lacking.

Table 28. Leprosy in Europe, including imported cases

Country	Year	No. of cases	Notes on importation
Austria	1975	2	
Belgium	1979	30 (38 in 1978)	
Bulgaria	1975	31	
Czechoslovakia	1975	2	
	1981	2	
Finland	1975	3	
France[a]	1979	1800–3000	748 imported (1952–1979)
Germany, Federal Republic of	1979	10–15 (53 in 1973)	180 in 1975, imported 43
Greece[a]	1979	1143–3000	690 in centres/hospitals 1970–1977; 8–20 new cases yearly
Italy[a]	1977	538 (545 in 1980)	94 imported
Malta[a]	1975	240 (206 in 1977)	
Netherlands	1979	600 (under treatment)	1970–1977; 39–116 yearly
Norway	1979	3	last case 1953
Portugal[a]	1975	2540	1970–1975: 32–42 yearly
Romania[a]	1975	101	
Spain[a]	1981	6000	3725 active between 1970 and 1977; about 10 new cases yearly
Sweden	1975	1	
Turkey[a]	1977	3900–15 000	1970–1976; 200–261 yearly
USSR[a]	1979	6000	
United Kingdom	1979	1054	20–50 new cases yearly
Yugoslavia[a]	1975	9	
Algeria[a]		?	
Morocco[a]	1980	6000 (3469 in 1975)	

Source: Government reports to WHO, published papers, and various reports of the WHO Regional Office for Europe.

[a] Countries with autochthonous cases.

Romania, Spain, Turkey, the USSR and Yugoslavia. Not all cases are classified according to the Ridley Jopling classification, nor is there a uniform definition of "case" or agreement about what to report: all cases or only positive or active cases. Including those imported, 16 986 cases were reported to WHO in 1976. However, the information available in the WHO Regional Office from various other official documents, WHO reports, and published papers gives a total of 32 188 cases in 22 countries, including Morocco but not Algeria and several other countries (Table 28). Leprosy and, particularly, leprosy epidemiology are neglected fields in Europe.[a] In general, leprosy infection rates are 200 times greater than the rates for clinical disease. Why so many of those who are infected do not develop the disease is a question that awaits immunological clarification.

---

[a]For more details, see *Proceedings of the First International Workshop on Leprosy in Europe, 1980*. Bologna, Associazione Italiana Amici dei Lebbrosi, 1980.

Leprosy was prevalent in historical times in the whole of Europe and as far north as Norway, where today there are three patients left, the latest two having been taken ill in 1951. The disappearance of leprosy from Europe is the subject of many interesting hypotheses, including immunity relations with other mycobacteria, the rise in living standards, and improved hygiene, which cannot be discussed here. However, the number of cases imported into European countries is constantly increasing.

Ancylostomiasis

The number of people in Europe suffering from ancylostomiasis (hookworm disease) is at present unknown. It was estimated after the Second World War at 4.2 million (24). Although newer data on the current prevalence are lacking, that estimate is certainly not valid now. The countries most highly infected by *Ancylostoma duodenale* are Algeria and Turkey. In recent decades *Necator americanus* has been introduced into certain countries (Italy, Portugal, Turkey). Ancylostomiasis is generally found in small well localized foci. The contamination of earth by human excreta (owing to the absence of latrines and the use of human fertilizer) and insufficient hygiene are thought to be the main reasons for the persistence of the disease. In Portugal the main focus was in the region of Coimbra; some 25 years ago the prevalence in some villages reached 66% (25). Although 1926 cases were notified in 1975 and 532 in 1977, it is estimated that about 6500 infected people returned to Portugal from tropical areas in those years. In 1979 there were only 57 cases. The infection rates in 1981 were insignificant and are further declining.

In Italy the disease is caused by *N. americanus* and is present in different regions. In the Fondi area in Latium the age group 21–30 years was found to be the most severely infected, and the prevalence was higher in rural than in urban areas (4.77% among 2157 persons examined compared with 1.67% among 1460) (26). In northern Italy it is reported that *A. duodenale* has been eradicated at present, but *N. americanus* is still found among horticulturists in the Veneto and Avellano regions (27). Both species, *A. duodenale* and *N. americanus*, are found in Turkey; the health statistical yearbook gives a total of 1452 cases for the years 1968–1972. In Algeria the prevalence among schoolchildren aged 6–16 years varies from zero to 33% in different localities.

Poor sanitation in some camping sites along the major land routes in Europe, particularly in the warmer areas, may create a hazard and facilitate the spread of certain geohelminths. This possibility requires investigation. Hookworm was formerly common in a number of mines, but improved sanitation has practically eliminated this risk in most countries (3).

Schistosomiasis

Schistosomiasis is of limited public health importance in the WHO European Region. However, prevalence rates of 40–85% of *Schistosoma haematobium* have been reported in a few foci in northern Algeria and the Djanet oasis. In Morocco the disease occurs mainly in nine areas on the

Saharan slopes of the Atlas mountains and parts of the Atlantic coast, where the prevalence rates vary considerably. In 1973, 13 416 cases were reported (12 774 in Agadir province alone) and in 1981 some 9621, of which 68% were in Beni-Mellal province, while the number of cases in Agadir province dropped to 725. There is an active control programme in Morocco. In the Nusaybin area of Turkey, adjacent to the endemic zone in Syria, a prevalence rate of 2% has been reported in the past, but the present situation is unclear. *S. haematobium* was once endemic in the Algarve province of Portugal but, in spite of the importation of about 10 000 cases from Africa between 1970 and 1977, the parasite has not become re-established in the country. However, one documented case in a tourist from Hamburg was reported in 1982, indicating that the focus has not died out. The intermediate host in the Mediterranean basin is *Bulinus truncatus*, with *Planorbis metidjensis* occurring as a potential secondary host in Morocco and Portugal (*3*).

The main importance of schistosomiasis lies in the danger of spread of infection following the development of irrigation in areas where the molluscan hosts are present, as in Morocco and Turkey. One important factor to consider in possible importation from outside is the capacity of schistosomes to develop in the indigenous snail population. The presence of *S. bovis* in cattle or of cercarial dermatitis in man is said to be a useful indicator of the potential risk of transmission of *S. haematobium* in an area such as Corsica or Sardinia (*3*).

Fascioliasis
Human infection with *Fasciola hepatica* appears to be very uncommon in Europe. A few small outbreaks have occurred, for instance in France and the United Kingdom, owing to the consumption of watercress grown in the vicinity of contaminated pastures. However, fascioliasis is common in sheep in Europe, and human infection appears to be increasing in France, where several thousand cases have been reported in recent years (*3*).

Opisthorchiasis, clonorchiasis and paragonimiasis
Human infection with *Opisthorchis felineus* is relatively common in eastern parts of the USSR, where raw fish is consumed, but has not been reported from other parts of Europe except in refugees from South-East Asia. In 1982 it was found in about 10–14% of Vietnamese refugees in the north of France.

Filariasis
Most European countries are outside the presumed endemic limits of filariasis, but a number of cases and even of small foci of bancroftian filariasis have been reported along the Mediterranean coast (*28*). In 1959 Sipahioglu reported finding microfilariae of *Wuchereria bancrofti* in 32 out of 312 persons examined in Antalya on the Mediterranean coast of Turkey (*29*). Three cases of early elephantiasis were also seen. A 1960 study (*28*) revealed a well established focus of population infected with *W. bancrofti* at Elazig, a town near the Euphrates river in east central Turkey. Although

the vector was not definitely identified, it was presumed on epidemiological grounds to be *Culex molestus*. Conditions propitious for filariasis transmission exist in the USSR on the Black Sea coast (*30*).

The challenge of imported tropical diseases

International travel and population movements are constantly increasing in the European Region. This phenomenon facilitates the importation of tropical and other diseases, and was a major factor in the revival of interest in tropical diseases in Europe in the early 1950s.

Statistical information on the subject is inadequate for an assessment of the full amount of the challenge, both past and present. In many countries of Europe the number of travellers from tropical countries is known, as is to a lesser degree the number of nationals travelling to tropical countries. However, in most countries tropical diseases, except malaria, are not notifiable or only selectively notifiable, and to our knowledge only a few countries have a system for routine assessment and follow-up, for example Denmark, the Federal Republic of Germany, the Netherlands, Norway, Sweden, Switzerland and the United Kingdom. Leishmaniasis was made notifiable in Italy in 1956 and in Spain in 1982, and imported malaria became notifiable in France in 1980. Information is thus incomplete and,

Fig. 33. Migration of labour and refugees to Europe
over the last two decades

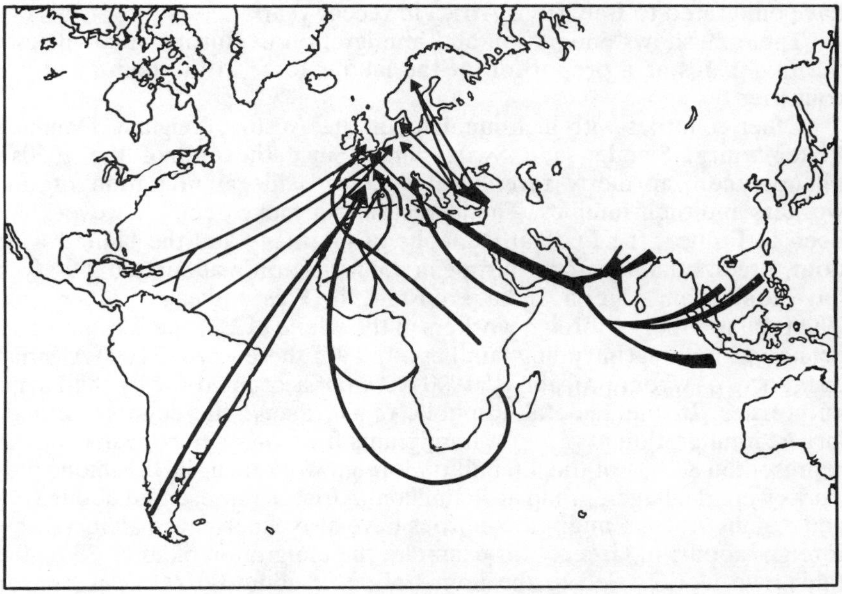

153

Table 29. Emigration and immigration in Europe as a percentage of the labour force

Emigration		Immigration	
Portugal	− 14.2%	France	+ 11.0%
Yugoslavia	− 8.5%	Germany, Federal	
Greece	− 7.8%	Republic of	+ 9.1%
Italy	− 5.6%	Belgium	+ 7.1%
Spain	− 4.7%	United Kingdom	+ 7.0%
Turkey	− 4.5%	Netherlands	+ 4.7%

Source: **Kidron, M. & Segal, R.** *The state of the world atlas.* London, Pan Books, 1981.

unfortunately, no routine statistics are sent to WHO from the tropical institutes to which most patients with tropical diseases imported into Europe converge. A proportion of diseases occurring in Europeans while travelling and treated on the spot do not appear in any statistics, either. of the travellers' country or of the country visited.

Immigration
The number of foreign workers entering the main receiving countries of Western Europe has been as much as 955 000 a year (Fig. 33). For example, in 1976 over 100 000 persons emigrated to Spain from Argentina, and in 1975 over 46 000 to France from Viet Nam. Over 440 000 people emigrated to Portugal from Angola and Mozambique in 1975, and over 500 000 people have emigrated to Italy from Africa in recent years.

Table 29 shows emigration and immigration in European countries in the mid 1970s as a proportion of the labour force in the home and host countries.

Other countries with high immigration are Austria, Belgium, Denmark, Luxembourg, Sweden and Switzerland. Since the end of the 1970s a phenomenon, formerly rare, was perceived: illegal migration of both workers and their families. The largest labour movements, however, have been to France, the Federal Republic of Germany and the United Kingdom, predominantly from European countries; only about 200 000 a year have come from Algeria, India, Pakistan, the West Indies and other areas. The total number of foreign workers in the whole of Europe is estimated at around 13 million (including families). In 1975 there were 871 000 Algerians in France, of whom probably 150 000 were not accounted for by the French authorities. In the Federal Republic of Germany, the country with the largest immigration at present, immigrants from other European countries represented 88.8% of the 4.6 million foreign workers in 1980. Among them Turks were the largest group at 1.5 million; Africans represented about 2.3% and Asians 7.8%. Emigrant countries have also experienced an increase in foreign labour; in Greece, for example, the emigration of some 280 000 of their own workers led to the immigration of about 80 000 workers from

154

Table 30. Tourist movements by region, 1981

Region	Tourist arrivals (domestic and international) (millions)	Percentage of the total
Africa	12.1	0.5
Americas	811.7	31.1
East Asia and the Pacific	65.3	2.6
Europe	1 697.3	65.1
Middle East	11.2	0.4
South Asia	9.0	0.3
Total	2 606.6	100.0

Source: World Tourism Organization.

North Africa. The health problems of migrant labour have been dealt with by WHO on several occasions.[a]

In 1977 there were about 570 000 refugees and displaced persons in Europe, and the flow has increased since. For example, in 1980 there were 108 000 requests for asylum in the Federal Republic of Germany, of which 26 000 were from Pakistan, an eightfold growth from 1974. Despite examination before arrival refugees, particularly those from South-East Asia, are likely to present high rates of infection, especially parasitic infection, and apart from falciparum malaria only clonorchiasis/opisthorchiasis, paragonimiasis and schistosomiasis are really tropical. Other protozoal and helminthic infections (amoebiasis, giardiasis, taeniasis, ascariasis, trichiuriasis, strongyloides, oxyuriasis, etc.), which are very frequently imported by refugees and usually seen in polyparasitic infestation, are not tropical diseases *sensu stricto* and are of importance mainly because they require costly organized treatment.

The largest population movements are, however, those of international tourism. The various published papers quote different and often conflicting numbers of tourists. Some general comments on overall travel trends are needed in assessing the risks of importing diseases not ordinarily prevalent in Europe.

Development of world tourism

Tourism has become a way of life of modern man in affluent countries. According to estimates by the World Tourism Organization, world tourist arrivals in Europe reached almost 1700 million in 1981, from 580 million in 1965. These figures include domestic tourist arrivals, i.e. travel by nationals

---

[a] *Health aspects of labour migration*, unpublished WHO document EURO 4003, Copenhagen, 1974; *Prevention of the inter-country spread of infectious diseases*, unpublished WHO document EURO 1002, Copenhagen, 1974.

Table 31. International tourist arrivals, 1980–1982, in thousands

Region	1980[a]	1981[a]	1982[b]	Percentage difference 1981/1980	Percentage difference 1982/1981
Africa	5 744	6 595	6 100	+14.8	− 7.5
East Africa	1 143	1 312	1 350	+14.8	+ 2.9
Middle Africa	199	198	200	− 0.5	+ 1.0
North Africa	3 346	4 066	3 500	+21.5	−13.9
Southern Africa	388	310	320	−20.1	+ 3.2
West Africa	668	709	730	+ 6.1	+ 3.0
Americas	56 070	56 698	53 500	+ 1.1	− 5.6
North America[c]	35 376	36 148	33 500	+ 2.2	− 7.3
Latin America	12 801	12 870	12 300	+ 0.5	− 4.4
Caribbean	7 893	7 680	7 700	− 2.7	+ 0.3
East Asia and the Pacific	14 264	15 338	15 800	+ 7.5	+ 3.0
South Asia	1 903	2 011	2 100	+ 5.7	+ 4.4
Europe	195 388	196 172	195 900	+ 0.4	− 0.2
Eastern Europe	39 017	36 930	34 500	− 5.3	− 6.6
Northern Europe	22 331	21 769	22 000	− 2.5	+ 1.1
Southern Europe	60 582	60 780	62 500	+ 0.3	+ 2.8
Western Europe	73 458	76 693	76 900	+ 4.4	+ 0.3
Israel	1 116	1 090	900	− 2.3	−17.4
Middle East	5 569	5 716	5 600	+ 2.6	− 2.0
World total	280 054	283 620	279 900	+ 1.3	− 1.3

Source: World Tourism Organization.

[a] Revised figures.
[b] Preliminary estimates.
[c] Canada and the United States.

within their own country, as well as international tourist arrivals. They therefore cover all tourist movements, whatever the motive, at the domestic and international level. Holiday travel accounts for almost 70% of all international tourist travel. The movements in the various regions of the world in 1981 are shown in Table 30.

It should be pointed out that Table 30 gives estimates based on incomplete figures. The data are nevertheless useful as a basis for analysing tourism both in the world and in the various regions. As the figures indicate Europe, with 65% of total arrivals, has the largest share of world tourism.

Tourism on the whole has increased at a rate of 4–8% per year for the past two decades, and it is now the second largest trade item in the world, surpassed only by oil. Its value was estimated at US $75 000 million in 1979, and it has not been more than momentarily affected by the energy crisis and the economic recession. It is also an important source of direct and indirect employment. In the Gambia, for example, one of Africa's fastest growing tourist resorts, it is claimed that for every 1000 tourist beds there are 5000 jobs. Tourism also has adverse consequences, such as the spread of prostitution and the dissemination of sexually transmitted diseases.

Total international tourist arrivals in the world in 1981 (excluding excursionists) were estimated at 283 million, an increase of 6% over 1979. Although it has not attained the growth rates recorded for 1977 and 1978, international tourism appears to have settled into a new rhythm of growth after easing off in 1973 and 1979.

Total international tourist arrivals in the various regions of the world during the period 1980–1982 are shown in Table 31.

In interpreting the figures for and the risk to health of international tourism by region, account must also be taken of the intra-regional element of these movements. The share of intra-regional tourism, i.e. travel between countries within the same region, is shown in Table 32.

It will be noted that international tourism in Europe is largely dominated by travel between countries of the region. The share of this in the total, not including Algeria and Morocco, is 84%.

Europe has thus continued to account for the largest share of the world tourism. Total domestic and international tourist movements in this region account for about 65% of total tourist travel. The largest volume of international tourism in Europe is from America. The information available on the breakdown of arrivals by country of origin for India and Sri Lanka indicates a significant increase in arrivals from European countries such as Belgium, France, the Federal Republic of Germany, the Netherlands, Switzerland and the United Kingdom.

The volume of tourism is evident from the fact that, for example, in 1979 some 22 million Germans visited the Mediterranean. Greece had over 5 million tourist arrivals in 1979 and Spain almost 40 million. In 1980 Italy had 48 million visitors, Yugoslavia 20 million and Portugal 2.7 million. In Mallorca at the height of the season there are 15 000 people per km^2, or 60 times more than in the Federal Republic of Germany. It is easy to imagine the possibility of a breakdown in standards of hygiene and pathogenic contamination of coastal waters. Since nothing stops the flood of tourists a progressive increase in the risk, particularly of enteropathogens and other bacteria, is to be expected in the future.[a]

Tourism within Europe itself, with rare exceptions, does not lead to the importation of tropical diseases, but it does lead to the importation of non-tropical diseases. Statistics on the increase in the volume of travel —

---

[a]It takes about 80 years for a natural exchange of water in the Mediterranean to take place, and some biologists believe that the Mediterranean has already lost up to 45% of its life-renewing capacity. The Mediterranean is singled out only because of its importance for tourism, but the same processes also apply elsewhere. The Baltic Sea receives about 2.3 million cubic metres of 40% treated sewage every day, and about 4.9 million cubic metres of industrial waste enter the North Sea every day. Worldwide about 450 cubic kilometres are released every year into lakes, streams and rivers, which account for only 0.01% of the total volume of water on the planet.

157

Table 32. Share of intra-regional tourism
in the different regions, 1967–1981,
as a percentage of total international arrivals

Regions	1967	1976	1981
Africa	16	12	24
Americas	94	85	75
East Asia & the Pacific	45	56	56
Europe	85	86	84
South Asia	20	18	24
Middle East	68	68	42

Source: World Tourism Organization.

passenger-kilometres, etc. — are of little value for assessing the health risk without clearer specification of the place and type of accommodation in the tropical countries visited. Most of the tourists or commercial visitors returning to Europe from tropical areas belong to a social class likely to have access to medical care in their own countries; this by itself reduces the risk of importing tropical diseases other than malaria. Nevertheless, the risk should always be kept in mind, particularly in view of the constant increase in tourist travel to Africa and Asia.

Tourist statistics do not give an exact picture of travel to the risk areas. For example, the flight destinations of citizens of the Federal Republic of Germany in 1978 included 80 000 for Asia and 650 000 for Africa. In 1980 some 5.8 million tourists travelled to Africa, a number that represents only 2% of the total number of tourists in that year; of these some 62% went to North Africa, 22% to East or Southern Africa, 11% to West Africa and 5% to Central Africa. The main risk group in international travel consists of nationals of European countries visiting tropical areas. Apart from tourists, there are members of voluntary aid groups, workers in industrial constructions, students, seamen, military personnel, etc.

The danger presented by imported tropical diseases is that they can be overlooked because the signs and symptoms are not familiar to European physicians even if they are typical, as often they are not. Imported tropical diseases are almost entirely of clinical, rarely of epidemiological, importance. It was estimated that in 1977 about 6 320 000 people from Europe visited malarious areas of the world: 2 250 000 to North Africa, 650 000 to Africa south of the Sahara, 1 200 000 to the Middle East, 1 300 000 to the Far East and the Philippines, 450 000 to India, 400 000 to Brazil, and 70 000 to Central America. The actual degree of risk to which they might have been exposed cannot be deduced from such data.

Which diseases are imported?
First place among imported diseases goes to *malaria*. Malaria, particularly that caused by *Plasmodium falciparum*, remains a major and increasing public health problem in the WHO Regions for Africa, South-East Asia and the Eastern Mediterranean, and in parts of the American and Western

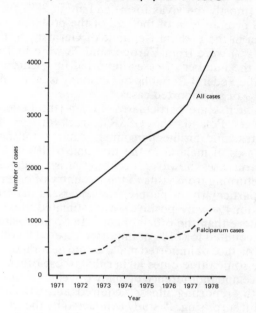

Fig. 34. Reported number of malaria cases
imported into Europe, 1971–1978

Pacific Regions. The problem is compounded by the alarming growth in the resistance of *P. falciparum* to drugs in the South-East Asia and Western Pacific Regions. In the jet age these regions are only hours away from Europe, and their malaria problem can indirectly add to the malaria problem in the European Region.

Malaria transmission originating from imported mosquitos has been reported in the vicinity of international airports in four otherwise malaria-free countries. In Zurich two soldiers stationed near the international airport at Kloten were infected by *P. falciparum*, most probably by an infected anopheline mosquito arriving in an aircraft; a third person was infected in the same area a year later. Eleven cases of falciparum malaria were described between 1969 and 1978 near the Charles de Gaulle airport at Roissy in the Paris area, and one case of vivax malaria is thought to have been due to local transmission by an indigenous mosquito. In 1978 and 1981 autochthonous cases of falciparum malaria were reported from the Netherlands in a village close to Schiphol international airport, and another in 1979 involved a 10-year-old girl who spent the night on a boat 1500 m from the airport. In 1982 a case was detected in Belgium close to the airport in a person who had never been outside the country. In 1979 importation of malaria into the United Kingdom reached an all-time high, even higher than in the years immediately after the Second World War. The pattern of importation follows that of travel. In the Federal Republic of Germany, for example, over half (58.7%) of imported malaria is from

Africa, followed by about 15.5% from India and 8.2% from Asia (excluding Turkey). In the United Kingdom 53% of the malaria cases imported were from Asia (mostly the vivax form) and about 28% from Africa. Fig. 34 and Table 33 give an idea of the size of the problem. Of 918 cases of imported malaria in the Federal Republic of Germany in the years 1977–1979 only 89 (10%) were from Europe, and 78 were in Turkish subjects (*31*). However, the number of cases imported into Europe from Turkey other than into the Federal Republic of Germany is minimal: only 31 cases in 1979, or 0.76% of all imported cases.

The persons at risk are particularly seamen (the Federal Republic of Germany, Greece, Poland, the USSR), truck drivers on long transcontinental routes, and airline personnel. Among Lufthansa personnel there were 70 cases of malaria in the first half of 1978 (*32*). The largest numbers of malaria cases, however, occur in tourists and businessmen, and in immigrants returning from visits to their country of origin. In France up to 2000 cases, particularly in people from overseas *départements* and in refugees (of whom 4% were positive), are estimated to be imported each year, which is more than the official figure. In Spain, visitors from Equatorial Guinea accounted for 81% of imported cases. The official figures do not give the full picture of imported malaria, the general opinion being that the numbers are some three times higher than those officially reported.

The ignorance and indifference of many travellers as regards protecting their own health, reporting illness acquired abroad, and following up treatment are still surprising. A study conducted by the Ministry of Health and Social Security in France (*33*) on the importation of malaria showed that 15% of travellers did not take any prophylactic drugs at all and only 1.5% of the 22% for whom drugs had been prescribed followed the prescription correctly. Nevertheless, the greater awareness of the medical profession has brought about a reduction in the fatality rate, which is now 1.2% in the United Kingdom, whereas formerly it had been 3–4%. In seamen in Hamburg eight deaths occurred from malaria and one resulted in dementia in the years 1961–1968 (*34*). Since 1978 the number of imported malaria cases in nationals of the Federal Republic of Germany has diminished, while travel to malarious countries has increased. In 1980 more than half of all cases were in foreigners and in people seeking asylum (*31*).

A special extension of imported malaria is transmission by blood transfusion. In France alone 79 cases were identified between 1960 and 1979, 60.7% from donors originating from Africa. Over half were falciparum infections.

Yellow fever was contracted by two French tourists on vacation in Senegal in 1979 in an area close to the border with the Gambia, where at that time an outbreak had occurred involving 24 known cases. (In the Gambia in 1978 there was an important epidemic with 8000 cases and 20% mortality.) They died in Paris, and the diagnosis was made histologically only post mortem and through isolation of the virus from blood taken before death. Vaccination against yellow fever was not required in Senegal for persons staying less than eight days.

Table 33. Malaria cases in Europe, 1973–1982

Country	1973	1974	1975	1976	1977	1978	1979	1980	1981	1982
Albania	0	0	0	1	3	0	—	0	0	1
Austria	7	6	11	31	33	94	35	44	54	60
Belgium	22	3	1	1	3	0	1	59	30	24
Bulgaria	13	32	45	60	90	101	101	128	420	—
Czechoslovakia	2	8	9	6	4	6	—	15	2	—
Denmark	38	59	62	46	49	54	—	70	120	102
Finland	4	16	4	22	2	12	13	13	14	33
France	43	58	143	197	232	494	25	111	77	108
German Democratic Republic	3	6	11	4	17	18	22	16	35	82
Germany, Federal Republic of	146	105	175	218	337	534	486	570	390	516
Greece	20	21	27	33	39	64	35	41	52	—
Hungary	6	5	8	2	4	8	13	6	34	25
Iceland	—	—	—	—	—	—	—	—	—	—
Ireland	2	2	1	6	58	11	32	22	25	—
Italy[a]	56	60	56	103 (132)	205 (228)	101 (259)	162 (105)	176	168 (143)	—
Luxembourg	—	—	—	—	—	—	—	—	7	4
Malta	0	0	0	0	0	0	0	0	1	—
Monaco	—	—	—	—	—	—	0	0	0	0
Netherlands	30	27	54	76	107	108	112	101	119	—
Norway	13	0	25	56	12	20	32	25	35	35
Poland	8	12	18	19	27	35	23	—	29	—
Portugal	594	903	971	482	133	52	45	25	27	—
Romania	3	3	10	7	17	17	13	12	22	—
Spain[a]	34	20	30 (19)	39 (28)	57 (27)	32 (29)	52 (47)	73 (90)	59	65
Sweden	49	52	59	62	78	79	104	97	123	121
Switzerland	11	37	85	49	48	112	93	95	138	130
USSR	226	272	275	310	350	408	399	386	304	—
United Kingdom	539	660	765	1 217	1 528	1 909	2 053	1 668	1 576	1 471
Yugoslavia	15	20	20	42	65	51	59	85	58	—
Total	1 884	2 387	2 867	3 089	3 498	4 390	4 045	3 838	3 919	
Deaths	42	19	25	13	28	40	9	21	19	25

a Two sets of official figures exist, the second set being shown in parentheses.

The importation of *dengue* occurs at the rate of about 20 cases a year.

A suspected case of imported bubonic *plague* has been reported only once in recent years, in a seaman arriving at Marseilles from Bombay in 1970. It was shown in fact to be lymphogranuloma venereum.

Filariasis was found in 51 of 2217 people returning from the tropics to Switzerland; slightly over half were members of development aid groups and slightly over a quarter tourists (*35*). In Portugal, out of 3206 military and civilians returning from Africa, filariasis was found in 14 (*36*). The clinic for tropical diseases in Amsterdam saw 100 patients in 13 years (1959–1971) (*37*). In London in 1966 and 1967 there were 14 cases out of 1000 reporting for examination, and in Liverpool about 65 out of 3140 specimens submitted for laboratory examination in one year were positive for *Filaria* spp. Between 40 and 67 cases were treated yearly in Antwerp in the period 1972–1980.

The importation of *trypanosomiasis* is exceptional. Only 109 cases were seen between 1904 and 1966, only 43 cases after 1912 (*38*), mostly among missionaries, military personnel and agricultural specialists, but recently also in tourists. In the 10 years up to 1977 there were two cases in Switzerland (*39*). In the Federal Republic of Germany two cases were reported over 26 years, in 1961 (*40*) and 1977 (*41*), and Chagas' disease was reported once. The Liverpool School of Tropical Medicine saw a case of sleeping sickness caused by *Trypanosoma rhodesiense*, contracted by a businessman while visiting a game park reserve in Zambia in 1978–1979 (*42*). Trypanosomiasis was also imported into Belgium and France (*43*), and in 1982 into Italy by a tourist visiting game parks in Zambia and Zimbabwe.

The importation of *schistosomiasis* occurs frequently. In 1970 there were about 20 000 cases in France in persons who had previously arrived from different countries. Between 28 and 122 cases were imported into Portugal yearly in 1975–1979, and 25–82 were treated annually in the clinical department of tropical medicine at Antwerp in the period 1972–1980.

Leishmaniasis is often regarded as an imported disease in Europe, although the disease is endemic in some European countries. Five cases of the cutaneous form seen in Alsace were imported from Mediterranean countries (*44*) and two cases in Lille were imported. Seven cases of kala-azar were seen in Hamburg (no date or period given) (*34*), of which six were contracted in Spain at Benidorm and Malaga. There have been seven cases of importation of leishmaniasis in recent years into the Federal Republic of Germany, from Elba, Rome, the east coast of Spain and Mallorca; two from Greece into Switzerland at Geneva; and seven others into Switzerland from the Balearics, the Costa Brava and Italy. Importations have been reported also into Sweden from Benidorm in Spain, and into the United Kingdom from Algeria, Corfu (Greece), and Spain. Leishmaniasis has also been imported from outside Europe: eight cases from Brazil into Italy (*45*), between two and six every year into France from North Africa, two into Belgium, two into England, and two into Yugoslavia from Kuwait and Libya.

Leprosy is imported into Europe with increasing frequency. In the

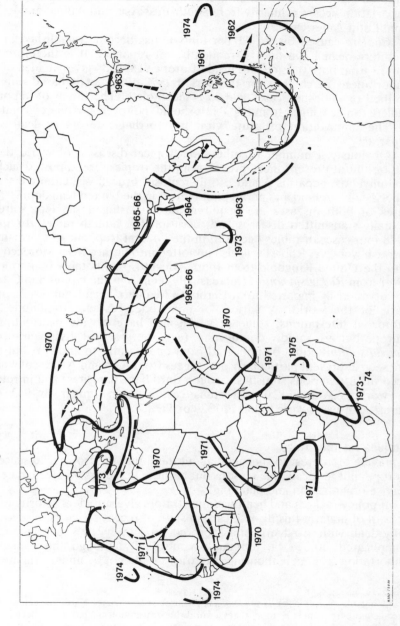

Fig. 35. Global spread of cholera from 1961 to 1975 (April)

Federal Republic of Germany 6–14 cases were diagnosed yearly in the period 1975–1980 (see Table 28, which includes also imported cases; it is safe to assume that all cases in non-endemic countries are imported). The importation occurs primarily from South-East Asia and Africa, and less so from Latin America.

Cholera caused by the El Tor biotype has become established in the Mediterranean basin and is frequently not reported. It is therefore imported from both outside and inside Europe. Table 34 gives an idea of the importations of cholera for the period 1972–1981 but is based only on notified or published cases and so is incomplete. The threat of imported cholera can be gauged from Fig. 35. It should, however, not be exaggerated.

The importation of acute viral haemorrhagic fevers is dealt with separately.

Obviously a number of other non-tropical diseases, of world distribution but at present more prevalent in the tropics, are imported such as poliomyelitis, hepatitis A and B, tuberculosis, brucellosis, enteric diseases (specifically typhoid and paratyphoid fever; in the United Kingdom 90% of cases of both diseases are acquired abroad), shigellosis, leptospirosis, sexually transmitted diseases and, occasionally, human rabies. In 1971–1978 four cases of rabies occurred in the Federal Republic of Germany in Turkish workers. Rabies was also imported into France from Morocco and into the United Kingdom from India. Rickettsiosis, notably boutonneuse fever from *Rickettsia conori* (increasingly seen), murine typhus and Q-fever are occasionally imported from European Mediterranean countries or other parts of the world. A variety of nematode, cestode, trematode and protozoal infestations, some of which also have a wide distribution in Europe but are rapidly diminishing[a] (e.g. the practical disappearance of *Taenia solium*) could be imported from one country to another, but they are seen at present particularly in refugees from Asia and Africa (of whom, according to various statistics, about a third have parasites) and in returning workers. Among 12 084 screenings carried out in Hungary in 1962–1982 parasitic diseases were found in 1329 or 11%.

Outlook for the future
It may be of interest to speculate about the future of "tropical" diseases in Europe, not for academic reasons but because of factors involved in health service organization and planning.

If policy-makers and health administrators give sufficient priority to the control of malaria this disease can, in spite of recent setbacks, be successfully dealt with in Algeria and Morocco. In Turkey the situation is more complicated; it can be ultimately controlled, although the danger of importation from neighbouring countries should not be underestimated as

---

[a]A notable exception is *Giardia lamblia*. The protozoan infection giardiasis seems to have become more frequent in Europe. It has a worldwide distribution and has always been present in Europe. It causes intestinal symptoms, particularly in institutions for children and the old. It is at present frequently associated with tourism.

Table 34. Cholera imported into Europe, 1972–1981

Year	Country	No. of cases	Cases imported from:[a]
1972	Germany, Federal Republic of	2	Angola, 2
	United Kingdom	2	Australia, 2
1973	Berlin (West)	1	Tunisia, 1
	France	4	Algeria, 2
			Ivory Coast, 1
			Tunisia, 1
	Germany, Federal Republic of	5	Italy, 1
			Tunisia, 3
			Turkey, 1
	Sweden	10	Tunisia, 10
	United Kingdom	5	India, 1
			Tunisia, 4
1974	France	3	Algeria, 1
			Portugal, 2
	Germany, Federal Republic of	3	Portugal, 3
	Spain	1	Portugal, 1
	Sweden	1	Portugal, 1
	United Kingdom	3	Pakistan, 1
			Portugal, 2
1975	France	3	Algeria, 2
			Portugal, 1
	Italy	1	Either Morocco, Algeria or Tunisia, 1
	United Kingdom	1	Iraq, 1
1976	France	5	Algeria, 1
			Morocco, 4
	Germany, Federal Republic of	2	Turkey, 2
	Netherlands	1	Morocco, 1
	Sweden	1	Tunisia, 1
	USSR	1	India, 1
	United Kingdom	1	Nigeria, 1
	Yugoslavia	3	Turkey, 3
1977	Germany, Federal Republic of	1	Either Iraq or Turkey, 1
	Italy	2	Tunisia, 1
			Turkey, 1
	Netherlands	1	Turkey, 1
	Switzerland	1	Turkey, 1
	Turkey	17	Saudi Arabia, 5
			Syria, 12
	USSR	1	India, 1
	United Kingdom	2	Iraq, 1
			Turkey, 1
1978	Netherlands	4	Indonesia, 4
	Switzerland	1	Thailand, 1
1979	France	7	Algeria, 1
			Morocco, 3
			Spain, 1
			Tunisia, 1
			Either Viet Nam or India, 1
	Netherlands	5	Morocco, 5
	Spain	5	Morocco, 5
	Sweden	1	Jordan, 1

continued

[a] Where known.

165

Table 34. (contd)

Year	Country	No. of cases	Cases imported from:[a]
1980	Belgium	1	Morocco, 1
	France	1	Morocco, 1
	Germany, Federal Republic of	4	Turkey, 4
	Spain	4	Morocco, 1
	United Kingdom	6	India, 4
			Indonesia, 1
			Sudan, 1
1981	Austria	2	Tunisia, 2
	France	19	Algeria, 11
			Either India or Japan, 1
			Tunisia, 5
	Germany, Federal Republic of	4	Tunisia, 4
	Netherlands	2	Tunisia, 2
	Poland	1	India, 1
	United Kingdom	11	India, 2
			Iraq, 1
			Pakistan, 3
			Tunisia, 2
	Yugoslavia	3	Tunisia, 1
1982	France	18	Algeria, 15
			Morocco, 2
			Tunisia, 1
	Germany, Federal Republic of	1	Ghana, 1
	United Kingdom	1	Tunisia, 1
1983	France	5	Algeria, 2
			Morocco, 3
	Netherlands	3	India, 3
	Spain	3	Algeria, 2
	United Kingdom	5	Either Hong Kong or Philippines, 1
			India, 2
			Pakistan, 2

[a] Where known.

long as the situation in those countries remains the same. However, control will be long and laborious, requiring a fresh look at the strategy and an organization firmly built on primary health services at the national level and vigilance activities able to take the necessary preventive and remedial measures, particularly in areas where the conditions for transmission are most favourable. Those conditions, which are the same for any country, include vulnerability to infection, meaning either proximity to malarious areas or likelihood of a frequent influx of infected individuals (as already seen in Algeria and Turkey) or of infected anophelines (as with the opening of the trans-Saharan highway in Algeria); it also includes receptivity through the abundant presence of vectors and the existence of other ecological and climatic factors favouring malaria transmission. All those factors are subject to change. The risk in other temperate areas appears to be low and, in relation to the possibility of the re-establishment of transmission in receptive areas by imported anophelines, has probably been overestimated. (The risk of ship-borne *Aedes* spread in the Mediterranean might be more serious.) Some of the risk factors related to malaria and the difficulties encountered, as seen from the European perspective, were summarized at a WHO conference in 1981:[a]

- resistance or increased tolerance of mosquitos to the available insecticides (an actual and potential problem in the Region)

- the possibility of importation of *P. falciparum* strains resistant to chloroquine (an increasing clinical problem)

- the possibility that African strains of *P. falciparum* may be transmitted by anopheline vectors coming into Algeria and Morocco (not thought to be much of a problem as European vectors are refractory to African strains)

- adverse side-effects of the 8-aminoquinoline group of antimalarial drugs in G6PD-deficient people, a problem existing in Turkey at present

- the relationship between drug addiction and malaria induced through the indiscriminate use of syringes

- the toxicity of insecticides to human beings, animals and the environment

- the difficulty, under given epidemiological circumstances, of defining an optimal strategy to stop transmission, using measures that are cheap, safe, effective, readily accessible, and acceptable

- the problem of administration of antimalarials at regular intervals to nomadic groups of people or migrant labourers

- the incapacity of health care systems, particularly at primary health care level, to cope adequately with imported diseases (from lack of training, of diagnostic facilities, and of means of treatment)

- the neglect of measures such as disinfection of aircraft and ships and provision of information to travellers

- the lack of coordination between departments within ministries of health (e.g. for communicable diseases and primary health care), between ministries (e.g. for health and the environment), and between government and private agencies (e.g. on the use of insecticides for pest control)

- the refusal of people to accept the small degree of inconvenience caused by periodic indoor residual insecticide spraying.

The vector mosquitos themselves have not been eradicated anywhere, and whenever they are brought in and conditions are suitable malaria transmission may and indeed does start again, as has happened on occasion

---

[a] *The role and participation of European countries in the fight against malaria in the world*, unpublished WHO document ICP/MPD 009, Copenhagen, 1981.

in Corsica, Sicily and Thrace. In those countries the health authorities have the means to bring any occasional transmission to a halt. Reintroduction and large-scale local transmission of malaria are unlikely in any country of continental Europe, provided that the epidemiological services function normally in receptive and vulnerable countries.

For leishmaniasis it is difficult to make a prediction as yet as the information is conflicting; some authors have reported an increase in its incidence and geographical spread. Quilici et al. (10) observed a steady increase of adult kala-azar in south-eastern France in the period 1970–1978, adult cases in the earlier years accounting for 90% of the total. With exact epidemiological delineation of the foci the detection and treatment of human cases is likely to be improved. If combined with careful control of leishmaniasis in dogs, so as not to switch the vector to humans by the indiscriminate destruction of dogs, it could be assumed that leishmaniasis in Europe will gradually diminish and eventually disappear from the continent, except perhaps in some parts of Asian USSR. The present trend seems to indicate a decline in kala-azar, but there is a certain persistence or increase of the cutaneous form, as in Algeria and Morocco. Increasing effort is now being made by WHO to develop a vaccine.

No extension or spread of schistosomiasis in the European Region is expected. The situation in Algeria and Morocco, however, particularly with the development of irrigation schemes, might present local problems, as is the case in eastern Turkey and the old focus in Algarve, Portugal.

A vaccine against leprosy is expected to be available by 1985 in sufficient quantity for trials to be undertaken in man. It will be necessary to wait another 20 years to know whether the vaccine is effective. By that time the incidence of leprosy will have further declined in Europe (there is no evidence that imported leprosy has been transmitted to indigenous populations with good standards of hygiene) and it is not likely that the vaccine will have any use in Europe except perhaps in families of patients with the disease.

General considerations

The problem of tropical diseases in Europe is, apart from malaria and leishmaniasis, one of adequate prevention before travel and early diagnosis and proper treatment after return. Both have weak points: lack of experience in a large part of the medical profession and laboratory personnel, lack of specific drugs except in special centres, and uncertainty about the correct dosage, particularly in children, when suitable drugs are available.

Although the big influx of tropical diseases expected after the 1950s, when the large-scale increase in travel started, did not materialize except for malaria, and although it is impractical to have special clinical departments outside the general infectious medicine wards (except in countries that have overseas territories and cities such as London and Paris with large numbers of imported or chronic infections) it is nevertheless wise to have in each country some people who keep up their knowledge of the relatively rare tropical diseases and have the experience and facilities for their diagnosis and management. As an illustration of the demand for services, almost 4000 specimens were received in the diagnostic laboratory of the Liverpool School of Tropical Medicine in the 12-month period 1 August 1980–31 July 1981 (42). Most of the 450 or so medical schools in Europe offer some teaching in tropical diseases, which no doubt should be compulsory, and there are about 24 special institutes or schools of tropical medicine or institutions of similar character registered by the Standing Council of European Schools of Tropical Medicine and Hygiene. The somewhat hasty tendency to establish new centres has now diminished, at least in Western Europe, and the existing institutions, lacking clinical material, are torn between their glorious past traditions (the first school for tropical medicine was established in Liverpool in 1898) and a new sophisticated pure research orientation requiring more and more highly specialized skills and expensive equipment. Some institutions depend on government development aid schemes or military or industrial funds for the maintenance of outposts in the tropics, or training sponsored by religious missions of doctors and nurses for work in the tropics. Many, however, are engaged in health planning, international health work, family planning, nutrition or general epidemiology.

There is a decline in the number of long-term residents from European countries in the tropics, and opportunities for a career in tropical medicine are shrinking. The department of tropical medicine in Edinburgh closed in 1972, and the universities of Heidelberg and Tübingen have not filled vacant chairs for tropical medicine in the 1980s. Budget cuts are hovering over even the most renowned schools, and the institutes of tropical medicine in Italy, Portugal and Spain are in partial eclipse. The question throughout the whole of Europe is whether the European commitment to tropical medicine should continue and what the consequences of discontinuing that commitment would be. Economic difficulties have already compelled some governments to withdraw from the WHO onchocerciasis control programme in Africa. The big boost to maintaining the interest in tropical diseases in Europe was the WHO Special Programme for Research and Training in Tropical Diseases, a UNDP, World Bank and WHO activity with an annual budget of about US $26 million. This programme involves over 2000 scientists from 78 countries, of whom 60% are from endemic countries. WHO provides 20.7% (£279 275) of the grants of £1 351 529 for research in tropical medicine in the United Kingdom. The European research commitment for the schistosomiasis programme is diminishing, 22% of research funds now coming from the United States. The fear has been voiced that the supply of trained scientists will decline and there might be no easy replacement in spite of WHO efforts to build up local capability in tropical countries, and also that the pharmaceutical industry will lose the possibility of testing new drugs for tropical diseases. While the discussion continues it is clear that, as Maegraith (2) said in 1969, the impact of European schools on the tropics must be made in the tropics.

In the present circumstances it might be desirable, not least for career prospects, to redefine the role of schools and institutes of tropical medicine and hygiene in Europe in relation to medical faculties and departments of infectious diseases. If the latter decided to integrate instruction on malaria and other imported tropical diseases into the undergraduate curriculum, the former could concentrate on courses at the higher, specialist research level and on collaboration in the training of teaching and research staff from tropical countries. This could be done either by establishing fellowships and posts in specialized institutions or by temporarily transferring teachers to institutes and universities in the endemic countries until they can assume a larger share themselves. This obviously could not be done overnight; a transitional period would be needed.

Tropical medicine today is predominantly medicine of the developing countries. It may be useful to regard it not only as a moral commitment (46) but also in the general socioeconomic context of the relationship of Europe with those countries.

Interest in tropical diseases in Europe will certainly continue, particularly in research (from a medium-term point of view) and in training. The long-term prospects are uncertain. If economic development and WHO plans for better health for all go well, and if tropical diseases are consequently greatly reduced at source, it would be logical to expect scientists in Europe to switch their interest to other fields of research. A breakthrough in immunotherapy, chemotherapy, strategies and methods could, if significant, speed up this process and thus reduce the importation of tropical diseases into Europe. But caution is warranted; the process is very slow and fraught with problems.

Much depends on international cooperation, development aid, and the commitment of governments, philanthropic foundations and private voluntary organizations; all of these again depend on the general economic outlook. Military action and civil strife affect control activities and add in many different ways to the probability of an increase in the diseases prevalent. Technical problems such as the spread of resistance of vectors to insecticides or drugs could compound the problems and lead to a reduction in control efforts. An epidemic resurgence would then be inevitable, as has been witnessed repeatedly in past decades. It is important to remember that the situation in the world is dynamic and that changes in relation to tropical diseases should be carefully monitored and taken into account in overall health development and planning. In any case, the possibility of tropical diseases being imported must be kept in mind in Europe and history-taking should in all cases of doubt start with Maegraith's question "Where have you been?".

The challenge of unusual diseases

While, with the increased rapidity and range of contemporary travel, virtually any disease can be imported from another country, a group of unusual diseases, formerly unrecognized and sometimes called "new", have attracted particular interest, although they may have existed already in specific geographical areas. The problem requiring special attention is that of the African viral haemorrhagic fevers or so-called "dangerous pathogens" or "special pathogens", classified by WHO as organisms for which no effective vaccine is available and which are so dangerous as to present great risk to the health of either laboratory workers or human or animal communities, so that material known to contain live organisms should not be accepted or kept in the country at all without authorization.[a] These pathogens are:

— Lassa fever virus

— Marburg (and Ebola) virus

— Crimean-Congo haemorrhagic fever virus

— Rift Valley fever virus (and Zinga virus which is identical or very similar).

"Unusual" means that these diseases are rare in Europe, in general uncommon globally, and unfamiliar to European physicians. A great many unusual diseases do not occur in Europe at all, or are strictly localized in small geographical foci. They do not receive much place in the already heavily charged medical curriculum, because the average physician is unlikely to encounter them during his medical practice. Yet they do occur occasionally and require early diagnosis, elaborate surveillance, emergency measures, and special diagnostic and isolation facilities. In addition, special training is needed for dealing with them, whether in diagnosis, clinical management, in the collection of specimens, or in the disposal of infected waste. This is particularly important as initially they do not present any typical signs and symptoms and the first three can be transmitted, with great risk of hospital spread since the clinical picture is similar to that of many commonly occurring diseases. As they cannot be recognized at the frontier but could occur in their early stages at any place of transit or at the final destination, it is useful to mention them briefly from the European perspective and experience, without going into any specific details about diagnostic methods or management.

Lassa fever

Lassa fever is a severe systemic febrile infection indigenous to Africa, a zoonosis recognized in 1969 in Nigeria and other parts of West Africa south of the Sahara, which is transmitted by contact with infected rodents (*Mastomys natalensis*) or people. It has an insidious onset, uncharacteristic symptoms, fever and haemorrhage, and can easily be confused with typhoid fever, streptococcal pharyngitis, diphtheria or malaria. In hospital patients a high fatality rate, 18–37%, has been observed so far. Secondary and tertiary cases can occur among hospital patients, hospital personnel and family members. Shedding of the virus in the urine may be prolonged: 42 days and longer have been observed. Five reported cases of Lassa fever

---

[a] *Herpesvirus simiae* should also be included in this group, as it requires special laboratory facilities. The South American haemorrhagic fevers are not included, as their importation has never been recorded and it is highly unlikely. Yellow fever, dengue fever, Kyasanur Forest disease and Omsk haemorrhagic fever are not included either.

were imported into the United Kingdom between 1969 and 1976, and there was a further case in a patient travelling through London's Heathrow airport to the United States. Three of the patients were ill on arrival, or soon after, and three were convalescent. No spread of infection took place. In 1976, two physicians from the Federal Republic of Germany working in Onitsha, Nigeria fell ill and one died. In 1980, Lassa fever was diagnosed in a Dutch diplomat travelling from Upper Volta to Amsterdam. In 1981 a teacher in the incubation period came to the United Kingdom on a scheduled flight. In 1982 Lassa fever was diagnosed in a Nigerian woman eight days after her arrival in London, and another case was imported in October 1982. Since none of the large number of contacts developed the disease, it seems that it is less infectious to contacts than originally thought.

Marburg and Ebola virus diseases[a]
Marburg virus disease was first described in 1967 when infected African green monkeys (*Cercopithecus aethiops*) or vervet monkeys were imported from Uganda to Marburg and Frankfurt in the Federal Republic of Germany and to Belgrade in Yugoslavia. A severe, formerly unknown disease occurred in people handling the tissues of one batch of infected monkeys or in their close contacts (*47,48*).

In these incidents there were 25 primary cases with 7 deaths (fatality rate 28%) and 6 secondary cases with no deaths. The clinical symptoms are those of yellow fever, typhoid fever, falciparum malaria or influenza-like illness, with which the disease can be confused. The haemorrhagic syndrome occurs 4–5 days after the onset. In fatal cases the patient dies between the fifth and tenth days. Transmission by close contact occurs, possibly by pharyngeal secretion or contamination with the patient's blood. Excretion of the virus in urine and in other secretions may be protracted; in one case evidence of sexual contamination occurred 80 days after the onset. As this virus is highly lethal to monkeys (almost 100%) the monkeys are thought perhaps only to have been the amplifier, not necessarily the reservoir, of the Marburg virus. In 1975 three cases occurred from an Australian index case returning from Zimbabwe via South Africa.

The clinically similar severe Ebola infection, caused by a closely related virus, has not yet been imported into Europe. The three recorded outbreaks occurred in southern Sudan (284 known cases, 151 deaths) and north-western Zaire (318 cases, 280 deaths) in 1976, and in southern Sudan in 1979 (33 cases, 22 deaths). The lethality rate, 53% in the Sudan and 88% in Zaire, is the highest known for any virus disease. Transmission in the Sudan and Zaire was by direct contact with patients and contaminated needles and syringes in hospitals. Casual contact does not seem sufficient to cause illness, but haematogenous transmission is highly invasive. Clinically, the disease is characterized by sudden onset, headache, muscle

---

[a]Marburg and Ebola viruses have recently been proposed as the type species of a new family, the Filoviridae (thread-like viruses) instead of the Rhabdoviridae, in which they have been included up to now.

and joint pains, and progressively developing fever, but about the seventh day prostration sets in with a dry cough, diarrhoea, vomiting and abdominal pain. There is no pharyngitis. Haemorrhagic manifestations were present in 91% of the fatal cases and in about 50% of those who survived. In the latter there was a very slow convalescence. Although the area of prevalence and the possible reservoir of these viral diseases are not yet well known, it may be assumed that all Africa south of the Sahara is an enzootic area. *Rattus rattus* and an insectivorous bat are suspected of playing a role.

Considering the extreme rarity of importation of these diseases as well as their clinical severity, a central world depot of convalescent serum for plasma immunotherapy has been established by WHO in Geneva, but the efficacy of this therapy is unclear.[a]

Rift Valley fever

This is a mosquito-transmitted, enzootic and epizootic Bunyavirus-like virus disease of domestic animals (particularly non-indigenous strains of wool-sheep, goats, cattle, horses and camels) in central sub-Saharan Africa along the Rift Valley, known as enzootic hepatitis but also able to cause human epidemics. It occurred in 1951, 1953 and 1957 in South Africa and in irrigated areas of Egypt, where the disease was introduced for the first time, probably by the cattle or camel trade, in 1977–1978 (18 000 cases with 598 deaths in people not usually associated with livestock). It has not yet spread north to other countries of the Eastern Mediterranean Region except to Sinai, but this is feared possible in view of the large volume of animal trade and the ubiquitous presence of *Culex pipiens*. WHO organizes courses on the diagnosis, surveillance and management of Rift Valley fever through the Mediterranean Zoonoses Centre, Athens. The clinical picture, as judged from Egyptian experience, is characterized after an incubation period of 3–6 days by sudden fever, nausea, vomiting, severe myalgia and ocular disturbances; in a small percentage of cases jaundice and haemorrhagic manifestations develop within 2–4 days and are the main cause of death. CNS involvement (encephalitis) is frequent. A clinical presentation that may be overlooked is post-infectious retinitis or encephalitis. Since these may follow a relatively benign acute illness by several weeks, they are of particular relevance to the issue of illness that may appear in the returning traveller. Diagnosis in the laboratory is by virus isolation or by haemagglutination inhibition, complement fixation and gel diffusion.

The mechanism of spread remains unclear; it is not known whether mosquitos — Culicinae, particularly *Culex pipiens*, *Aedes* spp., anophelines and others — are biological or mechanical vectors. Laboratory contamination occurs, possibly also by the respiratory route. Virus has also been isolated from the pharyngeal swabs and stools of patients, but no

---

[a]For more information see: *Marburg and Ebola virus infections. A guide for their diagnosis, management, and control*, Geneva, World Health Organization, 1977 (Offset Publication No. 36); and *Bulletin of the World Health Organization*, **56**: 245–294 (1978).

hospital infection has been seen so far. Control in animals is possible through immunization with live attenuated or formalin-inactivated vaccine, particularly of animals for export. A formalin-inactivated vaccine is available for persons exposed to high risk of infection such as veterinarians, butchers, herdsmen and laboratory workers. However, the vaccine is expensive and there are no readily available stocks. The vaccine may be obtained from the US Army Medical Research Institute of Infectious Diseases or from the Virus Disease Unit, WHO, Geneva. Live attenuated vaccines at low cost may become available in the future through genetic engineering techniques.

While the four haemorrhagic fevers mentioned above are not present in Europe, there are a few haemorrhagic diseases that have a focal distribution in some parts of the continent.

Crimean-Congo haemorrhagic fever

Knowledge of this disease was acquired from epidemics in 1944–1945 that were a consequence of the environmental disturbances caused by the Second World War in the Crimea and of improvement work in the swampy areas of virgin steppes for collective agriculture in the Moldavia and Rostov areas, the Caucasus, Astrakhan, Kalmyk ASSR, Dagestan ASSR, transcaucasian Turkmenia and other republics of the USSR (49). Epizootics occurred depending on the density of the tick *Hyaloma marginatum* and other species infesting people working in agriculture, forestry and other rural industries, or people gathering mushrooms or picnicking during the summer months. While there have been no recent cases in Moldavia, the disease has continued to occur sporadically in natural foci in the Crimea and Astrakhan area. The virus was isolated in 1967 and found to be identical with the Congo virus of the Bunyaviridae family, which causes a similar disease in Africa, and with a third member of the family, the tick-borne Hazara virus of India and Pakistan. The disease was identified in 1979 in several areas of Iraq (53 cases, 35 deaths), some on the border with Turkey (50).

Serological evidence of the circulation of the virus has been obtained in a wide range of animals — cows, horses, hares and birds — which are thought to be perhaps responsible for the geographical spread of the disease, as observed in recent times in Middle Eastern countries. Person-to-person transmission occurs by close contact with a patient and through blood or blood-contaminated material.

In Bulgaria[a] the disease was first observed in 1946 and is supposed to have been introduced by tick-infested horses or fodder during the Second World War. The disease was intensively studied between 1952 and 1968 (51) and the virus was isolated in 1968. The disease has continued to occur in Bulgaria sporadically in numerous foci in persons working in agriculture,

---

[a] A comprehensive book on haemorrhagic fevers (Crimean-Congo and haemorrhagic fever with renal syndrome): **Radev, M. et al.** *Hemoragichni treski*, Sofia, Medicina i Fizikultura, 1980 [in Bulgarian].

animal husbandry or forestry. Between 6 and 34 cases were registered yearly in the period 1970–1977. Specific globulin for treatment has been prepared, and selective vaccination is carried out in laboratory workers and in the exposed population in the focal areas. In Bulgaria the virus has been isolated from the ticks *Hyaloma plumbeum*, *Rhipicephalus sanguineus* and *Boophilus calcaratus*. Antibodies were detected in all domestic and in numerous wild animals, lagomorphs, field mice and other rodents. Foci have also been observed in Yugoslavia, with sporadic cases in humans in the period 1954–1967 and one epidemic in 1970. Serological evidence of the circulation of the virus has also been demonstrated in France, Greece, Hungary and Turkey. The existence of other silent foci in a wide range of ecological areas is possible. No importation into other parts of Europe is on record.

Contingency measures

The importation of haemorrhagic viral diseases into Europe, rare as it may be, has raised a number of questions concerning preparedness for epidemiological emergencies. With the speed of international travel, it is unlikely that an importation could be discovered at the port of entry. It could be discovered, however, at any time or in any of the destinations of the traveller; hence the need for surveillance systems that respond rapidly and handle diagnosis, transport, isolation and treatment. This is particularly difficult, as in many instances the symptoms are not characteristic and there is still incomplete knowledge of the pathophysiology, epidemiology and mode of transmission of the diseases.

The importation of acute viral haemorrhagic fevers has led to the creation in Europe of maximum security laboratories for virus isolation in three European countries.[a] Attention has also been given to isolation units for patients.

While the importation of known cases can be prevented by the decision of governments not to return patients to their home country until the risk of transmission is over, the possibility of their arrival home during the incubation period cannot be ruled out. Because they would rarely be used, if at all, it would appear wasteful to establish further maximum security laboratories requiring much capital and expensive maintenance in all European countries; thus regional cooperation and sharing are needed. This requires organizational steps to be taken in countries as well as

---

[a]The Microbiological Research Laboratory, Porton Down, Salisbury, United Kingdom, the Institute of Virology, Moscow, and the Institute of Tropical Medicine, Antwerp, Belgium. A laboratory for diagnosis and isolation exists in the Tropical Disease Institute, Hamburg. The above laboratories will provide help in identifying pathogens but they should be contacted through the WHO regional offices or WHO headquarters so that safe shipment and receipt of biological specimens can be arranged. Recently five more facilities have been established in the United Kingdom (Pill near Bristol, Manchester, Liverpool, Newcastle upon Tyne and Glasgow). The Netherlands is constructing a high-risk isolation unit in the De Lichtenberg Hospital, Amersfoort.

international and WHO cooperation for the early identification of cases, isolation in the units designated, and surveillance of contacts, who may be spread over several countries and create considerable logistic problems. On the other hand, adequate isolation of patients is more easily achieved by improving already existing infectious diseases clinics. Most countries have adequate facilities for the isolation of people with suspected or identified contagious diseases, but not necessarily high-risk units.

Suspected patients need to be put in high security rooms with filtered negative-pressure ventilation and separate facilities. The Class III Safety Biohazard Isolator Cabinet for the protection of personnel (as well as of the community at large) has been produced since 1980 as a flexible plastic-film isolator cabinet; in the past it was made of steel and aluminium. Similar cabinets with a minilaboratory are also available, as well as new versions of Trexler's bed isolators, which are now available in Belgium, Denmark, the Federal Republic of Germany, the Netherlands, the USSR and the United Kingdom. Smaller versions (stretcher transit isolators) can be used to transport patients by plane and in standard ambulances from airports or from small hospitals to designated special isolation units.

Countries should, however, establish contingency plans for such emergencies, including: the designation of the receiving facilities; a review of isolation wards and an appraisal of their suitability; arrangements for the disposal of wastes (including fluids); a sufficient quantity of the necessary equipment, such as high-efficiency particulate air filters, respiratory masks, plastic bags and gloves; decontamination facilities; staffing and training; and transport for suspected patients or of material (in tightly sealed primary and secondary containers to prevent breakage or leaking and a shipping container capable of resisting shocks such as a free fall from 10 metres).[a] The transport of patients in some countries is the responsibility of the air force, and some military authorities are wholly or partly in charge of emergencies of various kinds, including serious medical emergencies. Some countries, such as the United Kingdom, have separate codes, advisory groups on dangerous pathogens, and rules for the protection of laboratory workers.[b]

Arboviral disease in Europe

Among other unusual diseases two deserve special mention, not necessarily in the context of importation but as important, though rare, arboviral infections indigenous to Europe and not transmissible from person to person. These are haemorrhagic fever with renal syndrome (haemorrhagic

---

[a]See IATA's Packaging Note 695 on restricted articles (*Weekly epidemiological record*, No. 9, 1978, pp. 66–69).

[b]*Bulletin of the World Health Organization*, **58**: 249 (1980); *Weekly epidemiological record*, No. 22, 1977, pp. 185–192; and **Pattyn, S.R., ed.** *Ebola virus haemorrhagic fever.* Amsterdam, Elsevier/North Holland, 1978.

Fig. 36. Focal areas of haemorrhagic fever with renal syndrome in Europe

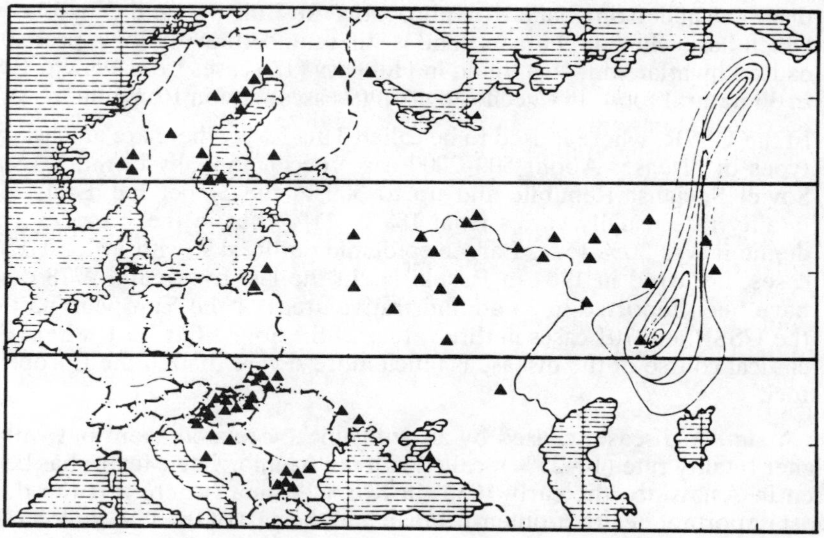

Source: **Vasilenko, S.V. et al.** *Haemorrhagic fevers.* Sofia, Medicina i fizicultura, 1980.

nephrosonephritis, epidemic haemorrhagic fever, epidemic nephritis, nephropathia epidemica) and Central European tick-borne encephalitis.

Haemorrhagic fever with renal syndrome
This is an acute infectious, primarily interstitial renal disease characterized by an abrupt onset of fever of 3–8 days' duration, headache, nausea, somnolence, tenderness over the kidneys, proteinuria, acute nephritis with thrombocytopenia, and haemorrhagic manifestations (in about 20% of patients with the European form of the disease), followed by proteinuria and hypotension. The renal symptoms are oliguria for a few days followed by hyposthenuria, which can continue for several weeks. Sometimes oliguria leads to anuria, azotaemia, renal failure and death. The disease is found in Europe in rural areas in early winter in three geographically distinct areas (Fig. 36).

● Scandinavia. In Finland, roughly north of the 60th parallel, it first occurred in the military in 1942–1943 with over 6000 cases. There are now about 10–100 cases per year. It was first described in Sweden in 1934 as nephropathia epidemica (279 cases in Umeå). In Denmark there were 7 cases in Svendborg. In Norway in 1949 there were about 46 cases in an area north of Oslo. There are cases in adjoining parts of the USSR (Murmansk and the Baltic republics). The disease has been encountered since 1957 with a periodicity of 3–4 years.

177

- Southern Europe. In Bulgaria in 1953–1978 there were 407 cases, and in Yugoslavia in 1951–1968 some 340 cases. Sporadic cases are found in Serbia. The disease is known as epidemic nephropathy and is to be distinguished from balkan nephropathy in Bulgaria and Yugoslavia, which has a chronic character and is still of uncertain etiology, probably caused by aflatoxin. It is found in Hungary (136 cases from 1952 to 1980 in 33 natural foci), in Czechoslovakia (9 cases) and in Romania.

- In the USSR, where it used to be called Tula fever, there are at least two types of disease. About 500–2000 cases occur annually in the Russian Soviet Socialist Republic and up to 300 in the Soviet Far East. The fatality rate usually varies from 1% to 11%, but in the Yaroslav epidemic it was 30% (52). Larger epidemic outbreaks, with at least 1500 cases, occurred in 1964 in Bashkiria. In the last five years, 9778 cases have been reported in 35 administrative areas of the European part of the USSR and 701 cases in three areas of the Soviet Far East, where the clinical course of the disease is much more severe than in the European foci.

A similar disease, caused by an antigenically related agent but with a higher fatality rate (10–25%), called Korean haemorrhagic fever, has been seen in Asia since the early 1930s in Korea, China (where it is the third most important health problem), Japan and the east of the USSR along the Amur River. The disease was recently observed in urban populations in the above countries.

After about 20 years of intensive search the etiological agent, the Hantaan virus, a non-cytopathic RNA virus similar to other Bunyaviridae (which are usually transmitted by arthropods) but without an insect vector, was identified in 1976–1978 by immunofluorescent techniques in the lungs of the field mouse (*Apodemus agrarius coreae*) and in humans. It was propagated in human cell lines in 1981, and purification and morphological identification were achieved in 1982. This has opened the way to demonstrating the similarity of the two forms of the disease, and to solving the question of whether they are a single entity with different antigenic sera or subtypes. Serological evidence indicates that the epidemic nephropathy and Hantaan viruses may coexist in South-Eastern Europe. Recently enzyme-linked immunosorbent assay (ELISA) and solid phase radio-immunoassay, tests that are more sensitive, have been developed. The antibodies persist for at least 34 years. The exact mode of transmission is not yet known, but it is assumed to be respiratory through dust contaminated by the excreta of a variety of *Apodemus* species, and possibly by contaminated food. Nevertheless an arthropod vector of Hantaan virus should be sought. The majority of cases occur in the rural population and especially farm workers. Laboratory infections have been reported. In Finland a similar antigen called the Puumala agent, which seems to be related to the Hantaan virus, has been detected in the lungs of the bank vole, *Clethrionomys glareolus*. On the basis of clinical and serological differences, Finnish authors postulate 2–3 virus serotypes. *Apodemus sylvaticus* and *A. flavicollis* in vegetable gardens invaded by voles, and

Rattus norvegicus in urban and port areas, are also thought to be hosts.[a] Person-to-person transmission does not seem to occur, although virus is excreted in saliva for one month and in urine for two years. Laboratory infections occur, however, in animal room personnel, as has happened in Belgium where there were six such cases in 1978–1983 and in France where one case was diagnosed in 1982. The disease is believed to be spreading slowly; in 1981 it was demonstrated serologically in healthy persons and patients with glomerular disease in northern Greece adjoining Bulgaria and Yugoslavia (*53*). Since the disease until recently presented diagnostic difficulties and was moreover not notifiable except in the USSR, the exact numbers of cases occurring in Europe are unknown. Cautious assessment of published material gives the impression that they are higher than assumed, since probably only severe cases come to the attention of the medical services. An evaluation of the size of the problem and the distribution of the disease, and a review of the as yet unanswered epidemiological questions in Europe are necessary, particularly of the transmission, virulence, persistence and pathogenesis of the disease in man. Special attention should be paid to the danger of spread of the disease to new areas.

Central European tick-borne encephalitis (TBE)[b]

This is clinically the most important European arbovirus infection (among 15 arboviruses whose occurrence in man in Europe has been definitely proved)[c] and was first identified in Siberia by Silber in 1932–1934. In subsequent years he also isolated the virus and discovered the vector, which is distributed throughout most of the USSR. It is a Flavivirus (formerly B group) arbovirus, transmitted in Europe by the common castor-bean tick *Ixodes ricinus* (in the Asian USSR partly also by

---

[a]New data on the geographical distribution of the Hantaan virus and related viruses indicate that it may be enzootic in the United States in *R. norvegicus*, and that it may have spread among rodents in northern Belgium. Antibodies to the Hantaan virus have since been recognized in many other parts of the world, where the classical disease has not so far been recognized.

[b]To be distinguished from tick-borne meningopolyneuritis, tick-borne erythema chronicum occurring in Scandinavia, Central Europe and the USSR, and the similar Lyme disease (erythema chronicum migrans followed by polyarthritis and meningeal syndrome within weeks or months). The last mentioned is a tick-borne spirochaetosis (**Burgdorfer, W. et al.** *Science,* **216**: 1317–1319 (1982)).

[c]There are, at present, about 408 known arboviruses in 51 antigenic groups and new ones are being discovered every year; the number rose from about 160 in 1960 to about 300 in 1970. About one quarter of the known arboviruses can infect man. Of the 15 demonstrated serologically in Europe, only a few have been linked definitely to the wide spectrum of clinical disease in man: tick-borne encephalitis, louping ill (in Scotland) and Tribeč (in Slovakia) involving meningoencephalitis; West Nile and Sindbis involving fever; Inkoo, Thogoto and Tettwang usually associated with mild fever and neurological involvement; Tahyna associated with atypical pneumonia; Crimean-Congo and Hantaan fevers with haemorrhagic symptoms; and the sandfly fever group of diseases (Neapolitan and Sicilian phlebotomus fevers). The clinical importance of Uukuniemi virus (Austria, Czechoslovakia, Finland, Hungary, Poland), Bhanja virus (south Italy), Pontèves virus (France) etc. is as yet unknown.

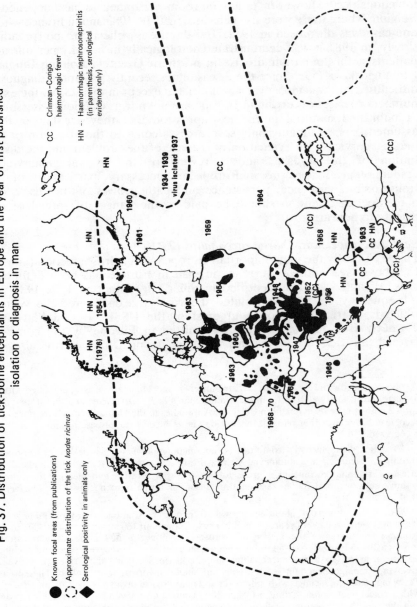

Fig. 37. Distribution of tick-borne encephalitis in Europe and the year of first published isolation or diagnosis in man

CC — Crimean-Congo haemorrhagic fever

HN — Haemorrhagic nephrosonephritis (in parenthesis, serological evidence only)

● Known focal areas (from publications)
◌ Approximate distribution of the tick *Ixodes ricinus*
◆ Serological positivity in animals only

180

I. persiculatus). It exists in small but numerous permanent natural foci in mixed deciduous forest, young forest, underbush and forest fringe habitats where the ecological conditions are suitable for ticks and small mammals such as field mice and voles, *Clethrionomys glareolus* and *Apodemus flavicollis* being the primary vertebrate hosts. Transmission to man is accidental by all three stages of free-living ticks, which remain infected for life. Infection can, however, also be transmitted by raw milk from infected domestic animals, particularly cows, goats and sheep, and by inhalation in laboratories. Those most often affected are forestry workers, hunters, holiday-makers and mushroom collectors. There is no transmission from person to person.

Although normally the radius of movement of small rodents is limited to about 150 metres, emigration of small young viraemic males from those microfoci, if ecological conditions are suitable, favours geographical spread and extension of the focal area. The role of birds in geographical spread is still not clearly proved. The disease occurs in two forms: the very severe taiga encephalitis, which is frequently lethal in the Soviet Far East, and a milder form seen in Europe. TBE occurs clinically in at least 14 European countries and has been shown serologically to be present in at least five others, in ticks, domestic animals and, without identified disease, man. In eight countries TBE is of particular importance (Fig. 37 and 38).

Fig. 38. Foci of tick-borne encephalitis in the USSR according to maximum incidence, 1952–1961

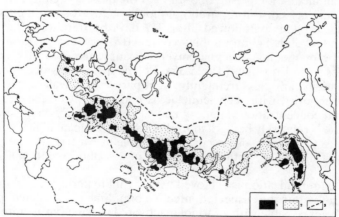

1 — High incidence
2 — Low incidence
3 — Isolines of the sum of effective temperatures of more than +10°C

Source: **Neronov, V.M. & Ivanova, L.M.** An attempt at a map of the habitat of tick-borne encephalitis in the RSFSR and some methodological compilation problems. *In: Metody mediko geograf. issled.* Moscow, 1965.

181

Table 35. Percentage occurrence of symptoms in the case histories and on admission to hospital of 105 patients with Central European tick-borne encephalitis

Case history		Admission to hospital	
Symptom	Percentage	Symptom	Percentage
Headache	73	Fever	86
Meningeal symptoms	30	Meningeal symptoms	86
Vomiting	25	Headache	81
Pain in the extremities	23	Vomiting	44
Chill	15	Photophobia	24
Pain in the back	13	Pain in the extremities	19
Nausea	8	Mental changes	16
Gastrointestinal symptoms	7	Paresis	16
Mental changes	7	Confusion	15
Photophobia	7	Chill	14
Nerve root pains	6	Nausea	11
Confusion	3	Gastrointestinal symptoms	7
Paresis	3	Pain in the back	7
		Tremor	7
		Nerve root pains	4

Source: **Möse, J.R.** *Bundesgesundheitsblatt,* **8**: 243–249 (1982).

After an incubation period of 3–14 days the disease is clinically characterized by diphasic or (more rarely) monophasic fever, seldom over 39°C, and headache. This is followed after 2–7 days by tremor of the hands, tongue and eyelids; photophobia; conjunctivitis; meningeal, meningo-encephalitic or meningoencephalomyelitic symptoms; dysarthria; dysdiadochokinesis; and myalgia (Table 35). Polyneuritic pains occur in up to 30% of patients and, less frequently, light pareses. Convalescence is slow (over one month), with such sequelae as persistent headache, insomnia, difficulty in concentration, memory and sight disturbances, and sweating. The disease is relatively benign, mortality usually being no higher than 1%. However, severe forms also occur, for example in Austria and the Federal Republic of Germany, with fatality rates of 2% and exceptionally up to 4.6%.

Passive immunization is achieved with 0.1 ml hyperimmunoglobulin up to three days after the suspected infective bite. Since 1976, active prophylaxis has been possible with a formol inactivated vaccine (virus cultivated in chick embryos) giving protection about six weeks after the first dose. It is given in 2–3 doses of 0.5 ml spread over 1–3 months and a further dose a year later. The immunity lasts about three years but can be extended by booster doses. In 7–10% of cases there is a local reaction, in 8–17% fever, and in 6–21% tiredness after immunization. The difficulty is to select the population at risk apart from those, such as forestry workers, who are clearly professionally exposed. The disease has been repeatedly observed in tourists, and cases have been imported into other countries.

Although there is a vast amount of excellent scientific literature, particularly on the virological, ecological and serological investigation of natural foci, ticks and animals, there is no ready information enabling the exact numbers of cases diagnosed yearly in affected countries and the trend to be determined, or the claim to be confirmed or disproved that the disease is spreading to the west. The ecology of TBE is extremely complex, and constant changes occur in the ecosystem as a result of human activity. Excellent reviews have been published by Hannoun (*54*) and Kunz (*55*), who have attempted to sum up the present situation in Europe.

The first description of TBE from *European USSR* was in 1939 (White Russia 1951, Ukraine 1964, Lithuania 1961) and it seems to be widely spread all over the forested parts of the country. Various clinical forms exist with late sequelae in about 20% of cases. About 500 cases occur every year. In *Czechoslovakia* the disease has been known and studied closely since 1948 (the virus was isolated in 1949/50) and is widely spread over the whole country: in Bohemia (except the north-west) but particularly in central, south-western and northern Moravia and the southern parts of the River Vah in Slovakia. The natural foci are in the immediate vicinity of the main towns (Prague, Brno and Bratislava) in the most frequented recreation areas. The morbidity, which is much higher in Bohemia, fluctuates; there are years with high rates and years with low rates, varying according to age group from 3 to 10.3 per 100 000 population. The lowest number of cases recorded per year was 170, the highest 2083. The highest morbidity — 21.3 per 100 000 population — has been observed in forestry and agricultural workers in the age group 15–39 years. Serological evidence suggests about 7% infection in those 6–19 years of age and up to 60% in those aged 50–64 years, mostly with no history of encephalitic involvement. About 0.3–8.3% of adult ticks are carriers of the virus (*56*); the figure is smaller for nymphs. The average infection rate of ticks is about 1%.

The disease, then of unknown etiology, had been clinically observed as early as 1927 in Lower *Austria*. In 1949 it started occurring in epidemic form in Styria and Carinthia (*55*). The history and serological evidence suggest that the disease has not been imported recently from the east but that it has existed in the country for many years. The virus was isolated in 1953. About 300 cases are diagnosed yearly in Vienna and Lower Austria and about 140 in Graz, particularly in children but with a shift to young adults in recent years. In the last ten years the highest number of cases (632) was in Carinthia in 1973. In the whole of Austria in 1979 there were 676 cases (237 in Styria alone) and 7 deaths. The foci are found around Vienna, in Lower and Upper Austria around the River Danube, in Burgenland, Styria and Carinthia, and in the north towards the borders with Czechoslovakia and Hungary (*57*). Some 15–38% of wild animals and a large proportion of the human population have been exposed to the virus, particularly those in close contact with forests. Even so, most infections are asymptomatic, particularly in children.

In *Hungary*, the virus was first demonstrated in 1952, and is found in deciduous forest throughout the country, particularly in the main hilly areas: from Budapest towards the north–south parts of the transdanubian mountains; towards Lake Balaton; the northern central chain of mountains towards Czechoslovakia; and east towards the Romanian border. In the south-west the foci merge with the Austrian and Yugoslav focal areas. Between 1959 and 1978 some 35.5% of the 5463 cases of acute central nervous system disease were caused by tick-borne meningoencephalitis. The foci show considerable stability: virus was isolated from ticks in 1973 on the same spot where it had been isolated 19 years before. Most cases of overt disease in man are found in young adults, 70% of whom are males. Cows in hilly areas are 15.7% seropositive, those in the prealpine region 3%, and those in flat country 1.8%.

In the *German Democratic Republic* TBE has been demonstrated serologically in patients with clinical encephalitis (in the Gera district of Thuringia west of Erfurt and south of Eisenach) and in domestic animals and rodents. Focal areas are found south of Schwerin, south of Stralsund, towards the border with Poland, south of Berlin, and west of the Oder. The seropositivity in this part of the country varies from 1.9% to 22.4%. About 400 cases are thought to have occurred between 1975 and 1978. In recent years all the northern areas (except one closely influenced by the Atlantic climate) and the central areas have shown little or no activity, while the hilly areas in the south are very active. Although maximum tick activity is in late May and early June, maximum morbidity is in August and September, with a small peak in May. There is thus a distinct risk for holiday-makers.

In the *Federal Republic of Germany* the disease made an appearance in the 1970s in lower Franconia and Bavaria (particularly along the rivers Danube, Paar, Isar, Vils, Rolt and Inn but not south of Munich and Augsburg towards the Austrian border), in south Baden-Wurtenberg, and in the upper Neckar valley. Isolation of the virus was made from the blood of patients and from ticks. About 150 cases yearly are recorded, but the number is probably much higher. Serological evidence indicates that 4–8% of the population in endemic areas have antibodies and 1.6% of the general rural population are reactors. The disease in South Baden is of marked severity, indicating possible changes in the virulence of the virus in nature (*58*).

In *Switzerland* the disease was demonstrated serologically in encephalitis cases in 1962 and by isolation of the virus from animals in 1970 and from ticks, particularly in Schaffhausen, Winterthur, Thun, Neuchâtel and Zurich. Between 31 and 55 confirmed cases per year occurred in the period 1973–1978. Serologically, an incidence of 0.5% has been found in humans and 3.6–5.6% in dogs (*57*).

In *Italy*, serological surveys demonstrated circulation of the virus in the animal population of Gorizia on the border with Yugoslavia in 1966, and in five human cases in a focus north of Florence in 1975 (*59*). The virus was isolated in 1978 from *Ixodes ricinus* in areas where infection had presumably occurred. The disease is of no practical importance in Italy.

184

In *Greece* the only evidence of the disease is serological and through isolation of the virus from goats.

In *Yugoslavia* the disease has been known clinically since 1946 but the presence of the virus was not demonstrated until 1953 (*60*). It has spread over the whole of the central and eastern part of central-western Slovenia and Croatia, with sporadic foci in Istria and Dalmatia (north of Dubrovnik, Zadar, Sibenik, Brac) together with isolated cases in Bosnia and Herzegovina. About 85–150 cases occur yearly, but there are epidemics approximately every three years. The virus has also been isolated from the tick *Dermacentor pictus*. In the focal areas up to 40% of the population have antibodies and up to 60% of the domestic pasture animals are seropositive.

In *Bulgaria* TBE was demonstrated serologically and epidemiologically in 1954 in man and animals and the virus was isolated from ticks. Data on human morbidity are not available but it does not seem to occur.

The virus was isolated in *Romania* in 1958; about 10–17% of the population of Moldavia are seropositive.

In *Poland* the virus was isolated in 1954 and several foci have been described: near Gdansk, Lower Silesia (Opole), Bialystok, Lublin, Bielowieza forest and Mazuria (Olsztyn). Some 27–54 cases are seen each year, particularly between June and September. The seropositivity of forest workers in Lublin province was found to be 19%. In 1970 a new natural focus was discovered in the province of Lodz. The disease was found in the Olsztyn area in a population having no contact with the forest area, and was presumed to have been caused by drinking cow's milk.

In *France* the virus was isolated in 1968–1970 in the Illkirch forest near Strasbourg (*54*). Rare sporadic cases occur. Surprisingly, during the investigation there, a focus was discovered of Tahyna (Bunyaviridae) virus transmitted by mosquitos.

In *Finland* the virus was isolated and found to be endemic in two focal areas: the Aaland archipelago in the south-west and the eastern part of the country (on the border with the USSR). There are about four cases a year and it is not a public health problem.

In *Sweden* the disease has been known since 1954 from serological evidence in encephalitis patients. Thirty cases were diagnosed in 1956 in Stockholm and a further 38 were classified as suspects. About 20 clinical cases occur every year. The seropositivity in animals, including the elk, is 14–17%.

In *Denmark* the disease has been demonstrated clinically on the island of Bornholm, but never in any other part of the country.

In *Norway* there is only serological evidence for the disease in 20% of persons in the foci. Virus has been isolated from ticks in several focal areas in the western part of the country.

The disease and serological proof of the circulation of virus have been demonstrated in recent years also in *Albania* and *Turkey*.

The occurrence of arboviruses in Europe, and in particular of TBE virus, creates a challenge that should be met not only by the epidemiological systems in the countries but also through multidisciplinary investigation. Although much work has been done in individual foci, valid ecological generalizations are still lacking. The questions to be answered are as follows:

- Are all the geographical areas where TBE occurs defined? Are the many blank spots on the map correct?

- What is a typical biotope in ecological terms? Is it a focus composed of one or a number of different ecological biocoenoses in which the virus circulates independently?

- Are the foci temporary or permanent? Temporary foci lasting several years have been seen, for example, in Sindbis virus importation and implantation; do TBE foci have similar characteristics? Foci lasting 20 years can still be only temporary. If it is assumed, however, that tick-borne arboviruses date as far back as the last glacial period (61), then they are permanent where the biotopes in all the synecological inter-connections among vector, host and causal agent have been favourable over innumerable centuries and correlate with the climate, flora, fauna and various geographical factors. The encounter with man (and thus disease) is always accidental and is not related to the maintenance of the focus.

- Are the foci linked with the two tick species only? The transmission potential of *Haemaphysalis concina* has been demonstrated, for example in southern Austria.

- Finally, is TBE spreading? Is the apparent spread to the west somehow conditioned by later seroepidemiological inquiry in some countries, or is some type of human activity interfering with conditions in nature that have changed the spatial distribution of foci — the reduction of forests, transformation of the landscape, more fringe habitats, changes in the balance of small mammals, spread of housing to the rural areas, sporting activities, etc.?

There is a need for systematic mapping of tick distribution and for delineation of the focal areas: clinically, serologically and by isolation of the virus in man, ticks and small mammals. Such studies should then be followed by detailed zoological and virological studies to demonstrate the critical mammalian carrier host(s) responsible for the maintenance of the focus.

Other unusual diseases

Among other unusual diseases in Europe are the recently observed (1974 and 1981) new Pogosta disease in Finland caused by an arbovirus similar to Sindbis virus, presumably carried by the *Culex* mosquito and perhaps imported by migrating birds. Another is Ockelbo disease, first observed in 1960 and occurring annually in late summer, which is an epidemic poly-arthritis with an exanthem, found in Sweden just north of the 60th parallel and associated with a Sindbis-like virus (many cases occurred in the east-central part of the country in 1981).[a] A third is epidemic haemorrhagic conjunctivitis (Apollo 11 disease).

Since it was first recognized in Ghana in 1969 and in Indonesia, the Philippines and Singapore in 1970, epidemic haemorrhagic conjunctivitis has been repeatedly imported into Europe, for example to France, Morocco, the United Kingdom and Yugoslavia. Outbreaks have probably also occurred in other European countries. It is caused by several picornaviruses: enterovirus 70, which is very resistant to heat and ultraviolet light, coxsackievirus A 24, and adenovirus 11. Transmission is rapid by direct or indirect contact with infected persons after 1–2 days incubation or so, particularly in schools, military barracks and other overcrowded conditions, or by objects contaminated by conjunctival discharge. In autumn 1981 epidemic outbreaks involving many thousands of cases occurred in Arab and Caribbean countries and in the United States, but few cases were imported from Europe.

Epidemic haemorrhagic conjunctivitis is to be distinguished from the iatrogenic infection epidemic keratoconjunctivitis, caused by adenovirus type 8, the mode of spread of which by hand or by instruments during eye examination has been well known to ophthalmologists since the early 1950s. Epidemic keratoconjunctivitis is a follicular conjunctivitis with nonpurulent exudate and preauricular lymphadenitis, followed after about a week by subepithelial punctate keratitis (keratitis maculosa, keratitis nummularis) which takes months or years to clear. Known also from industrial outbreaks in shipyards and factories because of its frequent association with eye injuries and community outbreaks, it is dreaded in hospitals where cross infection occurs, particularly in ophthalmology units, the infection usually being transmitted by tonometry examination. It can also affect hospital staff by person-to-person spread.

The *British medical journal* recently devoted an editorial (*62*) to this disease, on which again no exact information exists in Europe because of the epidemiological problems it raises: "Firstly the adenovirus responsible is unusual, for type 8 is not one of the common adenoviruses which are endemic in most communities; secondly, despite its mode of spread and the means of prevention being known, outbreaks of the disease continue. Just how adenovirus type 8 maintains itself in the community between epidemics — which are usually several years apart — remains something of a mystery". There would appear to be insufficient numbers of sporadic cases of infection to ensure its survival in the population. Although the virus can be cultured and the infection can be serologically diagnosed and is theoretically preventable, the editorial concludes: "the disease seems likely to continue: epidemic keratoconjunctivitis will survive". Epidemiological information is also lacking about the prevalence of adenovirus type 19, which can also cause outbreaks of classical epidemic conjunctivitis.

---

[a]**Skogh, M. & Espmark, A.** Oral communication at the VIII International Congress of Infectious and Parasitic Diseases, Stockholm, 7–11 June 1982.

The situation is no better with *Chlamydia* infections, partly because the classical infection, trachoma, is rarely seen outside Algeria, Morocco (25 272 cases in 1976, 19 185 cases in 1980) and Turkey, partly because they may be reported in a few countries as ornithosis/psittacosis. Only in Sweden and the United Kingdom do laboratory reports give some indication of the prevalence of the disease.

The new and mystery diseases

The question of "new" diseases has been with us now for 20 years or so.[a] Whether some of the diseases are new or merely newly described cannot now be decided, and probably never will. Some, like Reiter's disease or myalgic encephalomyelitis, have ceased to be new, but have not been clarified etiologically, a number of microbial pathogens still being incriminated.

It may well be that some already existed but were not diagnosed or reported. Once described they have scientific appeal and the medical press is filled with case reports, followed by descriptions of the diagnostic, physiological and pathological characteristics and sequelae. In this rush of publicity a proper perspective may not be obtained unless a national epidemiological surveillance system is there to assess the trends over time. The definition of new disease is usually based on severe cases that have attracted clinical attention and been described. In the absence of specific tests the question of diagnosis and classification of milder cases arises. Among the new diseases whose etiology has been clarified may be mentioned legionnaires' disease and staphylococcal toxic shock syndrome.

Legionnaires' disease[b]
Since their first identification in the United States in early 1977, *Legionella* infections have been observed sporadically in many European countries — Austria, Denmark, the Federal Republic of Germany, the USSR and Yugoslavia — and in outbreaks as well as sporadically in France, Italy (up to 300 cases), the Netherlands, Portugal, Spain, Sweden and the United Kingdom.

Accurate data on the incidence are not available because the diagnosis is not yet sufficiently widespread. From American experience it seems that the annual incidence is 12 per 100 000 population. Recent studies in Europe indicate that the causal agent, the previously unknown bacterium *Legionella pneumophila*, is responsible for less than 3% of the atypical

---

[a]The idea of new infectious diseases is disturbing to lay minds shaped by the euphoric 1950s and 1960s. It is exploited with preference by novelists, but also by astronomers speculating on the arrival of pathogenic material from space, e.g. **Hoyle, F. & Wickramasingh, H.C.** *Disease from space*, London, Dent, 1979.

[b]For a more detailed account of current knowledge about this disease see *Legionnaires' disease: report on a Working Group*. Copenhagen, WHO Regional Office for Europe, 1983 (EURO Reports and Studies No. 72).

pneumonias admitted to hospital.

Legionella has also been identified as the cause of formerly unexplained respiratory illness. Seven serologically different species have been identified so far, *L. pneumophila* being the organism mainly responsible. It has itself six serotypes. *Legionella* stains very faintly with Gram's stain. Its epidemiological associations with the hotel and tourist industry in the tourist season makes it of economic importance, and reports in the press have generated a considerable emotional charge in relation to the disease.

Clinically the disease is characterized by fever, headache, sweating, rigor, cough, chest pain, dyspnoea and, as a complication, respiratory failure, particularly in older persons. (A different clinical picture is found in Pontiac fever, a shorter but more severe illness of which only two outbreaks have so far been noted in the United States.) The diagnosis of legionnaires' disease is by isolation of the organisms or, serologically, by indirect immunofluorescence. Antigen can be demonstrated in respiratory secretory tissue or urine.

Legionella is ubiquitous in watery environments, ponds, lakes, air-conditioning cooling towers, condensers and domestic potable water. It is destroyed by continuous chlorination at $1.5–3.0\,mg/m^3$ and by temperatures above 50°C. The building up of slime and algae in cooling water systems should be prevented chemically. The organism is sensitive to erythromycin and rifampicin and these two antibiotics seem to provide effective treatment.

Two WHO collaborating centres for *Legionella* have recently been established in Lyon and Stockholm. Systems for the surveillance of this new pathogen are necessary in all European countries.

Two examples of the so-called mystery diseases are Reye's syndrome and Kawasaki disease, both known for almost 15 years and both not yet clarified etiologically. New diseases with unknown etiology have recently appeared: acquired immune deficiency syndrome (AIDS), Värö disease in Sweden, and an unexplained haemorrhagic disease in the United Kingdom. These diseases are mentioned to show that, without standardized regional surveillance and a central collecting point of information for the whole of Europe, there may never be sufficient valid data to draw statistical inferences or elucidate their epidemiology and trends.

Reye's syndrome
Reye's syndrome is still a mystery. A serious life-threatening disease, formerly called viral encephalopathy, it was described in 1963 by the Australian pathologist R. Douglas Reye and is now being increasingly seen in all parts of the world. It affects predominantly children and young people up to about 17 years of age, the annual incidence being 1–2 per 100 000. It is characterized by intractable vomiting, disorientation and liver disturbance (particularly of its ability to detoxify ammonia), and it goes on to coma, increasing intracranial pressure and, not infrequently, death from involvement of the respiratory centres. About 15% of patients have mental retardation or other permanent brain damage, and relapses occur. In the

United States national surveillance was introduced by the Centers for Disease Control (CDC) in 1976 and some states have made the disease notifiable. This has helped in the establishment of a definition of the disease, as follows, and the preparation of a standard investigation and report form (63).

1. Acute onset of non-inflammatory encephalopathy demonstrated by either:
   (a) an acute change in mental status with cerebrospinal fluid (if available) containing 8 white blood cells per mm³, or
   (b) an acute change in mental status with subsequent histological sections of brain obtained at autopsy or by biopsy showing cerebral oedema without perivascular or meningeal inflammation.

2. Hepatic involvement shown by either:
   (a) microvesicular fatty change in liver in sections obtained at biopsy early in the illness or at autopsy, or
   (b) a greater than threefold rise above the upper limits of normal SGOT or SGPT or above the control value for serum ammonia.

3. No other more plausible explanation for the neurological or hepatic changes.

The clinical stages outlined on the case investigation form are:

— vomiting, lethargy, sleepiness

— delirium, combativeness, hyperreflexia

— coma, hyperventilation, pupils equal, round and reactive to light, good doll's-head reflex

— decerebration, fixed dilated pupils, loss of doll's-head reflex

— seizures, areflexia, flaccidity, brain death.

Reye's syndrome has been described in almost all European countries. In some, for example Sweden, it seems to be extremely rare. The only investigation in Europe was carried out in the United Kingdom in 1979, and it found 37 cases of Reye's syndrome over a three-year period. A two-year surveillance scheme started in 1982. Most cases are reported from France and Spain, but they have also been reported from Czechoslovakia, Finland, the Federal Republic of Germany, Italy, Switzerland and Yugoslavia.

In the United States, although greatly under-reported, the incidence is estimated at about 0.88 per 100 000 population, with a lethality rate of 22%, for the years 1979 and 1980. In 11% of survivors there was residual neurological damage; 69% of patients had a prodromal illness, 64% an influenza-like one or respiratory symptoms, 16% had clinical evidence of preceding varicella, 14% had gastrointestinal symptoms only, and 6% had various other prodromal illnesses or no recognized prodromal illness at all (64).

The etiology of Reye's syndrome is unknown, but it seems to be multi-

190

factorial. It has been geographically and seasonally related to influenza B, but also to a lesser extent to influenza A, varicella, coxsackie B2 virus, herpesvirus and dengue. It predominates from January to March, and its association with viral infections, usually mild, has been definitely established. An association with the ingestion of salicylates, taken for influenza and other fevers, has also been demonstrated (64). Other theories consider it a metabolic response to an acute subcellular mitochondrial insult, contamination with the fungus *Aspergillus flavus* (aflatoxin), margosa oil poisoning, etc.

Clinical management at present is not without heroics and the optimum therapy is not yet clear. There is evidence that patients treated by exchange transfusion, peritoneal dialysis and brain decompression have no better a prognosis than those receiving supportive care alone. Steroid treatment was associated with poorer survival in all the clinical stages. Other treatments — surgical insertion of cranial pressure monitors, mannitol administration, drug-induced coma and craniotomy — have still to be evaluated.

Data in Europe, consisting mainly of clinical reports in the medical press or metabolic descriptions, lack uniformity and are mostly poor in epidemiological information (e.g. in relation to salicylates) that could be tentatively related to etiology. The chances of better treatment and a better prognosis or avoidance of brain damage, renal failure, and intellectual and psychological sequelae will depend not only on early recognition of the syndrome but also primarily on understanding of the etiological factors involved and epidemiological studies. The ICD classifies Reye's syndrome under code 331.8: "Other cerebral degeneration", a classification that will not help in assessing the real incidence.

Kawasaki disease: a new infection?
In the 1960s a new disease was observed in children under five years of age, similar to scarlet fever but not responding to antibiotics. It was described by the Japanese paediatrician Kawasaki in 1962 and 1967 (65) as an acute febrile mucocutaneous condition accompanied by swelling of the cervical lymph nodes. The disease started increasing in Japan, particularly in 1967, and by 1978 had reached over 3500 cases a year. More than 41 000 cases had been reported by 1982, although it seems to have started to decline since then.

Apart from Japan, the first cases were diagnosed in Hawaii. Some 65% of the 195 cases observed there in 1981 were in Japanese Americans, although their proportion of the total population is only 14%; white Americans, with 38% of the population, accounted for only 4% of cases — a highly significant statistical difference (66). Kawasaki disease, which was formerly also referred to as "mucocutaneous-lymph-node syndrome", is now increasingly diagnosed also in the continental United States (750 cases as of June 1981) (67), Austria, Belgium, Czechoslovakia, Denmark, France, the Federal Republic of Germany (over 3000 cases since 1978), Greece, Hungary, Italy, the Netherlands, Norway, Spain, Sweden, Switzerland, Turkey and the United Kingdom, and in other parts of the world (68).

Table 36. Symptoms and signs in Kawasaki disease

Principal symptoms
1. Fever of unknown etiology lasting 5 days or more
2. Bilateral congestion of ocular conjunctivae
3. Changes of lips and oral cavity
   — Dryness, redness and fissuring of lips
   — Protuberance of tongue papillae (strawberry tongue)
   — Diffuse reddening of oral and pharyngeal mucosa
4. Changes of peripheral extremities
   — Reddening of palms and soles (initial stage)
   — Indurative oedema (initial stage)
   — Membranous desquamation from finger tips (convalescent stage)
5. Polymorphous exanthema of body trunk without vesicles or crusts
6. Acute nonpurulent swelling of cervical lymph nodes of 1.5 cm or more in diameter

Other significant symptoms or findings
1. Carditis, especially myocarditis and pericarditis
2. Diarrhoea
3. Arthralgia or arthritis
4. Proteinuria and increase of leucocytes in urine sediment
5. Changes in blood tests
   — Leucocytosis with shift to the left
   — Slight decrease in erythrocyte and haemoglobin levels
   — Increased ESR
   — Positive CRP
   — Increased α_2-globulin
   — Thrombocytosis
   — Negative ASO
6. Changes occasionally observed
   — Aseptic meningitis
   — Mild jaundice or slight increase of serum transaminase
   — Swelling of gall bladder

Source: Japan Red Cross Medical Center, Tokyo.

As there are no specific laboratory tests, the diagnosis is made on the clinical picture. This is characterized by fever up to 41°C lasting over five days and not responding to antibiotics, cutaneous changes affecting the extremities and trunk, a polymorphous exanthem, congestion of the conjunctiva, changes in the mucous membranes, and non-purulent swelling of the cervical lymph nodes. In a large proportion of cases the patients present with arthralgia, arthritis and cardiac involvement — myocarditis, pericarditis, coronary aneurysms (20–30%), heart murmurs and electrocardiographic changes. Kawasaki disease is a major cause of heart disease in children. Meningeal signs and mild icterus are also seen. The symptoms are also described in Table 36 and epidemiological and etiological data in Tables 37 and 38. There is high leucocytosis, thrombocytosis, and raised serum globulin. The treatment is supportive and symptomatic, antibiotics being ineffective. Aspirin therapy (30–100 mg per kg of body weight per day) is given, similar to that for juvenile rheumatoid arthritis. Steroids are not recommended. The lethality rate has recently declined from 1–2% to

Table 37. Differential diagnosis of Kawasaki disease
from Stevens–Johnson syndrome and scarlet fever

	Kawasaki disease	Stevens–Johnson syndrome	Scarlet fever
Age	Under 5 years	3–30 years	2–8 years
Eyes	Congestion of ocular conjunctiva without pus; pseudomembrane formation	Shut with thick pus; pseudomembrane formation	No effects
Lips	Marked redness	Black with crusted blood	No marked redness
Oral cavity	Strawberry tongue; diffuse reddening of oral cavity	Vesicles; ulceration; pseudomembrane formation	Strawberry tongue; streptococcal tonsillitis
Peripheral extremities	Pronounced reddening of palms and soles; indurative oedema; membranous desquamation from finger tips	No effects described	Membranous desquamation from finger tips
Exanthem	Polymorphous erythema	Polymorphous erythema with vesicles and crusts	Diffuse, finely papular and bright red erythema
Swelling of cervical lymph nodes	Frequent, not purulent	Occasional	Occasional, sometimes purulent
Genitals	No marked effects	Vesicles and ulceration sometimes	No effects
Penicillin therapy	Not effective	Not effective	Effective
Throat culture	Non-specific	Non-specific	Haemolytic streptococcus group A (+++)
Seasonal variation of occurrence	Not clear but slightly high in summer	Not described	Higher in winter and spring
Autopsy findings of coronary artery	Marked changes	No effects	No effects

0.4%. Half of those who die do so within a month and 95% within six months of the acute onset. Pathological findings show a periarteritis of coronary arteries and aneurysm with thrombosis.

Kawasaki disease is now distinguished from scarlet fever, measles, rubella, Stevens–Johnson syndrome, juvenile rheumatoid arthritis and acrodynia (69). In the opinion of many clinicians its incidence is definitely increasing, and not only because of greater awareness of the disease; there

Table 38. A summary of the epidemiological features of Kawasaki disease in Japan

Epidemiological features	Comments
1. Prevailing throughout Japan, very few in neighbouring countries	Common sources specific to Japan
2. Area differences not clear	Scarlet fever more in north Japanese encephalitis more in south
3. Increase since 1968	New sources (foods, drugs, heavy metals, agricultural chemicals)
4. Age distribution: peak at 1 year	Infectious agent widespread, baby foods, articles for daily use
5. Seasonal variation not distinct	Infectious diseases usually distinct
6. Time–space clustering	Usually observed in infectious diseases
7. Occurrence in siblings (close time interval, initial case elder sibling)	Common sources in family (infection, disposition, family environment)
8. Previous history of pharyngitis (patient, siblings, parents)	Streptococcal infection
9. Allergic reaction in parents and siblings	Host factors
10. Weight at birth and birth order not unusual	Exposure after birth
11. Use of drugs during pregnancy	Unfavourable conditions during pregnancy
12. immunization not unusual	Mercury preservative in vaccine not responsible
13. Artificial feeding and baby foods not unusual	Trace substances in foods not responsible
14. Prevailing urban and rural, all occupational groups	Sources common anywhere in Japan
15. Consistency with drug production (tetracycline, chloramphenicol, steroid)	Drug-induced disease
16. Inflammatory findings in clinical pictures	Infection most probable
17. Antibiotics not effective	Virus, chemical substances, allergy

is a growing consensus that it is genuinely new. The disease is now being exceptionally recognized also in young adults.[a] Close geographical and social relations among those who fall victim to the disease were demonstrated in an investigation of an outbreak of nine cases within a month on a small island in Japan (71).

---

[a]**Shigematsu, I. & Tamashiro, H.** *Kawasaki disease.* Paper presented at the meeting of the International Epidemiological Association, Edinburgh, 1981. See also (70).

All efforts in Japan, the United States and Europe to establish the etiology have so far been unproductive. Clues have been sought in toxic chemicals, detergents, carpet shampoo, mercury and other toxic substances without success. Are there some new factors in the environment acting directly, triggering a modified host response in children with a genetic disposition, or providing a new sequela to a common bacterial or viral illness? Is Kawasaki disease an infection, as has repeatedly been said? (72) A microbial etiology has been strongly suspected — streptococci, staphylococci, *Leptospira*, rickettsiae, echovirus and Epstein-Barr (EB) virus. An association with a history of a recent virus-like illness has been repeatedly observed, but no virological or serological identification of an etiological agent has so far been made. The *Lancet*, in its second editorial on the subject in 1981, said: "It is difficult to believe that no cause or effective treatment can be found for a disease whose pathology contains elements of acute inflammation and hypersensitivity, but such is the case with the syndrome described in 1967 by Kawasaki" (73). Beyond widespread acceptance of the criteria for diagnosis and recognition of the frequent and sometimes severe cardiac manifestations, little progress has been made on the etiology, prevention, treatment or long-term outlook since the first *Lancet* editorial in 1976 (74). Association with pharyngitis, exanthema subitum, or infantile eczema in the family or previous personal history has not yet been ascertained to be causal, nor has a relationship to previous immunization. Some investigators have a strong suspicion that there may be a causal relationship with pyogenic exotoxin C secreted by *Staphylococcus aureus*, which they found in 10 or 11 of 13 children investigated. There is, however, no evidence of person-to-person transmission. Successive infection in relatives and siblings and clustering seem to have been observed in some cases. There is a higher incidence in the late winter and spring months. In 1981 and 1982 attention was again focused on rickettsia-like bodies found in mites collected from dust in the rooms of patients (75). An antigen associated with mites may be a causative agent, since serum levels of antimite-specific IgG are increased in the early stages of the disease (76).

Indeed almost every conceivable etiology has been looked into, even the possibility of exposure to wild or sick birds, but so far nothing definite has been established (66). Further multidisciplinary studies may eventually succeed in clarifying this mystery, but at present it is felt that epidemiological investigations have the best chance of finding the answers. Physicians should be encouraged to report suspected cases, and the disease should be made notifiable. Since 1979, Kawasaki disease has had its number in the ICD (446.1) but not as an obligatory or recommended notification under infectious diseases. Thus we do not know much about the true numerical incidence, the geographical, social, urban/rural or age distribution, or the trend of the disease. National registers are in operation in Japan and the United States, but not yet in Europe. The prominent Japanese epidemiologist Shigematsu has pleaded (67) for the establishment in Europe of a system of surveillance and epidemiological investigation. Some centralization of information on Kawasaki disease at national and regional centres and international collaborative studies are obviously necessary.

Acquired immune deficiency syndrome (AIDS)

This newest disease, probably secondary to an as yet unknown infective agent, made its sudden appearance in the United States in 1981, although retrospective enquiries showed that cases had occurred there as early as the autumn of 1979. It has attracted wide attention under the press name "gay epidemic", since the first cases were noted in young homosexual men with histories of promiscuity. It soon became apparent that it can also affect bisexual men and women, intravenous drug users, haemophiliacs, Haitian immigrants to Canada and the United States (and West Africans and Zairians in Europe).[a] It has recently also been found in babies born to sexually promiscuous mothers, in female sex partners of drug users, and in monogamous contacts of AIDS patients, suggesting the possibility of horizontal and vertical transmission of an infectious agent. There are also 20 cases in children under investigation. The case of a dustman in New York, collecting garbage in an area where many drug addicts live and denying homosexuality or drug abuse, is a perplexing example of the difficulties that can be met in investigation.

The definition used by CDC for reporting purposes is a person who has had a reliably diagnosed disease that is at least moderately indicative of an underlying cellular immune deficiency, but who, at the same time, has had no known underlying cause of cellular immune deficiency nor any other cause of reduced resistance reported to be associated with that disease. This general case definition may be made more explicit by specifying the particular diseases considered at least moderately indicative of cellular immune deficiency and the known causes of cellular immune deficiency, or other causes of reduced resistance reported to be associated with particular diseases.

Diseases at least moderately indicative of underlying cellular immune deficiency	Required diagnostic methods with positive results
Protozoal and helminthic infections	
Cryptosporidiosis, intestinal, causing diarrhoea for over 1 month	Histology or stool microscopy
Pneumocystis carinii pneumonia	Histology, or microscopy of a "touch" preparation or bronchial washings
Strongyloidosis, causing pneumonia, central nervous system infection, or disseminated infection[b]	Histology

---

[a]Retrospective studies indicate that there might have been cases in Europe and Africa in 1976.

[b]Disseminated infection refers to the involvement of the liver, bone marrow or multiple organs, not simply the lungs and multiple lymph nodes.

196

Toxoplasmosis, causing pneumonia or central nervous system infection	Histology or microscopy of a "touch" preparation

Fungal infections

Aspergillosis, causing central nervous system or disseminated infection[a]	Culture or histology
Candidiasis, causing oesophagitis	Histology, or microscopy of a "wet" preparation from the oesophagus, or endoscopic findings of white plaques on an erythematous mucosal base
Cryptococcosis, causing pulmonary, central nervous system, or disseminated infection[a]	Culture, antigen detection, histology, or India ink preparation of CSF

Bacterial infections

Atypical mycobacteriosis (caused by species other than *Mycobacterium tuberculosis* or *M. leprae*) causing disseminated infection[a]	Culture

Viral infections

Cytomegalovirus, causing pulmonary, gastrointestinal tract, or central nervous system infection	Histology
Herpes simplex virus, causing chronic mucocutaneous infection with ulcers persisting for more than 1 month, or pulmonary, gastrointestinal tract, or disseminated infection[a]	Culture, histology, or cytology
Progressive multifocal leucoencephalopathy (presumed to be caused by papovavirus)	Histology

Cancer

Kaposi's sarcoma	Histology
Lymphoma limited to the brain	Histology

Known causes of reduced resistance	**Diseases possibly attributable to them**
Systemic corticosteroid or other immunosuppressive or cytotoxic therapy	Any infection that began during or within 1 month of such therapy, if the therapy began before signs or symptoms specific to the infected

---

[a]Disseminated infection refers to the involvement of the liver, bone marrow or multiple organs, not simply the lungs and multiple lymph nodes.

anatomic sites (e.g. dyspnoea for pneumonia, headache for encephalitis, diarrhoea for colitis); or cancer diagnosed during or within 1 month of more than 4 months of such therapy, if the therapy began before signs or symptoms specific to the anatomic sites of the cancer.

Widely spread cancer of lymphoid or histiocytic tissue, such as lymphoma, Hodgkin's disease, lymphocytic leukemia, or multiple myeloma (this does not include cancer that is entirely localized to one site, such as primary lymphoma of the brain)	Any other cancer or infection, regardless of whether diagnosed before or after (because a lymphoma may have been present before, even if diagnosed after)
Age 60 years or older at diagnosis	Kaposi's sarcoma
Age under 28 days (neonatal) at diagnosis	Toxoplasmosis, cytomegalovirus, or herpes simplex virus infections
An immune deficiency atypical of AIDS, such as one involving hypogammaglobulinaemia; or an immune deficiency of which the cause appears to be a genetic or developmental defect (e.g. thymic dysplasia)	Any infection or cancer diagnosed during such immune deficiency

The disease has received such wide press coverage that it is now well known to the professional and even to the lay public. It is viewed with grave concern by the medical community. As at October 1983 there had been 2200 cases in the United States, mostly in California and New York State, but the disease has spread to 35 states and 16 other countries. The overall fatality rate so far reported is 37.6–60%, but these are provisional figures; it is expected to rise further, as less than 14% of AIDS victims have survived more than three years after diagnosis, and no patient has recovered fully. Average survival after diagnosis is estimated at about seven months. Most patients are in the 20–45 years age group. In Europe AIDS has been reported from 15 countries: Austria, Belgium, Czechoslovakia, Denmark, Finland, France, the Federal Republic of Germany, Ireland, Italy, the Netherlands, Norway, Spain, Sweden, Switzerland and the United Kingdom. As at October 1983 there were 268 cases of which 59 were in Africans (45 of them from Zaire). (For a complete breakdown by country see Annex 10).

The immune deficiency is cellular and irreversible; humoral immunity is not affected. The observed changes in T-regulating cells are initially a relative and later absolute decline in T-helper cells and an increase in T-suppressor cells. The normal ratio of T_H/T_S is above 1.4 but in all patients this ratio declines to <0.9 and the reversal is persistent and progressive. There is also an overall lymphopenia and consequent decline in response of T-helper lymphocytes, with loss of tuberculin hypersensitivity (anergy).

The cause of AIDS is as yet unknown, but there is strong evidence that it is a transmissible blood-borne infectious disease (similar to hepatitis B), presumably of viral origin. There are many hypotheses about the agents: cytomegalovirus, retroviruses such as human T-cell leukemia-virus (HTLV) or adult-TL virus, although there is no firm evidence to support this so far in spite of extensive virological research. Suggested causes other than a new virus include immunological exhaustion after heavy antigenic overload and stimulation, and provocation of immune regulatory defects permitting reactivation of EB-virus autoantibodies and the destruction of thymic epithelium. The role of formerly suspected "recreational" drugs (amyl- and butylnitrites) as an etiological factor has now been discarded although they may in some cases contribute to the risk.

The disease appears to present itself in three stages.

1. Incubation. There is indication of a "latent period" of several months up to five years between exposure and recognizable illness, which suggests that thousands of people may now be in incubation. Diagnosis in this phase is not possible. CDC points out that careful taking of histories and physical examination alone will not identify all persons capable of transmitting AIDS, and only risk assumptions may be made.

2. Lymphadenopathy — cervical, axillar, inguinal or generalized. This is usually accompanied by malaise, fatigue, sweating, weight loss and nonspecific prodromes: dry cough, diarrhoea, bleeding mucosa, thrush, anorexia and severe, progressive wasting.

3. Repeated opportunistic infections and tumorous manifestation such as an aggressive, disseminative and invasive form of Kaposi's sarcoma (*Sarcoma cutis multiplex haemorrhagica Kaposi*, a rare skin cancer[a] formerly seen almost exclusively in older persons), squamous cell carcinoma, and B-cell lymphomas similar to African Burkitt's lymphoma.[b]

The transition between the stages is not strictly delineated and diagnosis is by exclusion. There is no specific marker or diagnostic test as yet, but the identification of regulatory T-cell imbalance found in all AIDS patients is possible. Testing for β_2 microglobulin is promising but it still has to be evaluated.

All attempted forms of treatment have been unsuccessful and interferon has brought only temporary remission. Some individual symptoms can be treated but they eventually recur.

In the United States a special task force has been established at CDC in Atlanta to study the problem. Several European countries have also established special AIDS committees, and the WHO Regional Office in Copenhagen has started a voluntary surveillance scheme in compiling

---

[a]First described in Vienna a hundred years ago.

[b]In Zaire at least a five- to tenfold increase in Burkitt's lymphoma has been observed in the 1980s compared with the 1960s. There has also been a marked increase in cryptococcosis in Kinshasa hospitals.

available information. A special meeting held in October 1983 agreed on a common surveillance mechanism, to follow the spread in Europe, and to observe any possible extension of the risk groups. The formation of a committee or special group is envisaged. The main risk groups (next to homosexuals or their bisexual contacts) are patients with classical haemophilia, who receive lyophilized factor VIII concentrates (which is made from the pooled plasma of up to 20 000 donors) and plasma transfusion recipients (large quantities of plasma used in Europe are imported from the United States). It has been recommended that all new haemophilia patients not treated before with lyophilized concentrate receive cryoprecipitate (made from pooled plasma of about 40 donors only) and that all mild cases of factor IX deficiency should be treated with frozen plasma whenever possible.

There is as yet no evidence that AIDS can be acquired by casual contact with patients.

Recent evidence suggests that HTLV infection occurs in patients with AIDS. HTLV has been isolated from peripheral blood T-lymphocytes from several patients with AIDS, and a retrovirus, related to but clearly distinct from HTLV, has been isolated from cells from a lymph node of a patient with lymphadenopathy syndrome (LAS), a syndrome that may precede AIDS itself. Also, HTLV nucleic acid sequences have been detected by nucleic acid hybridization in lymphocytes from 2 (6%) of 33 AIDS patients. In addition, antibodies to antigens expressed on the cell surface of HTLV-infected lymphocytes have been detected by an indirect immunofluorescent technique in sera from 19 (25%) out of 75 AIDS patients, including patients with Kaposi's sarcoma alone (10 out of 34), *Pneumocystis carinii* pneumonia alone (7 out of 30), or patients with both diseases (2 out of 11). Similar antibodies were detected in 6 (26%) of 23 patients with LAS (77).

None of the theories propounded to date answers either fully or satisfactorily the epidemiological picture of AIDS. It is possible that multiple factors, rather than a single novel virus, induce AIDS. As the pattern of spread resembles that of hepatitis B (intimate contact involving mucosal surfaces or parenteral spread) the avoidance of contact with blood, excretion, secretions and the tissue of patients or of those presumed to suffer from AIDS and proper laboratory/pathology precautions are necessary. A disinfectant solution such as 0.5–1% hypochlorite or 2.5–5% chloramine T is recommended.

Värö disease

A disease of unclear etiology has been reported by the Swedish epidemiological services. This disease appeared first in November/December 1982 and again in January/February 1983. The main symptoms are pains in the hip joints on exertion and limping, preceded in 75% of cases by respiratory infection.

By early March 1983, 160 children had been admitted to Varberg hospital, 134 girls and 26 boys. The average age was 12 years. Several reports have been received from different parts of the country of patients with similar symptoms. In 80% of cases the symptoms lasted for less than two weeks, and there were relapses in approximately 15% of cases. It seems clear that the disease is infectious: close friends at school, particularly those who were also in close contact in their free time, and relatives were involved. A decrease in new cases over the Christmas period, when schools are closed, also points to an infectious disease, but the spread pattern indicates that it is not very easily transmitted. There was laboratory evidence of a slight rise in sedimentation, never more than 20 mm, a positive CRP in 50% of cases, and lymphocytosis. Virological investigations are in progress. There was no evidence that the infection was imported: in spite of 4½ months' duration, the illness was limited to two small towns. Antibiotics are of no help and anti-inflammatory drugs have no effect. There is no evidence of resulting hip handicap. A similar disease in the United States is known as transient synovitis of the hip, usually one side only. There is as yet no clear case definition.

Haemorrhagic shock and encephalopathy
A new and as yet unexplained disease was observed in the United Kingdom during 1982. Seven infants aged 3–7 months were admitted to a London hospital with a fulminant and usually fatal illness, characterized by severe shock, haemorrhage and encephalopathy. All had an abrupt onset of convulsions, high fever, watery diarrhoea and profound shock, and very large volumes of colloid or blood were required to restore the circulatory volume. Hypernatraemia and acidosis were always present on admission, suggesting pooling of fluid in the gut. All had severe disseminated intravascular coagulation, thrombocytopoenia and bleeding. Renal and hepatic function were markedly deranged, but plasma ammonia was always normal. Intensive support resulted in improvement, but gross neurological disorder persisted. Five children died, and the two survivors have severe neurological handicap. The cases were scattered geographically and temporally.

The disease affecting these children is distinct from previously recognized syndromes, but has features in common with the viral haemorrhagic fevers and toxin induced shock. Extensive bacteriological and virological investigations have failed to identify a specific cause (78).

References

1. **Macdonald, G.** Presidential address. *Transactions of the Royal Society of Tropical Medicine and Hygiene*, **59**: 611 (1965).
2. **Maegraith, B.** Tropical medicine today. *Transactions of the Royal Society of Tropical Medicine and Hygiene*, **63**: 689–707 (1969).
3. *Receptivity to malaria and other parasitic diseases:* report on a WHO Working Group. Copenhagen, WHO Regional Office for Europe, 1979 (EURO Reports and Studies No. 15).

4. **Bettini, S. et al.** Isolation of *Leishmania* strains from *Rattus rattus* in Italy. *Transactions of the Royal Society of Tropical Medicine and Hygiene*, **72**: 441 (1978).

5. **Pampiglione, S. et al.** Studies on Mediterranean leishmaniasis. I. An outbreak of visceral leishmaniasis in northern Italy. *Transactions of the Royal Society of Tropical Medicine and Hygiene*, **68**: 349–359 (1974).

6. **Pampiglione, S. et al.** Studies on Mediterranean leishmaniasis. III. The leishmanin skin test in kala-azar. *Transactions of the Royal Society of Tropical Medicine and Hygiene*, **69**: 60–68 (1975).

7. *Annuario di statistiche sanitare.* Rome, Istituto Centrale di Statistica, 1956–1973.

8. **Rioux, J.A. et al.** *Ecologie d'un foyer méditerranéen de leishmaniose viscérale. Essai de modélisation.* Paris, Colloques internationaux du C.N.R.S., 1977 (No. 239) p. 295.

9. **Rouque, J. et al.** Les leishmanioses du sud-est de la France: écologie –épidémiologie–prophylaxie. *Acta tropica*, **32**: 371–380 (1977).

10. **Quilici, M. et al.** Persistance de la leishmaniose viscérale dans le sud-est de la France et fréquence marquée de l'affection à l'âge adulte. A propos d'observations récentes. *Bulletin de la Société de Pathologie exotique*, **72**: 118–124 (1979).

11. **Léger, N. et al.** La leishmaniose en Grèce: résultats d'une enquête entomologique effectuée en juin 1977. *Annales de parasitologie humaine et comparée*, **54**: 11–29 (1979).

12. **Biocca, E. et al.** *Distribution des différentes espèces de phlébotomes en Italie et transmission des leishmanioses et de quelques arboviruses. Ecologie des leishmanioses.* Paris, Colloques internationaux du C.N.R.S., 1977 (No. 239).

13. **Busuttil, A.** Kala-azar in the Maltese islands. *Transactions of the Royal Society of Tropical Medicine and Hygiene*, **68**: 236–240 (1974).

14. **Lecour, H. et al.** Kala-azar. *Medico*, **86**: 595–600 (1978).

15. **Hörder, M. et al.** In Europa erworbene Kala-azar. *Medizinische Welt*, **30**: 280–284 (1979).

16. **Gil Collado, J.** *Phlébotomes et leishmanioses en Espagne.* Paris, Colloques internationaux du C.N.R.S., 1977 (No. 239).

17. **Urbano Jiménez, F.J. et al.** Kala-azar en el adulto: Revisión a propósito de los nuevos casos. *Revista clínica española*, **147**: 307–311 (1977).

18. **Genis, D.E.** Epidemiological features of visceral leishmaniasis in the northern part of the distribution area, Kzyl-Orda region of the Kazakh SSR. *Meditsinskaya parazitologiya i parazitarnye bolezni*, **47**: 15–21 (1978).

19. **Addadi, K. & Dedet, J.P.** Epidémiologie des leishmanioses en Algérie. 6. Recensement des cas de leishmaniose viscérale infantile entre 1965–74. *Bulletin de la Société de Pathologie exotique*, **69**: 68–75 (1976).

20. **Bobin, P. et al.** La leishmaniose cutanée en Algérie. *Médecine tropicale*, **38**: 424–429 (1978).

21. **Meyruey, M. et al.** Les leishmanioses au Maroc. *Bulletin de la Société de Pathologie exotique*, **67**: 617–622 (1974).

22. **Benallégué, A. & Tabbakh, E.** La leishmaniose viscérale en Algérie. *Archives de l'Institut Pasteur, Alger,* **52**: 85–94 (1977).

23. **Mazzi, R.** Kutane Leischmaniose: autotochner Fall in der Schweiz. *Dermatologica,* **153**: 104–105 (1976).

24. **Stoll, N.B.** This wormy world. *Journal of parasitology,* **33**: 1–18 (1947).

25. **May, J.M.** *The ecology of human diseases.* New York, MD Press, 1958.

26. **Ricci, M. et al.** *In: Proceedings of the International Congress on Parasitology, Rome, 21–26 September 1964.* Oxford, Pergamon Press, 1966, Vol. 2, p. 747.

27. **Carneri, J. de.** Spreading of *Necator americanus* in Southern Europe. *In: Proceedings of the Third International Congress on Parasitology, Munich, 25–31 August 1974.* 1974, Vol. 2, pp. 778–779.

28. **Yücel, A. & Deschiens, R.** Dépistage d'un foyer de filariose à *Wuchereria bancrofti* en Turquie orientale. *Bulletin de la Société de Pathologie exotique,* **53**: 885–891 (1960).

29. **Sipahioglu, H.** Filariasis in Turkey. *Transactions of the Royal Society of Tropical Medicine and Hygiene,* **53**: 151–153 (1959).

30. **Mihailova, Y. et al.** [First case of depetalonematosis in a Soviet specialist returning from Equatorial Guinea.] *Meditsinskaya parazitologiya i parazitarnye bolezni,* **1**: 116 (1978) [in Russian].

31. **Weise, H.J.** Malariaeinschleppungen in die Bundesrepublik Deutschland einschliesslich Berlin (West) unter besonderer Berücksichtigung der letzten 5 Jahre (1973–1977). *Bundesgesundheitsblatt,* **22**: 1–7 (1979).

32. **Weeber-Baark, G.** Untersuchungen der Malaria-Erkrankungen beim Bordpersonal der Deutschen Lufthansa. *Lufthansa Ärztetagung,* 24–28 September 1978.

33. **Bruaire, M. & Cassaigne, R.** Paludisme d'importation en France métropolitaine. *Médecine et maladies infectieuses,* **11**: 346–348 (1981).

34. **Mohr, D.** Einschleppung von Krankheiten durch Reisende und Einwanderer. *Medizinische Wochenschrift,* **11**: 1477–1484 (1969).

35. **Stürcher, D. & Degremont, A.** Filariosen bei Tropenrückkehrern. Beobachtungen an 64 Fällen. *Schweizerische medizinische Wochenschrift,* **106**: 682–688 (1976).

36. **Coutinho da Costa, F.A.** A metropole portuguesa e.a. importação de doenças parasitarias trópicas. *Annales Azevedos,* **21**: 9–45 (1971).

37. **Smith, A.M. & Zuidema, P.J.** Onchocerciasis als import-ziekte in Nederland; een overzicht van 100 patienten. *Nederlands Tijdschrift voor Geneeskunde,* **117**: 1225–1230 (1973).

38. **Duggan, A.J. & Hutchinson, M.P.** Sleeping sickness in Europeans: a review of 109 cases. *Journal of tropical medicine and hygiene,* **69**: 227–230 (1966).

39. **Boller, K.** Afrikanische Schlafkrankheit in der Schweiz (Trypanosomiasis rhodesiense). *Schweizerische medizinische Wochenschrift,* **107**: 1706–1708 (1977).

40. **Mohr, W.** Zur Differentialdiagnose und Therapie eines Falles von Schlafkrankheit (Trypanosomiasis). *Therapie der Gegenwart,* **100**: 227–230 (1961).

41. **Recht, K. et al.** Importierte ost-afrikanische Trypanosomiasis (Schlaf-krankheit). *Medizinische Welt*, **28**: 1378–1381 (1977).
42. **Liverpool School of Tropical Medicine**. *Annual report.*
43. **Moretti, G.** La trypanosomiase africaine dépistée en France. Diffi-cultés du diagnostic. *Presse médicale*, **77**: 1404 (1969).
44. **Callot, J.M. et al.** Leishmaniose cutanée d'origine méditerranéenne en Alsace. *Bulletin de la Société de Pathologie exotique*, **62**: 131–138. (1969).
45. **Bettini, S. et al.** Leishmaniases in Tuscany (Italy) IV. An analysis of all recorded human cases. *Transactions of the Royal Society of Tropical Medicine and Hygiene*, **75**: 338–344 (1981).
46. **Diesfeld, J.** Die Krise der deutschen Tropenmedizin. *Auslandskurier*, **6**: 27–28 (1980).
47. **Martini, G.A.** Marburg agent disease in man. *Transactions of the Royal Society of Tropical Medicine and Hygiene*, **63**: 295–302 (1969).
48. **Martini, G.A. & Siegert, R., ed.** *Marburg virus disease.* Berlin and New York, Springer, 1971.
49. **Chumakov, M.P. et al.** [New data on virus causing Crimean haemor-rhagic fever]. *Voprosy virusologii*, **13**: 377 (1969) [in Russian].
50. **Al Tikrity, S.K. et al.** Congo/Crimean haemorrhagic fever in Iraq: a seroepidemiological survey. *Journal of tropical medicine and hygiene*, **84**: 117–120 (1981).
51. **Hoogstraal, H.** The epidemiology of tick-borne Crimean-Congo haemorrhagic fever in Asia, Europe and Africa. *Journal of medical entomology*, **15**: 307–417 (1979).
52. **Casals, J. et al.** A current appraisal of hemorrhagic fevers in the USSR. *American journal of tropical medicine and hygiene*, **15**: 751–764 (1966).
53. **Lee, H.W. & Antoniadis, A.** Serological evidence for Korean haemor-rhagic fever in Greece. *Lancet*, **1**: 832 (1981).
54. **Hannoun, C.** Les encéphalites à tiques en Europe. *Médecine tropicale*, **40**: 509–519 (1980).
55. **Kunz, C., ed.** *Tick-borne encephalitis, proceedings of an international symposium in Baden/Vienna, 19–20 October 1979.* Vienna, Facultas Verlag, 1981. *See also* **Kunz, C. & Hoffman, H.** Arboviren in Europa, Fortschritte der geomedizinischen Forschung 47–62 geogr. Ztoch. (Beiheft). Wiesbaden, Steiner Verlag, 1974.
56. **Blaskovic, D. et al.** An epidemiological study of tick-borne encephalitis in the Tribeč Region 1953–63. *Bulletin of the World Health Organiz-ation*, **36**(Suppl.): 89–94 (1967).
57. **Kunz, C. et al.** Feldversuche mit einem Impfstoff gegen den Fruh-sommer-meningo-encephalitis (FSME). *Zentralblatt für Bakteriologie, Parasitenkunde, Infectionskrankheiten und Hygiene*, **234** (I Abt): 141–144 (1976).
58. **Boemann, H. et al.** Schwere und ungünstige Verlaufsformen der Zecken-encephalitis (FSME) 1979 in Frieburg. *Deutsche medizinische Wochenschrift*, **105**: 921–924 (1980).

59. **Balducci, M. et al.** Tick-borne meningoencephalitis in Italy. *American journal of tropical medicine and hygiene*, **16**: 211 (1967).
60. **Likar, M. & Komet, J.** Virus meningo-encephalitis in Slovenia. IV. Isolation of the virus from the tick *Ixodes ricinus*. *Bulletin of the World Health Organization*, **15**: 267–279 (1954).
61. **Smorodintsev, A.** [Tick-borne spring-summer encephalitis.] *Progresi virologii*, **1**: 210 (1958) [in Russian].
62. *British medical journal*, **283**: 629–630 (1981).
63. **Morens, D. et al.** Surveillance of Reye syndrome in the United States 1977. *American journal of epidemiology*, **114**: 406–416 (1981).
64. Reye syndrome. *Morbidity and mortality weekly report*, **29**: 532, 537–539 (1980).
65. **Kawasaki, I. et al.** A new infantile febrile mucocutaneous lymph node syndrome (MLNS) prevailing in Japan. *Pediatrics*, **54**: 271–276 (1974).
66. **Kangilaski, I.** Kawasaki disease termed "rising pediatric dilemma". *Journal of the American Medical Association*, **246**: 819–821 (1981).
67. **Shigematsu, I. et al.** Worldwide survey on Kawasaki disease. *Lancet*, **1**: 976–977 (1980).
68. Kawasaki disease. *Morbidity and mortality weekly report*, **29**: 61–63 (1980).
69. **Kawasaki, I.** Acute febrile mucocutaneous syndrome with lymphoid involvement with specific desquamation of the fingers and toes in children: clinical observation of 50 cases. *Japanese journal of allergology*, **16**: 178–222 (1967).
70. **Nahmias, A.J.** Kawasaki disease: from children to adults. *Annals of internal medicine*, **92**: 563–564 (1980).
71. **Yanagawa, H. & Shigematsu, I.** Epidemiological features of Kawasaki disease in Japan. *Acta paediatrica japanica*, **25**: 1–13 (1981).
72. **Melish, M.E.** Kawasaki disease: a new infectious disease? *Journal of infectious diseases*, **143**: 99–106 (1981).
73. Kawasaki enigma. *Lancet*, **2**: 456–457 (1981).
74. Kawasaki disease. *Lancet*, **1**: 675–676 (1976).
75. **Hamashima, Y. et al.** Mite-associated particles in Kawasaki disease. *Lancet*, **2**: 266 (1982).
76. **Furusho, K. et al.** Possible role for mite antigen in Kawasaki disease. *Lancet*, **2**: 194 (1981).
77. Acquired immune deficiency syndrome (AIDS). *Weekly epidemiological record*, **58**: 158–159 (1983).
78. *Communicable disease report*, No. 82/51. London, Public Health Laboratory Service, 1982.

5

Epidemiology and control of foodborne diseases in Europe

B. Velimirovic

Foodborne diseases occur in all countries of the world and some are on the increase, although there is a considerable variation in different climatic and socioeconomic areas. It is estimated that foodborne diseases in Europe rank second or third among the causes of short-term illness.

A round table conference held in 1980 jointly by WHO and the World Association of Veterinary Food Hygienists on the salmonella problem,[a] noting the extensive worldwide research that had taken place over the previous 25–30 years, asked whether it had led to any improvement in the situation and concluded that the major part had not progressed beyond categorization of the organisms. An enormous number of publications exist on the prevalence of salmonellae in all kinds of animals, but there are very few epidemiological evaluations and even fewer on proposals for the control of salmonellosis, the most important group of foodborne diseases. This applies to a lesser degree to other foodborne diseases.

Although the authorities are becoming more and more aware of these diseases, reporting is insufficient because the short duration and mild symptoms of most attacks prevent their true magnitude from being appreciated. The economic cost of these diseases is growing but, since it is a cost felt particularly by the food-producing sector, it does not carry much weight with the health authorities in the generally rising costs of the health services. However, the growing concern about foodborne diseases is shown by recent resolutions of the World Health Assembly (WHA31.48 and WHA31.49) and by the World Congress on Foodborne Infections and Intoxications in 1980 sponsored by FAO and WHO (*1*).

Definitions

Foodborne disease is any disease of an infectious or toxic nature caused or assumed to be caused by the consumption of food or water. A more precise

---

[a]Unpublished WHO document VPH/81.27, Geneva, 1981.

definition used by WHO in Europe (2) reads: "Food-borne diseases can be defined as those diseases which, with present knowledge and methods, can be traced (a) to a specific food, substance in the food, or dish which has been contaminated by noxious organisms or substances, or (b) to a particular food-producing or food-dispensing establishment where a contamination has occurred.

"Food-borne infections and intoxications include diseases which in some instances may be transmitted by food and those which are usually conveyed by food."

Food poisoning or food intoxication is a generic term applied to illnesses acquired through the consumption of contaminated food or water. In order to accommodate a variety of organic and inorganic substances that may be present in natural food (such as certain mushrooms, mussels and scombroid fish, as well as heavy metals and other substances) WHO in Europe has adopted the following definition of food poisoning: "Harmful effects following ingestion of food resulting from contamination with pathogenic bacteria, toxic products of fungi and bacteria, allergic reaction to certain proteins or other components of food, or chemical contaminants."

This definition must be regarded as superseding earlier definitions adopted by the Joint FAO/WHO Expert Committee on Meat Hygiene (1955), the WHO Expert Committee on Environmental Hygiene (1956) and the European Technical Conference on Food-Borne Infections and Intoxications (1959), which preferred the term "foodborne intoxication". The term "food poisoning" is also commonly applied to salmonellosis and various other bacterial enteric infections. The overwhelming majority of foodborne diseases are of bacterial origin, however, and should be referred to as food infections. Unfortunately the classifications in the ICD are not quite clear and, indeed, are sometimes rather confusing, e.g. for staphylococcal infections. Thus foodborne diseases include those classified as intestinal infectious diseases (001–009), tuberculosis of the intestine (014), other infections (021, 025, 027.1, 039), some of the group of viral diseases (047, 048, 070, 078.4), spirochaetal diseases (100), some of the helminthiases (120–129), some parasitic diseases (130, 131, 133), as well as intoxications due to metals (985), and accidental poisoning by agricultural and horticultural chemical and pharmaceutical preparations (E865), and plant fertilizers (E866). This list could include hormones (E932) if used as animal feed, but exclude accidental poisoning by drugs, biologicals and alcohol.

Epidemiology, distribution, and prevalence of foodborne diseases

Notification to the local health authority that foodborne disease exists within a particular jurisdiction is the first step toward surveillance and control. Administrative practices on notifiable disease and ways and frequency of notification vary greatly from country to country, this lack of a standardized methodology having been noted whenever any attempt has been undertaken to assess the situation from a regional perspective. It is generally agreed that most foodborne diseases are not reported, as studies in countries with good surveillance mechanisms have indicated. The data obtained from various countries cannot therefore be considered as representative or compared internationally. Although most countries in Europe have legislation on reporting some foodborne diseases (typhoid fever, paratyphoid fever, dysentery, hepatitis A, salmonellosis, gastroenteritis, or the group called food poisoning), the statistical base for assessing foodborne diseases is limited and the reporting, even in the most developed countries, less than adequate. Nor is there any immediate prospect that this situation will change. Fear of losing tourist or food trade has seriously affected the notification of a whole range of diseases even in Europe (and from the international perspective food hygienists can sometimes derive more information from surveillance of the food chain) which in turn tends to increase the tendency towards restrictive practices. It may be safely postulated that complete reporting is the sign of good epidemiological services and of the self-confidence of the health authorities, and an indirect indication of the stage of their development.

National statistics are eventually consolidated in WHO's statistical reports. For most countries of Europe the numbers of foodborne infections given therein are less than the numbers known to exist, e.g. from published scientific papers. WHO occasionally receives unofficial or confidential reports that cannot be used. Furthermore, private medical sectors provide incomplete reports. No comprehensive picture is therefore available in most countries of a number of agents whose role in foodborne diseases has only recently been recognized, such as *Escherichia coli*, *Bacillus cereus*, *Yersinia enterocolitica*, *Vibrio parahaemolyticus*, *Campylobacter jejuni* and rotavirus, although reports on them are published with increasing frequency in the scientific literature and several countries included them in their epidemiological notifications in 1979 and 1980. WHO is not aware of the extent to which outbreaks of foodborne diseases in the armed forces are reported to national authorities. In some countries they are not.

Chemical food poisoning is not dealt with in this volume.

Interpretation and validity of data

As a rule only serious cases of foodborne disease are reported. Sometimes, as for cholera, a case is reported from the country into which it has been imported, but not from the originating country. The definition for surveillance purposes of gastroenteritis, enteric disease, diarrhoeal disease, alimentary intoxication, toxi-infection, food poisoning, etc. varies, so most countries report only typhoid and paratyphoid fever and bacillary dysentery.

Reporting and control of infection (e.g. salmonellosis) in animals is usually the responsibility of the state veterinary services. Excellent laboratories or institutes exist in the majority of European countries, but they often lack statutory or administrative provision for investigations, funds, personnel or a central reference point. Although good surveillance has been established in several countries, in many others investigation depends on the scientific interest of individual workers or is limited to major outbreaks; full investigation of reported outbreaks and sporadic cases is not done and is rarely possible. In most European countries trained epidemiologists, formal university training, a proper career structure, and links with the veterinary profession are insufficient, a precondition if the full picture is to be understood. At the intermediate level a wide variety of personnel should participate in epidemiological investigation, but sometimes no such personnel exist. Only a few countries have guidelines for the investigation of foodborne diseases, and systematic training of managers and personnel in the food production sector is far from what is needed.

Surveillance services may or may not include control or food safety in their mandate. For example, in Eastern Europe the same service is responsible for epidemiological surveillance and a wide range of sanitation activities, including food control. In the USSR this service, directed by the Ministry of Health and the ministries of health in each republic, operates through more than 4000 sanitary–epidemiological centres. Each centre is directed by an epidemiologist–physician and has multidisciplinary staff, and each has its own laboratory. In other Eastern European countries there are independent veterinary services responsible for the hygiene of meat and other food of animal origin. Various other forms of organization are met, usually under the responsibility of local authorities; the federal units, regions, cantons or health boards often have a large degree of autonomy, with some overall coordinating and supervisory function at the national level. In most countries, however, the veterinary profession is placed under another administrative body, and the investigative part of the surveillance of foodborne diseases tends to be separate from the inspection, supervision and practical control of food. Whatever the pattern, it is obvious that for the surveillance and epidemiological analysis of foodborne diseases there needs to be a focal point for all the available information (other than the central statistical office) and an adequate distribution of the information to those who need to know.

There is no definition of an "outbreak" valid for the whole of Europe. In some countries outbreaks with a common source are scrupulously investigated but those originating at home and sporadic cases are not investigated or notified. Information is lacking on whether the diagnosis has been confirmed in the laboratory; thus in the United Kingdom non-foodborne salmonellosis is not a notifiable disease and microbiological investigation is not necessary for a case to be recorded as *Salmonella* food poisoning or non-foodborne salmonellosis if there is good epidemiological evidence for the diagnosis.[a] A routine reporting system on all general or household outbreaks of foodborne diseases and an early warning system have existed in Scotland since January 1980. In at least three countries only laboratory-confirmed cases are given in the statistics forwarded to WHO. Reporting on some non-contagious toxin-producing foodborne infections (e.g. clostridial diseases) is often combined with the reporting of other poisonings, for example chemical food poisonings. Only a few countries

---

[a]**Charles, R.H.G.** *The epidemiology and control of salmonellosis in the United Kingdom.* Unpublished WHO document VPH/WP/SAL/80.8, Geneva, 1980.

Table 39. Infectious enteric diseases in Europe as notified to WHO, 1973–1977

Disease	1973	1974	1975	1976	1977
Salmonellosis	20 406	16 053	60 115	81 586	47 282
Other gastrointestinal infections	143 422	123 791	162 284	605 556	583 056

provide information on foodborne diseases of undetermined or presumed infectious etiology. Only the United Kingdom reports on etiological agents suspected to be the cause of foodborne diseases and subsequently isolated, such as *Streptococcus* group D, *Citrobacter*, *Enterobacter*, *Klebsiella*, *Pseudomonas* or rotavirus. Even with the good system of surveillance existing in the United States, in 30–60% of foodborne disease outbreaks reported to the Centers for Disease Control (*3*) the responsible pathogen was not identified. The figures for Europe vary but are between about 12% and 40% of all outbreaks investigated.

Analysis of data

An analysis of the data submitted to WHO does not allow even approximate conclusions to be drawn. This unsatisfactory situation is reflected in the reports to WHO presented in Table 39, which must be viewed with the utmost scepticism. The data are a rough estimate of severe cases and may reflect only the pattern of notification in countries. They represent at best the minimum number of diseases serious enough for the patient to be treated or hospitalized and thus identified by the health authorities; in some instances they reflect the coverage of laboratory services and the organizational strength of the health system. All that can be hoped for at the moment is that the errors and incompleteness are consistent in countries from year to year. An example of a more realistic assessment is given in Table 40, which presents the situation in the German Democratic Republic in 1978.

The services in WHO collaborating centres and various reports indicate that the number of outbreaks and of individual cases is increasing in most European countries, in spite of the preventive and control measures in most of them. It is estimated (for example in the Netherlands) that the number of *Salmonella* cases reported is only 1–5% of the real incidence. In the United States it is estimated[a] that for every laboratory case an average of 29.5 are identified when a thorough investigation is made. In the Federal Republic of Germany there was a twentyfold increase in the period 1962–1979; about 200 000 cases of foodborne disease occur yearly. In Yugoslavia it is reported that foodborne diseases increased five times

---

[a]**Bryan, F.L.** *Epidemiology and control of salmonellosis in the United States and Canada.* Unpublished WHO document VPH/WP/SAL/80.10, Geneva, 1980.

Table 40. Foodborne diseases
in the German Democratic Republic, 1978

Disease	No. of cases	Trend
Typhoid fever	49	declining
Paratyphoid fever	31	declining
Salmonellosis	8 814	increasing
Dysentery	2 801	declining
Amoebic dysentery	9	stationary
Coli-enteritis	2 364	declining
Diarrhoeal diseases	315 978	increasing
Brucellosis	45	declining
Listeriosis	34	increasing
Taeniasis	16 338	increasing
Botulism	2	stationary
Food intoxications[a]	13 904	declining
Mushroom poisoning	390	increasing

Source: Annual report, 1978, of the Epidemiological Centre, State Hygiene Inspection, German Democratic Republic.

[a] Only common source infections.

between 1964 and 1978 (4). In Spain about 661 000 cases were reported in 1982.

Lack of epidemiological surveillance for communicable disease in some countries gives a distorted picture, particularly of the reported incidence of foodborne infections.

Important foodborne diseases in Europe

Salmonellosis
Although the genus *Salmonella* comprises about 2000 serotypes that can infect warm- and cold-blooded animals, only a small number of them commonly cause disease in man. Two broad patterns are recognized. One is associated with generalized infection of the reticuloendothelial system, bacteriaemia and prolonged pyrexia, i.e. "enteric fever", and is caused by *S. typhi* and *S. paratyphi* A and B. The other is also associated with septicaemia but in addition often with metastatic abscesses,[a] and is caused in particular by *S. sendai*, *S. cholerae-suis* and *S. dublin*. The classical manifestation, more common, is enteritis accompanied by fever, which is caused by a wide variety of serotypes.

Typhoid fever (see Chapter 3)
Man is both the only known reservoir and the natural host of *S. typhi*. The

---

[a] *Enteric infections due to Campylobacter, Yersinia, Salmonella and Shigella*. Unpublished WHO document CDD/80/4, Geneva, 1980.

infection depends on the size of the inoculum. Studies on volunteers have shown that when an inoculum of 10^7–10^9 organisms is ingested the attack rate for clinical typhoid fever approaches 100%, whereas a dose of 10^5 organisms causes clinical illness in only 25–50% of healthy adults. The critical inoculum in actual life is probably considerably less.

Typhoid fever is becoming a rare disease in Northern Europe and at present almost all cases result from infection acquired during travel to endemic areas. The disease is more prevalent in Southern and Eastern Europe but is also declining rapidly there. What proportion of cases are related to chronic carriers is not clear but documented cases are on record. Treatment with 2–4-week courses of intravenous ampicillin or higher doses (6 g) of oral amoxicillin achieves eradication of the carrier state in about 70% of cases. There is a natural reduction by 5–8% of typhoid carriers and of the disease per year, or by roughly 50% in 10 years.

The removal of chronic carriers from all occupations directly involving food handling and identification of the vehicle of transmission are at present the best methods of control, combined with the measures valid for all enteric infections such as general improvement of water supplies and sanitation. At present attention is being given to a newly developed oral vaccine prepared from an attenuated strain of *S. typhi* (Ty21a). A follow-up two years later showed no case in 15 000 vaccinated children in Egypt, while the incidence remained high in the control group (*5*).

Other salmonellae
Salmonellosis other than that caused by the *S. typhi* and *S. paratyphi* group is one of the most frequently occurring diseases in Europe and has shown a tendency to increase in industrialized countries such as the German Democratic Republic, the Federal Republic of Germany, the Netherlands, Poland, the USSR and the United Kingdom. The same tendency exists in Australia, Canada (an average of 150 000 cases yearly), Japan and the United States (an average of 740 000 cases yearly). In the Federal Republic of Germany the number of infections (47 360) increased 5–6 times between 1968 and 1979 (Fig. 39); they represent about 14% of all infectious diseases notified and 98% of all zoonoses (*6*) and it is estimated that their overall incidence of 50 per 100 000 population in 1968 had increased to 80 per 100 000 by 1980 (*7*). About 0.5% of the general population examined were found to be carriers of *Salmonella*. It has been calculated that salmonellosis cost DM 180 000 per 100 000 population in 1981 (*8*). Extrapolations of laboratory-confirmed data from England and Wales give an estimate of about 200 000 human infections. Of all reported foodborne diseases, 80% are caused by *Salmonella* spp. A large outbreak occurred in 1981 in Maastricht, Netherlands, affecting 700 out of 1000 guests at an international conference; the infection originated from potato salad and was caused by *S. indiana*, which is rarely found in the Netherlands. In the USSR the increase is eight-fold for the period 1961–1968. In the European part of the USSR it began in 1970–1971 and in the Central Asian part in 1974, with the rates in urban areas 2–5 times higher (this however might be because of better reporting in the cities). Salmonellosis in the USSR

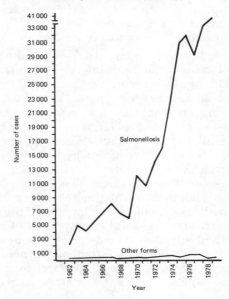

Fig. 39. Incidence of salmonellosis and other forms of enteritis
in the Federal Republic of Germany, 1962–1978

Source: **Weise, H.J.** *Bundesgesundheitsblatt,* **24**: 395–403 (1981).

represents about 8% of the total of identified intestinal diseases.[a] In
Poland, on the other hand, salmonellosis represents 42% of all enteric
infections and is reported to have increased since 1971 and particularly
since 1976.

Mortality from salmonellosis is low. The disease is, however, an
important cause of morbidity and of economic loss. The data suggest that
the highest incidence occurs in the first year of life, particularly the early
months, and infants may play an important role in the spread of salmonellosis in the household (9). The majority of infections originate from
consumption of contaminated food of animal origin, particularly chickens
(Table 41). Carriers or animals seem to be involved to a varying extent in
primary infections. The role of the carrier seems to be diminishing; in
Poland, however, where infection occurs in communal feeding, it is
thought that it may account for 50% of registered salmonellosis. In 40% of
cases carriers have been incriminated and in only 30% improper storage.
Only 10% of cases are thought to be attributable to primary meat contamination, with 90% due to secondary contamination by people in contact
with food.

What food will ultimately become the vehicle varies from country to

---

[a]**Shavakhalov, S.S.** *The epidemiology and control of salmonellosis in the USSR.* Unpublished WHO document VPH/WP/SAL/80.73, Geneva, 1980.

Table 41. Food responsible for *Salmonella* foodborne disease, 1972–1979 (percentages)

Food	France	Poland	USSR	United Kingdom	Federal Republic of Germany	Yugoslavia[a]	Greece
Meat products including poultry	44.4	52.2	99.6	76.8	54.6	35.7	60
Eggs and pastries	36			3.3	5		
Seafood	11	1.9		2.3	5		10
Ice cream and cakes		12–39.7					
Milk and dairy products		5.4–39.7		88	10.5	11.4	
Vegetable products					8.4	21.4	
Other				0.6		18.5	9

[a] Includes foodborne diseases other than salmonellosis.

country. In Scotland, for example, before 1983 some 10% of the people still consumed unpasteurized milk (*10*). On the other hand, in England only 3.3% of the people use untreated milk and milkborne salmonellosis is rare. No milkborne salmonellosis is seen in the Netherlands or the Scandinavian countries. In 1982 an outbreak in Norway was traced to black pepper from Brazil, and one in the United Kingdom to chocolate imported from another European country.

Salmonellosis is also a widespread infection in tourists. In Finland around 1970 imported cases accounted for about 10% of the total; by 1980 some 50–60% were of foreign origin and the total had almost doubled. A recent investigation of 369 faecal specimens of travellers returning to Switzerland from 57 different countries showed that 53 (14.4%) were positive for salmonellosis, although only nine persons noticed gastrointestinal symptoms (*11*). Only about 1% of notified cases in the Federal Republic of Germany are imported (*6,12*) but a study showed that of 15 000 passengers on international airlines 2400 became ill (*13*); in one well publicized outbreak connected with an air charter company in the Federal Republic of Germany there were 500 ill persons. An outbreak of *S. montevideo* infection was believed to have affected more than 500 children on a Mediterranean cruise in 1981. At present investigation is still not sufficiently prompt and, even if it is carried out, the patient often cannot give precise information. Thus in the United Kingdom the type of food associated with outbreaks was recorded in only 31% of reports, and in the Federal Republic of Germany in only 1 in 30 salmonellae isolated could the source be identified (*12*). Nevertheless it seems that meat and poultry are responsible for 44.4% of foodborne disease in France, 54.6% in the Federal Republic of Germany, 52.2% in Poland and 99.6% in the USSR (Table 41).

Recent studies in pathogenesis indicate that *Salmonella* spp. possess both invasive and cholera-like enterotoxic properties. Most infections are mild but serious disease may also be caused. Regarding antibiotic treatment, it has been demonstrated in the United Kingdom (*14*) that multiresistant strains of *S. typhimurium* now show increased virulence and a tendency to produce septicaemia, observed before only in *S. wien* (*6*). Eighteen centres participate in the WHO *Salmonella* surveillance scheme, often through a central *Salmonella* surveillance office such as that in the Federal Republic of Germany, which covers 90 institutions. A similar programme exists for the surveillance of animal salmonellosis.

To obtain meaningful *Salmonella* surveillance data, i.e. to discover the source and chain of infection, laboratory information is essential. *Salmonella* strains require serotyping, and some particularly prevalent serotypes such as *S. typhimurium*, *S. enteritidis*, and *S. panama* need the more precise phage typing. There are several distinct schemes for phage-typing *S. typhimurium*: one developed by the WHO collaborating centre in London, another by the National Institute of Public Health at Bilthoven in the Netherlands, and another in Sweden. They give different results and are not easily comparable, and some strains (about 1.5%) remain untypable. Lysotypes 12 and 17 have a predominant role in foodborne diseases.

Table 42. Main *Salmonella* serotypes isolated from man, 1980 (percentages)

Serotype	Austria	Belgium	Bulgaria	Denmark	Finland	France	Germany, Federal Republic of	Greece	Hungary	Italy	Luxembourg	Netherlands	Norway	Romania	Spain	Sweden	United Kingdom (England & Wales)	United Kingdom (Scotland)	Yugoslavia
S. typhimurium	27.6	56.5	24.2	21.5	32.1	27.7	56.5	8.4	23	22.2	68.6	53.9	38.1	15.9	46.3	17.3	31.1	32.7	32.8
S. enteritidis	15.8	2.6	34.6	43.5	20.1	5.4	6.5	18.6	25.7	5.1	34	1.9	13.4	27.6	32.1	12.9	7.3	7	22.7
S. infantis	7.7	2	—	2.7	13.3	4	3.5	3.2	9.6	5.5	2.4	2.7	2.9	0.8	—	4.5	1.8	4.5	2.3
S. hadar	7.3	0.8	2	—	1.3	2.5	2.1	1.6	4.6	—	2.4	2.7	4.9	0.7	—	3.4	15.3	3.4	6.8
S. heidelberg	5.2	0.7	—	1.4	3.6	3.1	1.3	1.2	—	5.4	—	—	3.7	9.2	—	—	3.8	6.7	—
S. saint-paul	4	—	—	0.9	1.8	2.7	0.7	—	4	1.8	—	—	—	—	—	—	2	1.6	—
S. bredeney	4	—	8.1	—	—	—	1.6	—	1.9	—	—	1.6	—	—	—	—	1.6	1.6	3.4
S. agona	2.4	1.1	—	3.6	2.9	2	1	4.4	—	2.5	2.4	1.2	2.3	2.9	3	4.6	2.8	0.8	1.2
S. montevideo	1.6	—	—	1.3	—	—	—	2	—	—	—	—	1.1	—	—	—	3.1	3.7	2.9
S. panama	1.5	—	0.5	—	1	11.7	7.7	—	7.5	11.2	8.4	12.1	2	14.2	—	—	—	1	—
S. newport	1.2	—	—	1.5	1.6	1.4	0.7	18.6	—	1.9	—	—	—	3	—	4.8	2.8	1.1	—
S. bovis-morbificans	1.1	—	—	—	—	—	—	—	—	—	—	—	0.8	3.5	—	—	—	—	—
S. derby	1.7	—	1.2	0.8	1.2	3.7	3	—	2.1	2.3	—	1.7	1.4	1.7	—	—	—	—	1.8
S. london	—	1.9	0.6	1.1	1	1.8	1.2	—	2.4	3.5	—	—	—	2.1	—	—	—	—	1.3
S. virchow	—	—	1.8	—	—	—	0.9	—	—	1.9	—	1.6	2.9	—	—	3	6	24.7	—
S. java	—	—	—	3.2	—	—	—	—	—	—	—	1.7	—	—	—	—	—	—	1
S. typhi	—	0.9	—	0.9	—	5.7	—	10.1	—	2.7	—	—	4.9	1.3	11.8	—	—	0.6	—
S. paratyphi B,C	1.6	—	—	—	—	1.5	—	5.6	—	—	—	0.9	2.9	—	2.5	—	1.9	0.7	0.7
Other identified	10.9	10.7	3.8	8.2	13.7	1.5	11.3	8.5	6.6	22.8	13.2	9	13.1	5.7	—	45.1	16.1	8	6.8
Total	2 746	3 567	1 791	841	1 999	10 039	55 335	247	11 190	8 657	83	9 114	343	9 184	424	3 135	11 473	1 593	10 424

Note: Not all identified serotypes are included in the table. Not listed are those that were isolated only very rarely or seen in a higher percentage in one country only, such as *S. isangi* 14.6% and *S. haifa* 4% in Bulgaria, *S. wien* 4.5% in Italy, *S. brandenburg* 4.2% in France and *S. branderup* 5% in Austria. The data, therefore, do not give 100% if related to the denominator.

Phage-typing shows a good correlation of *Salmonella* in humans and animals but not in birds (5). *S. typhimurium* is responsible for up to 50% or more of all human *Salmonella* infections all over the world and has held this position for some years (Table 42); its predominance, now challenged only by *S. enteritidis*, has not been satisfactorily explained. The rapid and continuous increase of *S. hadar* in the United Kingdom is interesting; although up to 1971 only 8 strains had been isolated, in 1975 it accounted for 3% and in 1979 for 15% of human isolations (spreading from the flocks of the largest turkey breeder in the country since about 1973–1974). Turkeys were the vehicle of infection in up to 46% of all the general outbreaks of foodborne diseases labelled as food poisoning. Although the numbers are small, a similar steady increase was observed from about 1976–1977 in Canada and the United States because of the importation of turkey breeding stock from England. However, *S. hadar* has been declining since 1979. Up to 1980 this *Salmonella* species had only rarely been reported from Southern Europe.

In October 1977 a large epidemic caused by *S. enteritidis* occurred in 28 schools in Stockholm, affecting 2865 persons. The vehicle was a remoulade sauce, and about 25% of infected people showed no symptoms. This outbreak demonstrates the risks inherent in mass catering (15), although no positive isolation was obtained from the kitchen personnel. In the course of investigation 27 000 faecal samples were examined, an indication of the costs such an outbreak may entail.

Salmonella also occurs as an important hospital infection. In the Federal Republic of Germany 1.8–11% of isolations occur in communal food establishments, of which 27.6% are in hospitals. In the United Kingdom the proportion of outbreaks in hospitals was 18% in 1979 but considerably higher in previous years (16).

The problem of salmonellosis can be seen as one of safe handling of animal wastes and feeds and of food of animal origin. Up to 30% of the intensively reared poultry in European countries are reputed to be infected with *Salmonella*. In spite of every effort to improve slaughterhouse hygiene and other control methods it has not yet been possible to achieve stocks of animals and raw meat, poultry and meat products free of *Salmonella*, nor can it be assumed that it will be achieved in the near future (although Sweden claims to have succeeded with poultry). The opinion of experts is that it is not possible to raise large numbers of *Salmonella*-free animals, but it is possible to reduce infection to levels consistent with the economic constraints. *Salmonella* is found not only in food animals and feeds but also in dust, water, manure, insects, birds, rodents and other mammals, fish, bone and fish meal, vegetables, soya beans, sewage and sludge. The organisms are highly adaptable, undemanding, and able to live in the most extreme ecological conditions. Strains that establish themselves in a hot climate, for example, develop highly heat-resistant mutants after a certain number of cycles.[a] It is not yet clear why there are some areas of pre-

---

[a]Skovgaard, N. *Special preventive and control measures. Control of Salmonella in the environment.* Unpublished WHO document VPH/WP/SAL/80.16, Geneva, 1980.

Table 43. Survival of salmonellae in various media

Medium	Survival time
Vegetables	20–40 days
Milk	2–4 days
Cheese	6 days–9 months
Fish flour	up to 2 years
Chocolate	at least 18 months
Butter	105 days
Poultry carcases (quick frozen at −37°C, stored at −21°C)	13 months
Dry meat	77–154 days
Eggs	several months
Egg powder	13 years
Pond water	115 days
Tap water	87 days
Sea water	24–32 days
Garden soil	28–280 days
Pasture soil	at least 20 days
Sand	12–16 months
Dry cow manure	30 months
Animal urine	52–112 days
Bird droppings	6 days–28 months
Bird feathers	1–4 years
Manure slurry	47 days
Finger tips	at least 10 minutes

Source: various, many cited in **Pretsch, C.** Salmonellosen. *In:* Blobel, H. & Schliesser, T., ed. *Handbuch der bakteriellen Infektionen bei Tieren.* Jena, Fischer, 1981.

dilection for *Salmonella* within what is apparently the same ecological area. Salmonellae can survive in soil for months (Table 43). The run-off from feed lots, manure heaps, or fields sprayed with fertilizer can reach watercourses; liquid wastes from slaughterhouses, processing plants and even human sewage are often discharged directly into streams or reach watercourses after minimal treatment; and fish, shellfish and aquatic plants can become contaminated by salmonellae from these sources (*17*). Wild animals and birds can acquire salmonellae from watercourses and transfer them to other streams, farms, land or animals. The organisms have been isolated from spring water within a few metres of its emergence from the ground. They are also found on aquatic vegetation and in river sediment, but not in nearby soil, forest litter, aquatic vertebrates, or aquatic or terrestrial invertebrates. Salmonellae may have a free-living existence apart from animal hosts (*18*). If this is so, the possibility becomes remote of achieving the goal of preventing infection in animals and contamination of foods, and thereby the eventual eradication of human salmonellosis.[a]

---

[a]**Bryan, F.L.** *Salmonella in foods and feeds and its control and consequences for international trade.* Unpublished WHO document VPH/WP/SAL/80.12, Geneva, 1980.

Table 44. Percentage removal of various organisms
by three sewage treatment procedures
and (in parentheses) the number of reports reviewed

Microorganism or pathogen	Treatment procedure		
	Percolating filter	Activated sludge	Anaerobic digestion
Total bacteria	70–95 (4)	70–99 (3)	
Salmonella	84–99 (2)	70–99 (2)	84–92.4 (1)
Escherichia	82–97 (4)	91–98 (1)	
Mycobacterium tuberculosis	99.66 (2)	88 (1)	69–90 (2)
Poliovirus		most (1)	
Coxsackievirus A	60 (1)		
Tapeworm ova	62–70, 18–26 (2)	little effect (1)	97 (1)

Source: **Kabler, P.W.** *Sewage and industrial wastes,* **31**: 1373–1382 (1959).

Salmonella spread by sewage or sewage-contaminated water used for irrigation survives fairly well on the crops; survival times of 10–53 days have been reported on root crops and of 1–40 days on vegetable leaves. Some authors (*19*) even report survival times of as long as 27 weeks on grass and in soil fertilized with contaminated sludge. Survival times on berries and fruit are only a few days. Outbreaks of cysticercosis and salmonellosis in cattle have been observed following the application of sewage sludge to grazing land in Scotland (*10*). Salmonellae are found in different countries in up to 5% of lettuces. There were 28 outbreaks of *Salmonella* infection resulting from environmental contamination affecting animals and/or human beings during the period 1973–1979 in Scotland (*20*).

Recycling occurs in various parts of the *Salmonella* chain. Sewage treatment greatly reduces but does not eliminate *Salmonella*. Utilization of sewage and sludge as fertilizers may subsequently result in animal carriers and cases of diseases, thus linking two important parts of the *Salmonella* chain: the feed cycle and the wastewater cycle. The presence of salmonellae in high numbers in sewage before and after biological treatment and in sludge is well documented; in raw sewage and mechanically and biologically treated sewage they are found to the extent of 100–2000 organisms per litre. Raw sludge may harbour as many as 10 000–100 000 salmonellae per litre, and stabilized sludge 100–1000 per litre. Although the reduction of salmonellae during sewage treatment may be large, the organism is still present after treatment. Table 44 shows the removal of pathogenic organisms by sewage treatment.

In the Netherlands, where 60% of wastewater is discharged to surface waters without treatment, it has been found that at least 10^2–10^4 salmonellae per 100 ml are constantly present in the effluent; almost every 100 ml sample of effluent will contain a certain number of salmonellae. Most of the serotypes isolated are important in human salmonellosis in the Netherlands as well as in the Federal Republic of Germany, which contributes by far the greatest volume of effluent to the Rhine. The same applies to the Meuse, which flows into the Netherlands from Belgium. The influence of environmental contamination was tested in a former island in the province of Zeeland, *Salmonella* being found in almost all material examined. Existence of a *Salmonella* contamination cycle has been postulated: from slaughter animal (infected from the environment and/or the feed) to meat, to the consumer, to a patient or healthy carrier, to effluent and surface water, to insects, rodents and birds, to slaughter animals, and to meat and possibly other foods. Salmonellae have constantly been observed in the sewage effluents of small villages even though the villages have no clinical salmonellosis and farms are unconnected to the effluents (*20*).

Escherichia coli

A variety of foods have been implicated in *E. coli* infections — milk, meat and salads. In the last ten years intensive research into the causes of acute diarrhoea has led to the recognition by WHO[a] of three groups of *E. coli* as important diarrhoeal pathogens: enterotoxigenic, enteropathogenic and enteroinvasive *E. coli*.

Enterotoxigenic *E. coli* (ETEC) is a major cause of diarrhoeal illness originating in the small intestine in children in developing countries, and is by far the most common cause of travellers' diarrhoea, accounting for 60–70% of diarrhoeal episodes in travellers from the industrialized countries who visit the developing world and often producing a severe dysentery-like or cholera-like disease. It is however rarely demonstrated, as the identification of enterotoxins requires specialized procedures that only a limited number of laboratories can perform. In the European Region it has been found in Morocco. A relatively large inoculum is required. In Sweden (*21*) bacteria producing heat-labile enterotoxin have been isolated from food suspected to have been the cause of secretory diarrhoeal disease — shrimp and mushroom salad, cold shop-sliced roast beef, cooked tongue, hot dogs, canned peas and carrots, canned bamboo shoots, home-made goat's cheese, cooked chicken and shredded beef — but human infections are rare except in tourists. Since many young animals (calves, lambs, piglets) also have severe diarrhoeal disease caused by ETEC (though the serotypes are different) there might perhaps be a relationship between the human and animal *E. coli* strains or the plasmids they carry.

Enteropathogenic *E. coli* (EPEC) causes disease of the duodenum, jejunum and upper ileum. Some serotypes long known as pathogens found in foodstuffs and infant nurseries have noticeably decreased in Europe, and since 1977 no serious epidemic has been seen. The reason for this

---

[a] *Escherichia coli diarrhoea.* Report of a subgroup of the Scientific Working Group on Epidemiology and Etiology. Unpublished WHO document WHO/DDC/EPE/79.1, Geneva, 1980.

marked decline in the frequency of EPEC outbreaks is unknown. Food-borne outbreaks in adults occurred in the United Kingdom in 1967 and 1973 and were traced to cold pork and pie, respectively.

Enteroinvasive *E. coli* (EIEC). Certain serotypes of *E. coli* have been isolated from the stools of older children and adults with fever and a dysentery-like disease located in the large intestine. Isolations have been made from sporadic cases and institutional outbreaks in the United Kingdom, and from waterborne outbreaks in Hungary. An extensive epidemic of gastroenteritis occurred in 1976 in a holiday camp on the Baltic Sea in the German Democratic Republic, with 152 cases among the 297 holiday-makers. Epidemiological investigations revealed secondary contamination of a mid-day meal (consisting mainly of potatoes) arising from damage to the camp's sewage disposal system (22). A large outbreak in 13 states of the United States was attributed to imported French cheese. Because of the biochemical and antigenic resemblance to *Shigella* infection and a classical picture indistinguishable from bacillary dysentery, it is likely that many EIEC outbreaks have been reported as shigellosis, particularly in laboratories with limited facilities. This is perhaps of little importance from the individual point of view, but for epidemiological purposes accurate etiological diagnosis is essential.

In 1981–1982 a newly recognized disease characterized by very severe abdominal pain was found to be caused by a serotype of *E. coli* (0157-H7) not previously associated with human disease. It seems to be linked with the consumption of undercooked meat, such as in hamburgers.

The distribution of the most frequently isolated serotypes in patients with *E. coli* infection seems to be comparable with the distribution of the same serotypes in food and water and on different surfaces. *E. coli* infection is reported separately in Belgium, France, the German Democratic Republic and Norway.

Staphylococcus aureus

After salmonellosis, staphylococcal infection is the most prevalent food-borne disease in Europe. In France it is reported as responsible for 37.4% of all known cases of mass foodborne disease (as against 42.4% for *Salmonella*). In Finland in 1978–1979 it was found to be responsible for about 20% of all outbreaks and 15% of all persons affected. Staphylococcal intoxication is common in all European countries but is rarely reported separately. It is considered that only larger outbreaks in industrial or institutional kitchens come to the attention of the health authorities, and that probably well under 1% of all cases have a chance of being reported.

Staphylococci are ubiquitous in nature and can be isolated from water, food, milk, dust, faeces and sewage and from the skin and mucous membranes of the nasopharynx; probably 30–50% of people are carriers. The onset of the illness is rapid (2–4 hours), the duration short (1–3 days) and the mortality low. Bacteriophage or lysozyme typing is therefore essential in epidemiological investigation as some carriers are harmless. Nevertheless, even with this procedure, it is often not possible to delineate epizootic strains if they are considered to be the cause of the outbreak. The

222

disease is typically transmitted directly to food by food handlers or kitchen personnel from the nose, the throat or skin lesions such as boils. Food is usually contaminated by handling, but raw substances of animal origin are thought by some authorities (23) to be the most common source of contamination, and eggs have been suspected. Staphylococci prosper under suitable conditions at room temperature and in a few hours produce toxin on food not rapidly cooled, ready-made dishes, non-acid salads, cream, bread, puddings, ice-cream, icing, ham, meat dishes, sandwiches, sausages, cheese, milk and, particularly, raw smoked fish. The organism tolerates salt well and thrives on salted protein food where salt inhibits the growth of competitors. Reheating destroys the staphylococci, but the toxin may remain in the food. The organism will not thrive at temperatures below 4°C. It can persist in fermented salami mixes, which could be about 50% contaminated. Occasionally staphylococci penetrate faulty cans wet-handled by carriers immediately after processing. The water-soluble enterotoxins (at least five in number) are produced by coagulase-positive staphylococci and cannot be destroyed by conventional cooking or heat processing of food.

The development of antibiotic resistance by staphylococci has been rapid and universal. At present they are susceptible almost to only the newest antibiotics.

Faecal streptococcal food poisoning occurs in the same way as staphylococcal food poisoning, but there is no way at present of evaluating it. Man is the reservoir (sore throat, impetigo, etc.) of the group β-haemolytic streptococci, although other groups have been found, in animals such as pigs and cows, that can occasionally be transmitted to man. These groups are a risk to those in close contact with live or slaughtered animals.

Shigellosis

The genus *Shigella* is subdivided into four subgenera or subgroups according to their biochemical reactions: *Sh. dysenteriae*, *Sh. flexneri*, *Sh. boydii* and *Sh. sonnei*. The first three may be further subdivided by serotyping but for *Sh. sonnei* colicin-typing is used, and less commonly phage-typing. There are 10 serotypes of *Sh. dysenteriae*, 8 of *Sh. flexneri* and 15 of *Sh. boydii*. *Shigella* causes bacillary dysentery, which typically presents with fever and watery diarrhoea, the latter often changing on the first or second day of illness to frequent stools of small volume containing blood and mucus. Although it has frequently been reported that *Sh. dysenteriae* 1 (Shiga's bacillus) produces the most severe disease and *Sh. sonnei* the mildest, in fact the disease caused by any of the subgroups has a wide spectrum. The typical case is of short duration (about four days) but exceptionally the symptoms may last for up to two weeks; host factors seem to play an important role in determining the severity and duration of the disease. In contrast to salmonellosis, extraintestinal complications are uncommon and *Shigella* is rarely recovered from blood culture. A long-term carrier state is exceptional but does exist.

Shigellosis has a global distribution, with the highest incidence in countries where hygiene is poor. As the general level of environmental and personal hygiene rises in a country the proportion of cases caused by *Sh. sonnei* increases and that of cases caused by *Sh. flexneri* falls. Thus in more developed areas *Sh. sonnei* infection is the most common, *Sh. flexneri* infection the next most common, and *Sh. boydii* and *Sh. dysenteriae* infections rare, while in many developing areas infection with the latter two subgroups is more common and *Sh. flexneri* infection more frequent than *Sh. sonnei* infection. This subgroup distribution pattern was exemplified by the frequency of the subgroups in travellers returning to the United Kingdom between 1972 and 1978; during that period about 80% of *Sh. dysenteriae*, 70% of *Sh. boydii* and 50% of *Sh. flexneri* infections occurred in persons who had recently returned from developing countries, while *Sh. sonnei* was most frequent in the indigenous population. *Sh. flexneri* has been isolated in recent years from travellers returning from Morocco, Romania and a few other European countries.

Man is both the reservoir and the natural host of *Shigella*; apart from man only monkeys and chimpanzees seem to suffer from natural infection. Infection is by the faecal–oral route, and the most common mode of spread is by person-to-person transmission owing to the low infectious dose (10^{10} organisms). In developing countries foodborne and waterborne transmission is also common, and in areas with inadequate excreta disposal facilities flies may be an important vector. Shigellosis is a declining disease in a number countries in Europe, most cases observed in Northern and Central Europe being imported. There is now a high degree of resistance of *Shigella* to sulfonamides, frequently combined with resistance to streptomycin and determined by a single plasmid. Multiple plasmid-mediated resistance to four or more antibiotics, in particular tetracycline, ampicillin and chloramphenicol, is now not uncommon. It has also been seen in developed countries, especially among *Sh. sonnei* infections, although recent information from the United Kingdom suggests that the incidence of drug resistance in *Sh. sonnei* may be decreasing. Outbreaks occurred recently among tourists on the Adriatic coast of Yugoslavia, caused by *Sh. boydii* type 1 and *Sh. sonnei*; 17 and 54 persons respectively were infected from the kitchen personnel (*24*). An outbreak in Scandinavia in 1982 was traced to contaminated cheese bought at a French airport.

Live oral vaccines using streptomycin-dependent strains in a polyvalent preparation, and given in three or four doses with preparations to neutralize gastric acidity, have given highly significant protection against clinical disease for 6–12 months. A single booster injection prolongs the protection for another year. This vaccine may be of use to travellers staying for rather longer periods of time in endemic areas.[a]

Other Enterobacteriaceae
The status of other Enterobacteriaceae and related organisms such as *Alkaligenes*, *Aeromonas*, *Pseudomonas* (over 200 species reported and so

---

[a]For a complete review of *Shigella* vaccines see *Bulletin of the World Health Organization*, **57**: 719–734 (1979).

far 29 species recognized taxonomically), *Providencia, Klebsiella* and *Proteus* is difficult to evaluate, particularly as some of them constitute part of animal faecal flora. If found on food they indicate gross faecal contamination, but the exact etiological role they play remains uncertain in spite of individual published reports. Recently particularly *Pseudomonas multivorans (Cepacia)*, a phytopathogen recognized only in 1950, has attracted attention in Europe rather as a source of waterborne and hospital infections than as a cause of foodborne infection.

Bovine tuberculosis

Bovine tuberculosis in man caused by infected milk or milk products has become extremely rare except for sporadic infections, particularly in rural areas. Where milk is pasteurized, and in countries where the eradication of bovine tuberculosis in cattle has been achieved or is in progress, it has disappeared altogether. No case of bovine tuberculosis in urban areas has been reported. Several cases of man infecting animal herds with *Mycobacterium tuberculosis* are on record in Europe.

Campylobacter jejuni

Since the pioneering work in Belgium in 1972 (*25*), evidence has been rapidly accumulating that *Campylobacter jejuni* is a major foodborne and waterborne zoonosis. Infections formerly attributed to *C. fetus* might have been caused by *C. jejuni*. The epidemiology has not yet been clearly elucidated, partly because of the absence of suitable methods for differentiating strains and of an internationally recognized scheme for serotyping and phage typing. Infection is by the faecal–oral route or through contaminated food or water, as in salmonellosis. It is known that campylobacters are found in the intestine of many animal species — birds (particularly poultry, which are heavy carriers), bovines, dogs, sheep and others — which serve as a source of infection. Contamination of fresh and frozen chicken carcases has been reported from several countries, and it is thought that consumption of contaminated poultry is one of the most common modes of transmission. *C. jejuni* can survive the grilling of chickens. Some human infections have been traced to contact with live birds on farms and the handling of dressed carcases in processing plants, butchers' shops and kitchens. Unpasteurized or insufficiently pasteurized cow's milk was incriminated in 1979 as a source of infection. However, the routes of transmission and the exact role of animals will be better determined after markers of the pathogenicity of strains have been found.

Campylobacter infections in Europe are most frequent in the warmer months. The incubation period is 2–5 days. *Campylobacter* produces an invasive type of infection and a variety of clinical pictures: enterocolitis, fever, vomiting, particularly colicky pain in the abdomen, and bloody stools. Usually it is a self-limiting disease, but it can sometimes be more severe. The organism is excreted in the stools for a few days following the illness, but in untreated cases for 2–7 weeks. The disease has been reported increasingly in Europe from Austria, Belgium, Denmark, Finland, France, the Federal Republic of Germany, the Netherlands, Sweden, and the

United Kingdom. In the United Kingdom an explosive outbreak traced to milk affected over 2000 children in schools in the Luton and Dunstable area. The increase in *Campylobacter* reports in that country illustrates the importance of this infection: there were 8577 cases in 1979, 9506 in 1980, and 12 496 in 1981. In Finland, *Campylobacter* was isolated from 340 patients in the 18 months ending in 1979; 98 were hospitalized, mostly in the warmer months, and half of them fell ill while abroad (particularly in the Mediterranean countries and Eastern Europe) (*26*). This indicates the presence of the disease in countries not yet reporting it and probably represents increasing recognition of *Campylobacter* as an enteric pathogen, but in at least two European countries there is an actual increase in incidence.

The organism is sensitive to aminoglycosides, erythromycin, clindamycin, tetracycline (particularly minocycline), chloramphenicol and furazolidone, and resistant to penicillin, cephalosporins, lincomycin, colistin and trimethoprim; ampicillin and the sulfonamides are intermediate. Although erythromycin is considered the antibiotic of choice, reports from Northern Europe (and North America) indicate that 2–10% of strains are resistant to it. Antibiotics should, however, be used only in severe or prolonged illness or to limit the duration of excretion of the organism. At present, unfortunately, many hospital and public health laboratories are still not able to diagnose the disease adequately. A WHO collaborating centre established in Brussels offers its assistance in this respect.

Botulism
The true incidence of botulism in man in Europe is unknown,[a] epidemiological information being more complete on the disease in animals. It is estimated that only 1 in 10 cases in man is being reported in the literature; however, data from France show that the numbers have tripled in the last 10 years. Between 1971 and 1978 there were 567 cases, an average of 70 per year. In 1981 there were 32 outbreaks, almost the same number as reported in the years 1971–1978. Many of the outbreaks originated from liver paste prepared at home. Still a relatively rare foodborne disease, it is showing a tendency to increase. Its seriousness and its fatality rate depend on the quantity of toxin ingested. The highly durable spores of *Clostridium botulinum* are widely but unevenly distributed in the soil and in stagnant or swampy water, which may be the source of contamination of foodstuffs. The standard chlorination treatment of water supplies is effective in inactivating any toxin that may enter drinking water. Large outbreaks in modern broiler farms in many European countries have been reported (*28*). Botulism occurs sporadically in all European countries; for example, 45 cases on average are reported in the Federal Republic of Germany yearly. Of the seven types existing, outbreaks in man are caused by type A,

---

[a]The last comprehensive report on botulism as a world problem was published in 1956 (*27*).

B or E. The non-proteolytic type B predominates in Western Europe, and type E has repeatedly been confirmed in Scandinavia and the USSR, mainly in the marine environment of the northern hemisphere. Fish is considered to be heavily contaminated and type F was isolated for the first time in Denmark (29). Type A is stated to be exceptionally rare in Europe except in the USSR, but it is frequent in the United States. Nearly all the type B strains found in North America belong to the proteolytic type. This distribution has some epidemiological significance.

The vehicle is usually vegetables of low acidity, mostly home-canned and home-preserved food, highly preserved or semi-preserved fish, vacuum-packed, dried or smoked sausages, smoked meat, home-made raw ham, pâtés, salted fish, and a wide variety of other insufficiently heated or pickled food such as olives, peppers and, recently, common low-acid tomatoes. In most outbreaks, however, the vehicle is not known. In an outbreak in 1980 in Izmir, Turkey three people became ill and two died, and in another outbreak in 1983, of seven people affected four died. Both incidents followed the consumption of canned peas. The toxin, one of the most lethal poisons known, is fortunately heat-labile and is easily destroyed by a temperature of 80°C for 15 minutes or 100°C for 3 minutes. E toxin is stable for more than four months at room temperature in salted fish products of low acidity such as marinated herring (pH 4.3–4.5) and salt-cured and spiced herring (pH 5.7–5.9) (29). Commercially canned food should thus be safe and if implicated a thorough investigation of the manufacturing process in the producing plant is required unless there is evidence of mishandling at home. However, in an outbreak in Belgium in 1982, tins of salmon from Alaska sold under different brand names were found to have been damaged in the canning plant and the total production of the series implicated was recalled. In home curing a ham-curing temperature of 8–10°C may fail to eliminate danger from psychotropic non-proteolytic strains if the salt concentration is not sufficient (30).

Recently identified infant botulism in the United States results from *in vivo* production of toxin after *Clostridium* has colonized the infant's gut. Honey is the only food source so far implicated. Since 1978 this form has also been described in Europe, in the United Kingdom. It usually occurs during the first six months of life.

Rapid investigation and tracing of persons who might have eaten the same food could prevent or limit the size of an outbreak, and antitoxin therapy could improve the prognosis of those already affected. It is essential that every country should provide information on sources of antitoxin or designate a central repository from which it could be obtained immediately, even after working hours and on holidays. Trivalent ABE antitoxin is usually given in cases where the toxin is unknown, and precautions are taken against the risk of anaphylaxis. Polyvalent ABCDEF antitoxin is produced in Europe only by the Statens Seruminstitut, Copenhagen and Behring Werke Marburg (Lahn).

Other clostridial diseases
Clostridium perfringens is an important and not infrequent cause of

227

foodborne disease, presenting either as enterotoxaemia and severe diarrhoea leading to collapse or as a severe, often fatal, necrotic enteritis. Food poisoning is caused by ingestion of food heavily contaminated by *C. perfringens* type A. The incubation period is usually 10–12 hours and the vehicle implicated is mostly meat or chicken. Spores withstand normal cooking and germinate and multiply in the food, producing four toxins (types A, B, C and E). Type E is pathogenic only for laboratory animals. The disease is also frequent in animals in Europe; in the Federal Republic of Germany 9% of slaughtered cattle and 8% of slaughtered pigs are infected (*31*). Outbreaks of *C. perfringens* disease have been recorded in recent years in Finland, the German Democratic Republic, the Federal Republic of Germany, Italy, the Netherlands, Norway, Sweden, the United Kingdom and Yugoslavia. In Finland *C. perfringens* was responsible for 30 outbreaks affecting 743 people in the years 1978–1979. This made it the largest single group of foodborne diseases, responsible for 20% of all outbreaks and 30.6% of all those affected (*32*). In the United Kingdom there were 29–84 outbreaks a year in the period 1970–1979 (*16*). In 1981 an outbreak affected 95 out of 490 people attending a reception and in 1982, of the 900 guests who attended a banquet at an hotel in London, more than half experienced diarrhoea and abdominal pains 6–8 hours after the meal. A seafood cocktail was suspected as the source of infection.

The investigation of many outbreaks is often inadequate. As *Clostridium* exists in sewage, soil, water and the gastrointestinal tract of man and animals, an exact typing of the strains is important for epidemiological (and sometimes legal) purposes. Serological typing has recently been developed in the United Kingdom, where it was used in the investigation of 524 outbreaks in the country and 37 outbreaks in other countries. Only Japan and the United States have developed such typing as an epidemiological tool. An international serotyping scheme is under discussion, but there is a need for national serotyping centres that would enable laboratories to serotype strains from every outbreak, which at present is not possible. It appears that some serotypes are more common in food outbreaks. Some strains are more heat-resistant and some cross-react with *Klebsiella* spp. and *Bacteroides fragilis*, whose antigens are also located in the capsule polysaccharides as in *C. perfringens* (*33*).

Necrotizing clostridial enteritis mainly attacks infants and those over 30 years of age (*34*). It seems in recent years to have been found predominantly in aged persons, at least in fatal cases.

C. difficile has been newly identified as the cause of pseudomembranous colitis in adults, pseudomembranous necrotizing enterocolitis in infants and, occasionally, neonatal pneumonia. It is uncertain whether this organism is transmitted by food.

Cholera and other vibrio-associated diseases
Cholera and other vibrio-associated diseases are foodborne or waterborne diseases. Europe is not receptive and large outbreaks are unlikely, but this

does not mean that cholera could not occur in the form of sporadic cases, imported cases or limited outbreaks.

The response to cholera by some health authorities, even in countries with excellent epidemiological services, is frequently emotional, and there is a tendency to apply excessive measures or require vaccination certificates for cholera, although this is not recommended by WHO. Because of that, and because of the somewhat uncertain state of the nomenclature and taxonomy of the genus *Vibrio*, the situation is described here in rather more detail than is warranted by the actual importance of vibrio-associated diseases.[a]

Epidemic strain V. cholerae 0-group 1 or V. cholerae 01
This has been isolated in recent years in Algeria, Morocco and Turkey, and occasionally in France (Corsica), Italy and Spain. All were El Tor serotype Ogawa. The example of Italy and Spain shows how effectively a good surveillance mechanism can contain an outbreak. A fairly large epidemic occurred in Algeria in 1982.

V. cholerae 01 can survive for varying periods and even multiply in various foods and water and in milk and milk products for 2–3 weeks at room temperature. It dies off rapidly if desiccated, but survival is possible up to three days on paper money, coins etc., up to eight days in shallow well water, and for one week on raw or cooked fruit and vegetables. Food and water have been incriminated as vehicles of cholera transmission. From volunteer studies and other epidemiological and clinical studies it has become quite clear that gastric acidity is a major factor in host resistance, the disease being more common in persons with hypochlorhydria. Susceptibility may also be increased by increased gastric emptying following the intake of large amounts of food and water. Volunteer studies with El Tor vibrio have established that the infective dose is lower when organisms are administered with food than when they are given in a small amount of water. It is not yet known if food itself acts by neutralizing the gastric acid or if the vibrios are protected from the acid by adhering to food particles, as seems to be indicated by the observation that adhesion of vibrios to chitin (crabshell) particles enhances their survival in an acid environment.

The major source of infection is from symptomatic and asymptomatic people whose stools reach and contaminate food and water. The organisms are probably also transported by moving bodies of water that have been contaminated with infected faeces. The possibility that other reservoirs of infection, such as infected shellfish or coastal waters, can maintain the vibrio for prolonged periods of time cannot, however, be excluded. Vibrios are halophilic and may remain viable for many weeks in salt concentrations as high as 2%. In the USSR, for example, following a cholera outbreak in

---

[a]Most of the information in the section on cholera has been extracted from *Cholera and other vibrio-associated diarrhoeas:* report of a subgroup of the Scientific Working Group on Epidemiology and Etiology. Unpublished WHO document WHO/DDC/EPE/80.3, Geneva, 1980.

Astrakhan in 1970, *V. cholerae* 01 El Tor was isolated from two small water basins near the Volga river for up to 14 months. These waters were not subject to known human faecal contamination. In 1975 El Tor vibrios were isolated from sulfurous spring waters in the region; the sources of contamination may have been tourists visiting the region from cholera-infected areas, but this was not proved. These observations were corroborated by similar findings in Louisiana, United States, and Australia.

Plasmid-encoded strains of high multiple resistance (to ampicillin, kanamycin, streptomycin, sulfonamides, tetracycline and gentamicin) have been found in Bangladesh.

Atypical *V. cholerae 01*

These organisms are non-toxigenic strains of *V. cholerae* 01 and are isolated primarily from environmental sources such as surface waters during cholera surveillance activities. They are only in exceptional instances pathogenic and have been associated in man only with extraintestinal disease or wound infection. In 1977 atypical *V. cholerae* 01 Ogawa strains were continuously isolated for five weeks from brackish agricultural drainage ditchwater in England, where the possibility of sewage contaminants was considered to be negligible. In the USSR many strains of *V. cholerae* 01 El Tor were isolated from various sources over a period of 11 years. Most of these atypical vibrios were not markedly sensitive to any of the classical or El Tor phages. In contrast, all known *V. cholerae* 01 associated with human infection have so far been sensitive to one or more of these phages.

Non-01 *V. cholerae*

These organisms have been associated with outbreaks and sporadic cases of rather short gastrointestinal illness. In Europe they have been isolated from the stools of persons with diarrhoeal illnesses in Bulgaria, Czechoslovakia, England, the Federal Republic of Germany, Hungary, Sweden and the USSR. It is believed that they could have been isolated also in other countries where investigations had not been carried out. No large epidemics have been reported. Transmission is probably exclusively by contaminated food and water. Non-01 *V. cholerae* can multiply in a variety of foods; in an outbreak in Czechoslovakia the vehicle was potatoes, in the United States oysters. Non-01 *V. cholerae* strains have been found to be widely distributed in the environment whenever they have been looked for. In ecological studies in the Federal Republic of Germany and the United Kingdom the organisms were generally found in brackish surface waters (rivers, marshes, bays and coastal areas), were more numerous during the warmer months, and were not associated with sewage contamination. The organisms are thus usually considered aquatic and are probably free-living in the environment. However, whether free-living strains cause disease in man is not known; pathogenicity may be restricted to strains adapted to the human intestine.

230

V. parahaemolyticus (35)

This organism, a halophilic marine vibrio known to cause food poisoning in Japan and first recognized in 1951, was long thought to be limited to the Far East. In Europe the disease has been reported from Romania, the United Kingdom (in 1972) and the USSR. *V. parahaemolyticus* appears to be transmitted exclusively by food, usually seafood but also cheese, probably contaminated by raw seafood or surface or sea water. It has, however, also been found in many cases in stools, food and water in Calcutta, in strictly vegetarian households with no history of seafood consumption or other marine exposure. The organisms multiply quickly, the generation time being reported to be as short as nine minutes and permitting the production of large infectious doses, but they are inhibited at temperatures below 15°C and die out at lower temperatures. *V. parahaemolyticus* is part of the normal flora of estuarine and other coastal waters throughout most of the world. In Europe it has been isolated from sea water, sea mud, or seafood in the Baltic Sea, Black Sea, Mediterranean Sea, North Sea, Denmark, Greece, Italy, the Netherlands, Spain, Turkey, the United Kingdom and Yugoslavia. In estuarine waters in temperate regions *V. parahaemolyticus* passes the winter in the sediment, is released from the bottom in the spring, becomes attached to zooplankton, and proliferates as the water temperature rises. Not all the strains are pathogenic.

Group F vibrios

These vibrio-like organisms, often mistakenly identified as *Aeromonas* spp., have been isolated in Europe from patients with diarrhoea only in Spain (and, nearest to Europe, in Tunisia). It is at present uncertain whether these organisms are diarrhoea-producing pathogens.

Other Vibrio species and related organisms

Occasionally isolated from man, *V. alginolyticus* and *V. metchnikovi* are not believed to cause diarrhoeal illness. *Aeromonas hydrophila* and *Plesiomonas shigelloides* have been isolated from man with diarrhoeal syndromes but the role they play is not clear.

Yersinia enterocolitica

Y. enterocolitica has recently been shown to cause foodborne disease, but its epidemiology has so far not been completely elucidated (see also Chapter 6). It is mentioned here because of its spectacular increase and the interest it has awakened, especially in Europe. Reports are published almost daily and come from practically all countries. The magnitude of the problem in Europe remains to be determined exactly, but it is evident that the disease is of considerable clinical importance. It is most prevalent in children, causing enteritis of 3–14 days' duration, often fever, and a clinical picture resembling acute appendicitis. In Scandinavia it is reported that 9% of cases diagnosed as appendicitis were *Y. enterocolitica* enteritis or lymphadenitis. In adults erythema nodosum, often discrete, normally follows a week or two after the enteritis, and a reactive arthritis frequently occurs lasting for more than a month. There is evidence from Denmark that *Y. enterocolitica* may be associated with certain thyroid syndromes, specifically Graves' disease and diffuse non-toxic goitre (*36*). Septicaemia and a wide variety of other complications (meningitis, myocarditis, hepatitis or hepatic abscesses, ophthalmitis, arthritis and glomerulonephritis) have occasionally been described.

According to studies in Belgium, Czechoslovakia, Finland, France, the Federal Republic of Germany, Hungary, Romania and Sweden, the organism has been isolated in 1–3% of acute enteritis cases, but further studies are needed.[a] In 1974 WHO established a collaborating centre for yersiniosis at the Pasteur Institute in Paris.

Y. enterocolitica is a psychrophilic organism that multiplies at refrigerator temperatures, and in milk even at 0–2°C. There are at least five biotypes and probably more than 34 serotypes, but only a limited number cause illness in man. Others are found only in various animals, particularly pigs, which consistently yield the bio-serophage types that are frequently isolated from humans. Outbreaks have been traced to contaminated packed meat, raw and pasteurized milk, chocolate, whipped cream, ice cream, vegetables and pig tongue. Studies in Belgium, Denmark and the Federal Republic of Germany have shown that 3–5% of pigs are intestinal carriers, but further epidemiological investigation is needed to clarify their exact role in human yersiniosis. Throat and tongue cultures have been positive in up to 53% of pigs. The organism is also isolated from a wide variety of environmental sources (*37*). In severe cases with complications antimicrobial treatment may be needed; streptomycin, tetracycline, chloramphenicol, nitrofurantoin, sulfonamides, trimethoprim-sulfamethoxazole, gentamicin and nalidixic acid could be used (*38*).

Bacillus cereus

The anaerobic spore-forming *B. cereus* was formerly considered a harmless saprophyte. It is now well documented that it can and does produce nausea, vomiting or a diarrhoeal illness if the infective dose is sufficiently large. It has been recently comprehensively analysed by Gilbert (*39*). Low numbers of *B. cereus* were found in 14% of single faecal specimens from 711 healthy adults. The question of the existence and nature of the enterotoxins produced among a number of extracellular metabolites of *B. cereus* appears to have been definitely solved in 1978–1979. Two thermolabile toxins destroyed at 56°C in 30 minutes have been recognized; emetic toxin responsible for the vomiting type of disease and intestinonecrotizing toxin responsible for the more severe diarrhoeal form. The organism has 23 recognized serotypes and a provisional typing scheme has been described by Taylor & Gilbert (cited by Gilbert, *39*). However, some 10–48% of the

---

[a]For more detailed information see *Yersiniosis:* report on a WHO meeting. Copenhagen, WHO Regional Office for Europe, 1983 (EURO Reports and Studies No. 60).

232

isolates are not yet typable. The relation of the clinical disease to a special serotype needs to be further studied. The incubation period is short: 1–5 hours after ingestion of contaminated food in cases where vomiting is the predominant symptom, 6–16 hours where diarrhoea is predominant. Various foods have been implicated: meat and chicken, puddings, rice, ice cream and milk; it has also been found in mishandled commercial infant formulae. Spores of *B. cereus* can survive temperatures up to 100°C and even to 135°C for several hours, some serotypes being more resistant to heat than others. The risk comes from storing cooked food at a kitchen temperature of 10–48°C, which permits germination of the spores and growth of the vegetative organisms.

Outbreaks of *B. cereus* disease have been documented in Norway in 1950 after four outbreaks involving 600 persons, in the United Kingdom since 1971, and in Denmark, the Federal Republic of Germany, Hungary, Italy, the Netherlands, Poland, Romania, Sweden and the USSR. In Finland 11 outbreaks affecting 705 people were reported in 1978–1979; a meat dish and vanilla sauce were implicated (*32*). Six outbreaks in the United Kingdom in 1981 were associated with the consumption of rice.

Leptospirosis is usually a waterborne disease transmitted by direct contact through abraded skin, but ocasionally it is transmitted through food contaminated with rodent urine. Although leptospirae are very sensitive to drying, survival on food has been found for up to 276 days.

Intestinal anthrax

Animal anthrax occurs in Albania, Algeria, Austria, Bulgaria, France, Greece, Italy, Morocco, Norway, Poland, Romania, Spain, Sweden, Turkey, the USSR, the United Kingdom and probably also other countries. Over 98% of anthrax occurs in the cutaneous form; visceral, pulmonary and intestinal anthrax are rare. Intestinal anthrax is a deadly foodborne disease, as seen in April 1979 in Sverdlovsk, a known endemic area in the USSR, where it was caused by the private sale of undercooked or semi-raw meat from diseased animals that had not passed through sanitary slaughter control (*40*). Soviet literature has established that outbreaks of intestinal anthrax can be expected at a rate of one every three years. For the situation of anthrax in general see Annex 7.

Tularaemia

Although enzootic in Europe over extensive areas, particularly in Northern Europe, Czechoslovakia, Hungary and the USSR, tularaemia is not a serious problem as a foodborne disease. Rather it is an occupational disease, sporadic cases being noted in hunters, processors of rabbit or sheep meat, butchers, etc. Tularaemia caused by the consumption of infected water or food is not known ever to have occurred in Sweden, where the disease exists, but this mode of transmission has in the past caused large epidemics in the USSR, where millions of people in recent decades have received the live vaccine in the context of the tularaemia control programme. Two outbreaks (one waterborne) occurred in the

Tuscany region of Italy in 1982 following the release of large numbers of rabbits from Eastern Europe for hunting.

Erysipelothrix rhusiopathiae
This bacterium is transmitted by animal products, particularly meat, but it is more an occupational than a foodborne disease. It is not reported and no information is available on its present prevalence in Europe, but it seems to be very rare.

Various pathogenic yeast-like fungi have been found in a number of basic foods and may also be transmitted through meat products, but infections are not usually seen.

Rotavirus
Rotaviruses have emerged as the most important viral agents associated with severe diarrhoeal disease and vomiting in infants and young children. First detected in Australia in 1973, rotavirus was isolated soon afterwards in the United Kingdom. Morphologically similar viruses showing certain common antigens are found in a number of animals and, particularly where young animals are congregated, the incidence of rotavirus infection frequently reaches 100%. The epidemiology of rotavirus in man and animals is not yet well understood. All the evidence to date indicates that rotavirus infection spreads by faecal–oral transmission, and this has been confirmed by volunteer and animal experiments.

The disease is more prevalent in cold weather and affects infants and younger children. Outbreaks of rotavirus infection have been documented in nurseries, especially those providing special care, and in a number of paediatric hospital wards. High antibody levels in later childhood and adult life were found in family studies in Norway, up to 55% of older siblings and household contacts showing evidence of infection, mostly asymptomatic and probably representing reinfection. The incubation period of rotavirus enteritis ranges from 1 to 7 days but is usually less than 48 hours, and the average duration of the illness is 5–7 days. In adults mostly only mild diarrhoea or asymptomatic infection occurs, probably because of acquired active immunity, but outbreaks have been noted, for example after a wedding party at a good hotel in Scotland in 1983. Rotavirus and other viruses have been isolated from the intestine and intestinal contents of animals, which can further spread the infection through products made from the intestine (sausage skins) or secondarily contaminate other products (41). Several approaches to the development of a rotavirus vaccine are now being undertaken.

Other enteric viruses
The role in foodborne disease of the new group of agents (such as Norwalk particle) found in association with outbreaks of generally mild gastroenteritis occurring in schools and in the community and family setting, has not yet been elucidated. Nor has that of astroviruses, first found in Scotland in 1975 in the diarrhoeal stools of infants and subsequently observed elsewhere in the United Kingdom, or of the caliciviruses, first detected in

Scotland in 1976 and by two other laboratories in the United Kingdom and tentatively associated with gastroenteritis and a school outbreak of "winter vomiting". The morphologically similar coronaviruses have been isolated from children, mice, pigs, calves, dogs, rats and cats, and cause a variety of clinical symptoms in certain animals, including diarrhoea.[a]

Enteric viruses persist for a long time, particularly in food consumed fresh or raw such as oysters, steak tartare and eggs. Their viability is prolonged by refrigeration (over weeks and months), freezing below −15°C (over years), and pickling and salting, the salt concentration reached stabilizing the viruses (42). Drying prolongs the life of the viruses over weeks and months without refrigeration.

Viral hepatitis A

Infectious hepatitis type A is usually spread by the faecal–oral route. Its exact importance among foodborne diseases is not easy to determine because of the difficulties inherent in investigation. Numerous foodborne outbreaks have been described in the literature. Careful epidemiological studies have incriminated raw food or food contaminated after preparation by persons who have been in the incubation period of the disease. Ingestion of raw shellfish or shellfish cooked in the shell is particularly known to have caused epidemics. This may also happen as a result of contamination of private or public water supplies (old pipes, old sewerage systems, low water pressure). There is no evidence that chlorination in the usual dosage always destroys the virus. However, waterborne outbreaks can be incriminated in only a small percentage of cases, probably less than 1%; most cases of hepatitis A are caused by person-to-person transmission, persons in the same household being at greatest risk. There is no animal reservoir. Hepatitis A outbreaks have been traced to contaminated strawberries in Central and Eastern Europe and to frozen raspberries in the United Kingdom. Outbreaks from a common source, such as contaminated jam or shellfish, have been reported recently from the United Kingdom (see Chapter 3).

In a suspected foodborne outbreak rapid establishment of the etiology is of particular importance because excretion of virus is of short duration, the maximum excretion being in the period of about two weeks before symptoms appear. Only about 10% of ill persons excrete the virus two weeks after the symptoms appear.

The reporting of sporadic cases is notably unreliable and not all infections are investigated. Laboratory investigation may become easier with the ELISA test now available. A WHO reference set of sera containing predominantly anti-HAV IgE and trace amounts of anti-HAV IgM has been prepared and is now being tested. There is strong evidence to

---

[a]For full information on this group of diseases see unpublished WHO document WHO/DDC/EPE/79.2, Geneva, 1980. Recently more viruses have been isolated: "small round viruses" closely resembling enteroviruses, and "small round structured viruses" associated with shellfish. Their role in foodborne disease is currently being assessed.

suggest that one form of non-A non-B hepatitis can also be transmitted orally.

The precautions taken against foodborne spread are usually late, and prophylaxis with immune serum globulin in a countrywide programme is not indicated. Among specifically identified persons with brief exposure such prophylaxis is not indicated if other cases have already begun to occur. On the other hand, where persons have been continuously exposed, some of whom may be in the first half of their incubation period, it may be worth an attempt at prevention.

Seafood poisoning

It is not possible to deal with all possible food poisoning here, as it is by definition non-infectious. Only scombrotoxic fish poisoning, paralytic fish poisoning, and shellfish poisoning are briefly mentioned because of their importance in a differential diagnosis of food infections and because of their increasing incidence in Europe, accompanied by alarming clinical signs, and the serious economic consequences that may result from public apprehension about eating fish when the alarm has been raised. Scombrotoxic fish poisoning occurs from the consumption of smoked or canned fish or fish paste from the family Scombridae (tuna, mackerel) that has become toxic as a result of bacterial contamination and decomposition without external appearance of spoilage. The illness was noted only sporadically before 1978, for example in the United Kingdom, but by the end of 1979 a total of 50 incidents affecting 196 persons had been reported in that country; in one outbreak 80 of the 150 people in a hotel were affected. Similar observations have been made in other countries (43). Fresh fish does not cause poisoning and it is assumed that the histamine concentration increases with spoilage, but the mechanism and exact role of this reaction are not yet quite clear.

Paralytic shellfish poisoning is caused by a group of neurotoxins similar to saxitoxins in crustaceans and bivalve molluscs — mussels, clams, oysters, cockles, scallops — feeding on phytoplankton. About 5000 people were affected in 1981 in Galicia and Murcia, Spain, but cases have occurred also in Belgium, France, the Federal Republic of Germany, the Netherlands, Norway and the United Kingdom. The quantity of the phytoplankton dinoflagellates belonging to the genus *Gonyaulax* (*G. tamarensis* var. *excarata*) along the Atlantic coast and in the North Sea increases sometimes so much as to colour the sea red ("red tide"). This had been observed occasionally before, but in the last few years, for unexplained reasons, it has been more frequent in summer along the Moroccan and Spanish Atlantic coasts, the North Sea coast of England, and in the Mediterranean.

Special monitoring of the toxin had to be established in the countries at risk and commercial gathering halted whenever the toxicity exceeded 400 mouse units per 100 g shellfish (44). The toxin is highly poisonous, but cooking of the shellfish destroys some 30% of it. The disease is manifested by tingling of the mouth and tongue, paraesthesiae, gastrointestinal symptoms, and rapidly progressing paralysis with respiratory death in

236

about 10% of those affected (*44*). There is no antidote. Fish are usually not poisonous, but can be killed by the saxitoxin in the "red tide".

Similar disease produced by other types of dinoflagellate and other types of toxin (ichthyotoxin), eaten by littoral fish and incorporated in their flesh, is known in the Caribbean and on the American Pacific coast as ciguatera (ciguatoxin and ichthyosariotoxin).

Foodborne parasitic diseases

A number of parasitic diseases are spread by the faecal–oral route, in many instances almost exclusively via food, although in some person-to-person transmission may also be possible. Waterborne outbreaks are not reported in Europe. In the European context only amoebiasis, giardiasis, balantidiasis, trichinosis and coccidiosis are important; trichinosis is of particular interest as a direct foodborne disease. Amoebiasis is not highly prevalent in Europe and, particularly in the central and northern part, is extremely rare.

In the United Kingdom the reported carrier rate for *Entamoeba histolytica* is between 2% and 5%, and the number of hospitalized cases of amoebiasis has been estimated at some 300 per annum.[a] However, the reports do not indicate how many cases were imported. Amoebiasis is somewhat more common in the countries of southern Europe, where it may be underdiagnosed. The influx of immigrants and refugees from Africa and Asia into European countries has stimulated interest in a better diagnosis of parasitic disease; in many countries examinations for them are carried out in this population group.

Giardiasis is at present one of the most commonly diagnosed intestinal protozoan foodborne infections, mostly seen in children and the old, in psychiatric homes and among tourists (1371 cases were found in Sweden in 1979). Giardia cysts survive for two months in water and are resistant to routine chlorination. Although it is a self-limiting infection, it can lead to long-standing symptomatic diarrhoeal disease in some persons.

The protozoan *Isospora belli* is described in Europe as a curiosity. On the other hand *Isospora* (*Sarcocystis*) *hominis*, causing a parasitosis called sarcosporidiosis or sarcocystiasis, has been described with increasing frequency. It is a common parasite of various animals with a carnivorous, feral or herbivorous intermediate host. Persons eating raw meat are those most often parasitized, but the infection is frequently asymptomatic.

The prevalence of human trichinosis caused by *Trichinella spiralis* in Europe is low. The disease occurs mostly in arctic areas such as Greenland, but also in Bulgaria, Czechoslovakia, France, Ireland, Poland, Romania, Spain, the USSR and the United Kingdom, sporadically in the Federal Republic of Germany, Hungary, Italy, Portugal, Sweden and Yugoslavia, and only exceptionally in other countries such as Greece and Switzerland.

---

[a] *Parasite-related diarrhoeas*. Report of a subgroup of the Scientific Working Group on Epidemiology and Etiology. Unpublished WHO document WHO/CDD/PAR/80.1, Geneva, 1980.

No human trichinosis has been seen for a number of years in Austria, Denmark, Finland and Norway (except in an employee of a zoo in Finland who ate meat from a captive wild pig in 1970), although those countries also have a large wildlife reservoir and a smaller pig reservoir. The highest prevalence among domestic pigs is found in Poland, and there the number of cases of human disease seems to have been the highest. An epidemic outbreak in 1976 in a suburb of Paris involved about 100 people (45). Recent outbreaks were recorded in Romania in 1970, in Yugoslavia in 1975, in Italy in 1971, in Hungary in 1980 and in Spain in 1982 (325 cases). The only large outbreak in the Federal Republic of Germany dates from 1967 and involved some hundreds of people. In the USSR the highest prevalence, some 90% of all the cases reported in the country, is in Byelorussia near the western border. In the Ukraine 33% of human cases were traced to lard and 31% to insufficiently cooked pork. In those areas salted lard containing streaks of muscle is consumed raw in the winter months. There is a large wildlife reservoir in the USSR (boars, bears, etc.) and rare sporadic infections occur in hunters (46). In 1975 an epidemic of trichinosis with 42 cases occurred in Reggio Emilia, Italy, and was attributed to horse meat imported from Poland or Yugoslavia. The parasite was identified as *T. nelsoni*, which is usually found in wild animals such as the wolf (47). Cases in other European countries have been extremely rare.

A temperature of −25°C for 20 days will effectively destroy all *Trichinella* cysts in pork. Smoking, curing and drying are not reliable methods for the prevention of infection. Trichinosis is classically a disease of raw or undercooked meat, but strict veterinary control has reduced it in Europe to being a local disease of insignificance. Outbreaks can occur from imported meat, as happened in 1980 in the Federal Republic of Germany, when privately imported air-dried camel meat affected five persons (48).

Echinococcosis (hydatidosis) can be transmitted by food infected from the faeces of dogs, cats, foxes and other carnivores. *Echinococcus* eggs can be destroyed only by heat; no effective chemical agent is available. The disease has been reported in human beings from Algeria (473 cases in 1980), Bulgaria (168 cases in 1978), the south of France and Normandy, Greece (989 cases in 1981), Italy (44 cases in 1980), Morocco (1488 cases in 1978), Poland (4330 cases in 1978), Portugal (100 cases in 1978), Romania (40 cases in 1981), Spain, Turkey (1542 cases in 1981) and Yugoslavia, and can cause considerable illness. It is, however, an occupational disease, related to the keeping of livestock and dogs.[a]

New trends in treatment

The treatment of foodborne infections depends on the causative agent. The presenting symptom in by far the largest number of foodborne in-

---

[a]See *Hydatidosis control (Mediterranean countries)*. Unpublished WHO document ICP/BVM 009, Copenhagen, 1981.

fections is the acute diarrhoeal syndrome. This syndrome places the biggest demand on primary care; incorrect treatment is often given and the economic cost is often considerable. Some advances have been made in separating useful from useless therapies. There is a special need for reorienting members of the medical profession, particularly paediatricians, hospital clinicians and general practitioners, many of whom are not yet aware of the new developments.

The most significant development in recent years has been the discovery that dehydration from acute diarrhoea of every etiology and in all age groups can be safely and effectively treated by the simple method of oral rehydration, using a single fluid consisting of glucose, sodium chloride, sodium bicarbonate and potassium chloride dissolved in water, in a mixture known as oral rehydration salts (ORS).[a] Dehydration should be prevented from occurring when it is not present. The prescription of antimicrobial drugs, including antibiotics and antidiarrhoeal agents, is at present almost a ritual, but in fact they are rarely needed in most uncomplicated foodborne diarrhoeas.

Many infectious diarrhoeal diseases, such as rotavirus gastroenteritis and staphylococcal food poisoning, do not benefit from antibiotics. Neither do some bacterial gastrointestinal infections such as salmonellosis, despite the *in vitro* sensitivity of the *Salmonella* strain concerned. For these reasons antimicrobial agents should only be prescribed (*a*) for selected gastrointestinal infections that have been shown to benefit clinically from specific chemotherapy, (*b*) if the epidemiological indication strongly favours a particular etiology such as giardiasis or cholera, or (*c*) for patients prone to septicaemia because of impaired defence mechanisms. Empirical chemotherapy may also be considered in severe cases if *Salmonella* food poisoning is suspected. The use of ampicillin, co-trimoxazole or chloramphenicol may prolong the period of excretion of salmonellae after clinical recovery. Most patients with a mild *Shigella* dysentery recover eventually without chemotherapy. Most acute diarrhoeas caused by *Escherichia coli*, *Vibrio parahaemolyticus* and *Campylobacter* do not need chemotherapy. The routine prophylactic use of antibiotics by travellers to developing countries is not recommended because of possible side-effects and the likelihood of inducing resistance.

Antimicrobial drugs are not indicated for the routine treatment of acute diarrhoea. Specific indications for their use include:

— cholera

— severe *Shigella* dysentery (particularly *Sh. dysenteriae*)

— amoebic dysentery (more often chronic than acute diarrhoea)

— acute giardiasis.

---

[a] *A manual for the treatment of acute diarrhoea.* WHO unpublished document WHO/CDD/Ser/80.2, Geneva, 1980.

Table 45. Antimicrobials used in the treatment of specific causes of acute diarrhoea

Cause	Drug(s) of choice[a]	Alternative[a]
Cholera[b c]	Tetracycline *Children* — 50 mg/kg/day in 4 divided doses × 3 days *Adults* — 500 mg 4 times a day × 3 days	Furazolidone *Children* — 5 mg/kg/day in 4 divided doses × 3 days *Adults* — 100 mg 4 times a day × 3 days Erythromycin[d] *Children* — 30 mg/kg/day in 3 divided doses × 3 days *Adults* — 250 mg 4 times a day × 3 days
Shigella dysentery[b e]	Ampicillin — 100 mg/kg/day in 4 divided doses × 5 days Trimethoprim (TMP)-sulfamethoxazole (SMX) *Children* — TMP 10 mg/kg/day and SMX 50 mg/kg/day in 2 divided doses × 5 days *Adults* — TMP 160 mg and SMX 800 mg twice daily × 5 days	Nalidixic acid — 55 mg/kg/day in 4 divided doses × 5 days (all ages) Tetracycline — 50 mg/kg/day in 4 divided doses × 5 days (all ages)
Acute intestinal amoebiasis	Metronidazole[f] *Children* — 30 mg/kg/day × 5–10 days *Adults* — 750 mg 3 times a day × 5–10 days	In very severe cases: dehydroemetine hydrochloride by deep intramuscular injection, 1–1.5 mg/kg (maximum 90 mg) for up to 5 days depending on response (all ages)
Acute giardiasis	Metronidazole[f] *Children* — 15 mg/kg/day × 5 days *Adults* — 250 mg 3 times a day × 5 days	Quinacrine *Children* — 7 mg/kg/day in divided doses × 5 days *Adults* — 100 mg 3 times a day × 5 days

Source: Unpublished WHO document WHO/CDD/SER/80.2, Geneva, 1980.

[a] All doses given are for oral administration unless otherwise indicated.

[b] A decision on the selection of an antibiotic for treatment should take into account the frequency of resistance to antibiotics in the area.

[c] Antibiotic therapy is not essential for successful therapy but shortens the duration of illness and the excretion of organisms in severe cases.

[d] Other choices include chloramphenicol and trimethoprim-sulfamethoxazole.

[e] Antibiotic therapy is especially required in infants with persistent high fever.

[f] Tinidazole and ornidazole can also be used in accordance with the manufacturers' recommendations.

240

The drugs of choice for treatment of these diseases are given in Table 45. Specific drug therapy may also be required when acute diarrhoea is associated with another acute infection, such as measles or malaria.

Neomycin causes damage to the intestinal mucosa and can contribute to malabsorption. The use of clioquinol is associated with severe neurological sequelae; moreover, the efficacy of this drug has never been documented in controlled trials. These two drugs should *never* be used in the treatment of acute diarrhoea.

Antidiarrhoeal agents, though commonly employed, are of no use in the prevention and treatment of dehydration and are not indicated in the routine treatment of acute diarrhoal disease. Adsorbents such as kaolin, pectin, activated charcoal and bismuth subcarbonate have not been shown to be of value in the treatment of acute diarrhoea. Opiates and opiate derivatives (e.g. tincture of opium, camphorated tincture of opium, codeine, diphenoxylate with atropine) may provide some transient relief from pain, but they may greatly slow peristalsis and delay the elimination of the causative organisms. They can be very dangerous, even fatal, if used in infants.

Other drugs used are stimulants, steroids and purgatives. Shock in acute diarrhoeal disease is generally due to dehydration and hypovolaemia and must be treated quickly with appropriate intravenous fluids. The use of stimulants such as epinephrine or nikethamide is not indicated. The use of steroids is never indicated; they can cause serious side-effects. Purgatives worsen diarrhoea and dehydration and should never be used.

Culture, education and legislation

The objective of health education in the prevention of foodborne diseases is to change behaviour patterns and practices. Health education not based on an intimate knowledge of habits conducive to foodborne disease has been singularly ineffective. A WHO meeting on salmonellosis control in 1980[a] concluded that: "there is no direct evidence that the issue of booklets on food hygiene has a significant effect on the occurrence of *Salmonella* infection", and it went on: "legislative measures alone seem to have had little effect except in some limited areas, e.g. pasteurization of milk and liquid egg, and preventing emergency slaughtered animals from entering the human food chain".

Health education must be directed towards food producers, food handlers and consumers. It seems, however, that it has only too often been based on premises that appear unrealistic.

- That one lives in a risk-free world. The industry or producer has the duty and the technological means to produce safe and wholesome products, but this is not always possible. The risks in certain food products or in certain modes of preparation are not fully appreciated by the public.

---

[a]Unpublished WHO document VPH/81.27, Geneva, 1982.

- That the consumer will not buy food from unhygienic shops or eat in unhygienic restaurants, so that dirty manufacturers and shopkeepers must then either improve their standards or go out of business. In fact the consumer is guided by the price; he will always prefer cheaper goods and will not know the hygienic standards of the kitchen or place of manufacture. Social pressure can be effected only through publicity, which again must be done extremely carefully if collaboration between the health authorities and the food sector is to be maintained. A high level of press exposure is a powerful but temporary means of assuring compliance, but also produces a negative reaction.

- That it is simple to convince managers that the cost incurred in achieving good hygiene is more than counterbalanced by the benefits. In fact the producer (except the large producer) is more concerned with the immediate cost to himself than with the cost to others or to the community as a whole. Producers, caterers and restaurant owners are more likely to be influenced by regulations, financial penalties, loss of a licence, fear of prosecution or litigation, or direct economic losses. Experience in the United Kingdom shows that most outbreaks of *Salmonella* infection arise from mishandling by the retail trade or catering outlets, or in the home.

- That the consumer is prepared to pay the cost for proper hygiene at the production level. In fact the consumer will do this only reluctantly or if the need is clearly explained and understood, and even then there is a point at which people will not accept the protective measures. The economic costs of changes must be within the capacity of the producer, and the social cost must not be seen as outweighing the perceived advantage.

The principles of food hygiene that need to be taught are very simple, and practical application of those principles is not very difficult, but imparting the motivation to apply them sometimes seems almost impossible. Teaching must start early in the primary school and be a continuous process, requiring a regular provision of material and regular updating. The impact need not be assessed by elaborate computer scoring, which has been found ineffective, but rather by visual observation of behaviour after teaching. For the education of the public the mass media, and particularly television, should be used and the public should be instructed where to report foodborne illnesses. It is, however, unlikely that deeply entrenched popular perceptions and beliefs related to food will be altered by argument or persuasion alone (*49*).

Paradoxically "culture shock", the introduction of new cash crops, changes in land tenure and in trade patterns, taxation, changes in the labour market, new equipment, and urbanization change food habits more radically than health education. The changes that occur are mostly those linked with prestige, status, and the adoption of different value systems. Such changes can sometimes be beneficial, as for example when they lead to eating more protein; often they result in the replacement of one disease-favouring habit by another unexpected and unwelcome one (*49*).

Behavioural and environmental changes reducing the risk of infection, including changes in eating habits and food storage and preparation, are not simple, "and to constantly pass them off as being well understood will do little to attract the kind of attention of sociomedical sciences they deserve and the kind of skills and dedication needed to solve them" (50). As an experienced food hygienist in Europe has remarked, the government that prohibited raw meat would not survive the next election. Studies of individual awareness of the different diseases and of risk-taking behaviour can contribute to partial understanding only of the occurrence of disease in a given area or population group (49). Food habits have first to be assessed in the context of the given sociocultural situation of the community and the individual disease potential identified. Second, one can pinpoint the areas where change is possible, impossible, or possible under special circumstances, and plan behavioural change so as to avoid creating another set of health problems.

Information, advice and warnings prior to legal sanctions are common practice, but enabling food laws and flexible bylaws are the best means at the disposal of the food control officer.[a] "Social pressure is always more effective than legislation though legislative action can both direct and reinforce social pressure".[b] There is a danger that the public might be inclined to perceive food hygiene as unimportant in the absence of legislative backing. For example, ever since specific legislation has been passed in the United Kingdom to deal with *Salmonella* infection associated with the consumption of frozen liquid egg, there has been no infection from this product.

Aspects of the control of foodborne diseases

The control of foodborne disease is the joint task of many professions: producers, marketing and retail personnel, veterinarians, epidemiologists, sanitary and environmental specialists, educators, the media, and the public in general. The maximum of collaboration is desirable. Many institutions are involved: local authorities, central bodies such as the ministries of agriculture, health, environment, industry and trade, the tourist industry, and the water services. A few of the measures needed are:

— improvement of sanitation in general and provision of safe water supplies

— strict implementation of rules of hygiene and of good manufacturing practices

— appropriate training and education of workers, food-handlers and consumers, as well as keeping health professionals up to date

---

[a]**Blomberg, B.** *Organization of food control.* Unpublished WHO document VPH/WP/SAL/80.4, Geneva, 1980.

[b]**Charles, R.H.G.** *The epidemiology and control of salmonellosis in the United Kingdom.* Unpublished WHO document VPH/WP/SAL/80.8, Geneva, 1980.

— improvement and/or better enforcement of existing legislation and harmonization of the legislation of European countries

— effective inspection and establishment of control points in the operation of plants.

The above measures are, of course, obvious and have been heard a thousand times. Some of the more specific measures needed in connexion with certain prevalent food diseases are:

— the prohibition of antibiotics used in human medicine as growth promoters in animal-rearing or as preservatives and additives in food

— careful scrutiny of the chemicals used in the food industry

— sterilization of animal feeds, irradiation, pelletizing, chemical decontamination of feeds with propionic acid, and pretreatment of feeds as far as possible for economic or health reasons

— improvement of animal husbandry and development as far as possible of pathogen-free herds with attention also to the pastures, the transport of animals and slaughterhouses

— pasteurization of all milk and liquid egg products

— immunization of animals against, for example, *E. coli*, *Salmonella* and *Brucella*

— care in rehabilitation procedures, if allowed, of foods with a slight contamination index

— separation of raw meats from cooked foods and salads in butcher's shops

— particularly, epidemiologicial surveillance of suspected cases and investigation of outbreaks of foodborne diseases to identify the contributing factors and mechanisms by which they occur; bacteriological examinations are indispensable.

Practices in food service establishments that frequently lead to outbreaks are summarized by Bryan (51) as follows: (a) improper cooling, such as keeping cooked foods at room temperature for long periods and refrigerating large quantities of foods in large containers; (b) improper holding of food at bacterial incubating temperatures; (c) lapse of a day or more between preparing and serving food (coupled with one or both of the improper storage practices cited above); (d) inadequate reheating of cooked food; (e) inadequate cooking of raw contaminated food; and (f) handling of raw contaminated food by workers who subsequently handle cooked food, or by equipment that is subsequently in contact with cooked foods before being thoroughly cleaned. Practices at home that frequently lead to outbreaks are the use of contaminated raw ingredients, improper cooling, cross-contamination and inadequate cooking.

Efforts at control have to involve the whole population. Even if only the people directly involved in the food industry are to be addressed the task is enormous; in the Federal Republic of Germany alone there are more than 873 000 persons involved (6).

244

Continuing research is needed into the technologies used in food hygiene monitoring. The controversy about what indicators of food pollution should be used is not yet satisfactorily resolved. There is a growing feeling that indicators such as the coliform count and standards based on total bacterial counts, transferred to food hygiene from water examination, are inadequate, their being unable to reveal anything about clostridia, salmonellae, staphylococci and other microorganisms, for example in the control of ice-cream (52). The differentiation of coliforms from other Enterobacteriaceae is based on their capacity to split lactose. The test thus screens lactose-positive and, at best, facultatively pathogenic bacteria, whereas the primary interest is in lactose-negative organisms. An examination should be made, therefore, for all Enterobacteriaceae and certain anaerobes, or specifically for *E. coli*, because of their closer association than the coliform groups with faecal contamination.

A critical appraisal of salmonellosis surveillance is also needed. While salmonellae are of course undesirable in any food, it has been repeatedly stated that a salmonellosis-free product is difficult to achieve. Present methods are so sensitive that salmonellae can be demonstrated even in amounts (for example 10–100 per 1–25 g of ice cream) that in most people would probably not cause illness, for which a 10^5–10^{10} or even a 10^6–10^8 concentration is needed (52). Understanding of these factors is needed when examining random samples of imported food for *Salmonella*, and it has been recommended that examination be discontinued, particularly when the presence of an identical degree of contamination is to be expected in domestic food of the same type.

The magnitude of the task is not to be underestimated. The authorities have been largely unsuccessful, for example, in preventing the rapid spread in European countries of butcher's shops selling at the same premises, and often by the same person, both unpacked raw meat and cooked food and salads.

There have, however, been recent successes worth mentioning. It was possible to reduce the *Salmonella* content of dust from halls in four rendering plants in the Netherlands from 25.3% in 1973 to 7.4% in 1978–1979. Samples of the products for the same period varied from 11.4% to 2%. The sale of raw meat sausage in the Federal Republic of Germany was prohibited after it was demonstrated that 15.6% of samples contained *Salmonella*, of which 39.4% were *S. typhimurium* (7).

Role of WHO in the field of foodborne diseases

Several WHO programme groups collaborate in the field of foodborne diseases: epidemiological surveillance, the global diarrhoeal disease control programme, and the veterinary public health unit. Their work is complementary and is expressed in the reports of scientific groups. At the regional level in Europe implementation is carried out by the communicable diseases unit and the food safety unit of the environmental health service, with the appropriate technology for health unit participating.

Close collaboration exists among WHO, FAO, the International Commission on Microbiological Specification for Food, the International Organization for Standardization, the International Dairy Federation, and the Association of Official Analytical Chemists.

A WHO programme of international surveillance of salmonellosis, based on national *Salmonella* reference laboratories (nine of them in Europe) started in 1967 but was terminated in 1976 owing to the reduction of staff. This programme, although aiming primarily at the identification of *Salmonella* serotypes circulating in different countries rather than at a thorough analysis of the dynamics of circulating pathogens, recorded an increase in the incidence of *Salmonella*, an increasing importation of rare serotypes, and the association of certain organisms with certain countries, certain animal or food sources, or a certain type of antibiotic resistance. In agreement with the WHO policy of full utilization of its system of collaborating centres, it was decided that this work would be more economically and comprehensively carried out if based not at WHO headquarters or in a Regional Office but in specially designated centres. At the same time the view was expressed by a number of countries in Europe that surveillance should cover not only salmonellosis but also other foodborne diseases. The function of the former WHO programme has in part been taken over by the collaborating centre in London until a regional foodborne disease surveillance centre can be created. A WHO surveillance programme for the control of foodborne infections and intoxications in Europe, based at the FAO/WHO collaborating centre for research and training in food hygiene in Berlin (West), was established in 1980. Fourteen countries are now participating in the programme.

The main objectives of the WHO surveillance programme are:

- to identify the causes of foodborne diseases and determine the factors contributing to the spread of these diseases
- to make available and distribute relevant surveillance information
- to cooperate with national authorities in the identification of priorities and use of resources to meet both emergency and other needs in the prevention and control of foodborne diseases.

Although surveillance is the central activity in the programme, the overall aim is action to prevent and control foodborne diseases. It is obvious that such action must be taken at the national level and that international involvement is needed to secure the necessary coordination and cooperation. The international involvement is intended to stimulate national effort and produce early and long-term benefits. The long-term benefits include:

— the strengthening of food control practices

— the improvement of epidemiological investigational procedures

— more efficient laboratory analyses of suspect food and water samples and clinical specimens

— improved reporting of foodborne diseases

246

Table 46. Agents of foodborne disease included
in the WHO surveillance programme for the control
of foodborne infections and intoxications in Europe

Bacteria, including their toxins:
  Bacillus cereus
  Clostridium botulinum
  Clostridium perfringens
  Salmonella typhi and *Salmonella paratyphi* A, B, C
  Salmonella (other than *S. typhi* and *S. paratyphi*)
  Shigella
  Staphylococcus aureus
  Vibrio cholerae and related vibrios
  Other bacteria, e.g. *Brucella*
                        Campylobacter
                        Escherichia coli
                        Francisella tularensis
                        Mycobacterium
                        Vibrio parahaemolyticus
                        Yersinia enterocolitica

Parasites and protozoa:
  Cysticercus/Taenia
  Echinococcus
  Trichinella
  Other parasites, e.g. *Entamoeba histolytica*
                         Giardia
                         Toxoplasma

Viruses and rickettsiae:
  Hepatitis A
  Rotavirus
  Other viruses, e.g. echovirus
  Coxiella burnetii

Toxic animals:
  Fish, e.g. scombroid poisoning
  Shellfish, e.g. paralytic shellfish poison
  Other animals

Toxic plants:
  Mushrooms. e.g. *Amanita* toxin
  Other plant poisons

Mycotoxins:
  Aflatoxins
  Other mycotoxins

Chemical contaminants and residues:
  Heavy metals, e.g. copper, lead, mercury, tin, zinc
  Organochlorine compounds, e.g. polychlorinated biphenyls
  Organophosphorus compounds, e.g. parathion
  Other chemical compounds, e.g. monosodium glutamate,
  polybrominated biphenyls

— identification of significant trends in foodborne diseases

— encouragement of research on new foodborne disease organisms, toxins and chemicals

— stimulation of surveys on foods regularly implicated in illness

— evaluation of the cost–benefit of foodborne disease control

— improved coordination among existing international collaborating centres

— improved health manpower training and utilization

— harmonization of legislation.

An international programme of this type must of necessity be based on surveillance activities at the national level, where the responsibility for investigating, collecting and analysing national data often lies with different government authorities. To avoid communication difficulties there must be effective liaison, particularly between the medical and veterinary services.

The collaborating centre functions as the international contact point in the programme. On behalf of FAO and WHO it collects data from participating countries through the national contact points and interprets them, with particular attention to regional and international trends and factors that influence the illness, the cost–benefit, and the specific control action taken.

The type of data required and collected should fulfil the main objectives of the programme and will depend on what countries are able and willing to provide. A proposed list of groups of causal agents for surveillance, with examples of individual agents, is given in Table 46. The information required on epidemiological and clinical investigation and on the vehicles responsible (food and water) is given in Table 47. Qualitative and quantitative data are integrated by electronic data processing, and the results will be presented to national experts for discussion. As the centre in Berlin (West) collaborates with four other WHO regions, the conditions are suitable for an expansion of the surveillance programme to the global scale at a later stage.

One of the aims of the programme is to provide an early warning report before trade restrictive measures are envisaged (which, in the absence of an effective international system, are all too often applied). Such early warning reports cover situations when (a) internationally distributed foods or feeds have resulted in incidents, or contaminated lots have been identified; (b) incidents occur associated with international caterers and carriers (by air, train or ship); (c) illness occurs among members of tourist groups or is introduced by tourists or immigrants; (d) incidents of unusual foodborne diseases are recorded in a country; (e) the incidents concern a disease of a severe nature; or (f) other matters are considered to be an emergency by the country making the report.

248

Table 47. Report of incident, WHO surveillance programme for the control of foodborne infections and intoxications in Europe[a]

1. Place of incident:[b] _____
2. Date and hour of onset of illness: first person _____ last person _____
3. Number of people: ill _____, at risk _____, hospitalized _____, died _____
4. Symptoms: per cent of total ill: nausea _____, vomiting _____, diarrhoea _____
5. Incubation times: shortest _____, longest _____, median _____
6. Duration of illness: shortest _____, longest _____, median _____
7. Food/vehicle involved: _____
    Confirmation:[c] epidemiological   laboratory   unconfirmed
8. Place where food prepared: _____ date and time: _____
    For commercial products: brand _____ lot No. _____
9. Methods of processing and preparation: _____
    _____
10. Place where food was contaminated:[d] _____
11. Place where food was eaten:[e] _____ date and time: _____
12. Source of food/water/vehicle, if applicable:[f] _____
13. Factors contributing to incident:[g,h] _____
    Interpretation: _____
14. Results of laboratory tests: (testing laboratory _____)

Specimens from	Number		Details/comments agent, count, concentration, types, etc.
	Tested	Positive	
Ill people			
Well people			
Food handlers			
Suspect food			
Other foods (specify)			
Environment (specify)			

Presumed causative agent: _____ ICD code No.: _____

16. Name of reporting centre: _____ date: _____
    Name of reporting officer: _____ telephone No.: _____

                    Signature _____

[a] Attach narrative report and other national forms, if appropriate.

[b] Indicate country, province/district and municipality (city, town, village, etc.) as appropriate.

[c] Confirmation of food/vehicle is based on epidemiological evidence, e.g. food-specific attack rates, or laboratory analysis, e.g. counts, toxin levels.

[d] Example of entries: farm, stream, food-processing plant (e.g. canning establishment), warehouse, vending machine, retail store, home, food service establishment (e.g. restaurant, cafeteria). More than one establishment may be listed, if applicable.

[e] Example of entries: restaurant, canteen, school, medical care facility, home, camp, picnic, goods or passenger carriers (airline, train, ship).

[f] Sources of water may include: public supply, semi-public supply, individual household supply, institution, bottled water, camp or recreation area supply, spring, stream.

[g] Example of entries for foodborne outbreaks: improper refrigeration, improper hot holding, preparing food a day or more before serving, inadequate cooling after heat processing, inadequate reheating, obtaining food from unsafe source, using a contaminated ingredient in an uncooked product, contamination by infected person, improper cleaning of equipment, toxic container or pipeline, addition of toxic chemical or natural toxicant. If more than one factor has contributed, list all that are applicable.

[h] Example of entries for waterborne outbreaks: overflow of sewage, seepage of sewage, flooding, use of untreated water, use of supplementary source, water inadequately treated, interruption of disinfection, inadequate disinfection, deficiencies in other treatment, processing, cross-connection, backsiphoning, contamination of mains during construction or repair, improper location of well or spring, use of water not intended for drinking, contamination of storage facility, contamination through creviced or fissured rock. If more than one factor has contributed, list all that are applicable.

References

1. *Proceedings of the World Congress on Foodborne Infections and Intoxications, Berlin, 29 June–3 July 1980.* Berlin (West), Robert von Ostertag Institute, 1982.
2. **Hogarth, J.** *Glossary of health care terminology.* Copenhagen, WHO Regional Office for Europe, 1975 (Public Health in Europe No. 4).
3. *Foodborne disease surveillance, annual summary for 1978.* Atlanta, GA, Centers for Disease Control, 1979.
4. **Kendereški, S.** The problem of alimentary intoxications and toxic infections in Yugoslavia. *In: Proceedings of the World Congress on Foodborne Infections and Intoxications, Berlin, 29 June–3 July 1980.* Berlin (West), Robert von Ostertag Institute, 1982, pp. 223–227.
5. **Germanier, R.** Present status of immunization against typhoid fever. *Boletín de la Oficina Sanitaria Panamericana,* **82**: 300–311 (1977).
6. **Weise, H.J.** Krankheitseinschleppungen in die Bundesrepublic Deutschland einschliesslich Berlin (West) 1976–80. *Bundesgesundheitsblatt,* **24**: 241–250 (1981).
7. **Brandis, H. et al.** Beitrag zur Epidemiologie von *Salmonella typhimurium,* dargestellt an Hand der Ergebnisse der Lysotype aus den Jahren 1969–1978. *Öffentliche Gesundheitswesen,* **42**: 75–128 (1980).
8. *Economic aspects of communicable diseases:* report on a WHO Working Group. Copenhagen, WHO Regional Office for Europe, 1982 (EURO Reports and Studies No. 68), p. 12.
9. **Schothorst, M. van.** Babies as a source of salmonella contamination in households. *In: Proceedings of the World Congress on Foodborne Infections and Intoxications, Berlin, 29 June–3 July 1980.* Berlin (West), Robert von Ostertag Institute, 1982, pp. 387–390.
10. **Forbes, G.I. et al.** Outbreaks of cysticercosis and salmonellosis in cattle following the application of sludge to grazing land in Scotland. *In: Proceedings of the World Congress on Foodborne Infections and Intoxications, Berlin, 29 June–3 July 1980.* Berlin (West), Robert von Ostertag Institute, 1982, pp. 439–440.
11. **Breer, C.** Salmonella infection in tourists. *In: Proceedings of the World Congress on Foodborne Infections and Intoxications, Berlin, 29 June–3 July 1980.* Berlin (West), Robert von Ostertag Institute, 1982, pp. 155–156.
12. **Pöhn, H.P.** Salmonellosis in man in the Federal Republic of Germany. *In: Proceedings of the World Congress on Foodborne Infections and Intoxications, Berlin, 29 June–3 July 1980.* Berlin (West), Robert von Ostertag Institute, 1982, pp. 334–339.
13. **Gork, F.P.** Foodborne infections and intoxication in international travel. *In: Proceedings of the World Congress on Foodborne Infections and Intoxications, Berlin, 29 June–3 July 1980.* Berlin (West), Robert von Ostertag Institute, 1982, pp. 126–133.
14. **Threlfall, E.Y. et al.** Spread of multiresistant strains of *Salmonella typhimurium* phage type 204 and 193 in Britain. *British medical journal,* **2**: 997 (1978).

15. **Hellström, L.** Food transmitted *S. enteritidis* epidemics in 28 schools. *In: Proceedings of the World Congress on Foodborne Infections and Intoxications, Berlin, 29 June–3 July 1980*. Berlin (West), Robert von Ostertag Institute, 1982, pp. 397–400.
16. Surveillance of food poisoning and *Salmonella* infection. *Weekly epidemiological record*, **56**: 1–4 (1981).
17. **Bryan, F.L.** Diseases transmitted by foods contaminated by wastewater. *Journal of food protection*, **40**: 45–56 (1977).
18. **Cherry, W.B. et al.** Detection of salmonellae in foodstuffs, feces, and water by immunofluorescence. *Annals of the New York Academy of Sciences*, **254**: 350–368 (1975).
19. **Hess, E. & Breer, C.** *Salmonella* Epidemiologie und Grünlanddüngung mit Klärschlamm. *Zentralblat für Bakteriologie, Mikrobiologie und Hygiene, I. Abt.*, **161**: 54–60 (1975).
20. **Reilly, W.J. et al.** Human and animal salmonellosis in Scotland associated with environmental contamination. *In: Proceedings of the World Congress on Foodborne Infections and Intoxications, Berlin, 29 June–3 July 1980*. Berlin (West), Robert von Ostertag Institute, 1982, pp. 344–346.
21. **Danielsson-Tham, M.L. & Wadström, T.** Gram-negative enterotoxigenic bacteria in food associated with outbreaks of food poisoning. *In: Proceedings of the World Congress on Foodborne Infections and Intoxications, Berlin, 29 June–3 July 1980*. Berlin (West), Robert von Ostertag Institute, 1982, pp. 306–308.
22. **Pohl, U. et al.** Eine Lebensmittelvergiftung durch *Escherichia coli* 0 124 (K72) H — in einen Ferienlagen. *Deutsche Gesundheitswesen*, **35**: 1195–1198 (1980).
23. **Raska, K. et al.** To the origin of contamination of foodstuffs by enterotoxigenic staphylococci. *In: Proceedings of the World Congress on Foodborne Infections and Intoxications, Berlin, 29 June–3 July 1980*. Berlin (West), Robert von Ostertag Institute, 1982, pp. 272–274.
24. **Cuculic, M. et al.** Observation on food poisoning among tourists in the Rijeka subregion. *In: Proceedings of the World Congress on Foodborne Infections and Intoxications, Berlin, 29 June–3 July 1980*. Berlin (West), Robert von Ostertag Institute, 1982, pp. 163–167.
25. **Dekeyser, P. et al.** Acute enteritis due to related vibrio: first positive stool cultures. *Journal of infectious diseases*, **125**: 390 (1972).
26. **Kosunen, T.** Gastroenteritis caused by *Campylobacter fetus* ssp. *jejuni*. *In: Proceedings of the World Congress on Foodborne Infections and Intoxications, Berlin, 29 June–3 July 1980*. Berlin (West), Robert von Ostertag Institute, 1982, pp. 309–313.
27. **Meyer, K.F.** The status of botulism as a world health problem. *Bulletin of the World Health Organization*, **15**: 281–298 (1956).
28. **Haagsma, I.** Clostridial diseases in Europe. *In:* Steele, J.H., ed. *Handbook of zoonoses*. Boca Raton, CRC Press, 1979, pp. 225–236.
29. **Huss, H.H.** Some aspects of the epidemiology of type E botulism. *In: Proceedings of the World Congress on Foodborne Infections and Intoxications, Berlin, 29 June–3 July 1980*. Berlin (West), Robert von Ostertag Institute, 1982, pp. 294–297.

30. **Hechelman, H. et al.** Relevance of *Cl. botulinum* to fermented sausage and raw ham. *In: Proceedings of the World Congress on Foodborne Infections and Intoxications, Berlin, 29 June–3 July 1980.* Berlin (West), Robert von Ostertag Institute, 1982, pp. 823–825.

31. **Wiegand, D.** About the frequency of *Clostridium perfringens* in animals. The bacteriological and toxicological characterization of the isolated strains and the resulting consequences for bacteriological meat investigation. *In: Proceedings of the World Congress on Foodborne Infections and Intoxications, Berlin, 29 June–3 July 1980.* Berlin (West), Robert von Ostertag Institute, 1982, pp. 287–293.

32. **Raevuori, M.** Foodborne disease outbreaks in Finland in 1978–79. *In: Proceedings of the World Congress on Foodborne Infections and Intoxications, Berlin, 29 June–3 July 1980.* Berlin (West), Robert von Ostertag Institute, 1982, pp. 241–243.

33. **Stringer, M.F. et al.** Application of serologic typing to the investigation of outbreaks of *Clostridium perfringens* food poisoning, 1970–1978. *Journal of hygiene*, **84**: 443–456 (1980).

34. **Wilson, G.S. & Miles, A.** *Principles of bacteriology, virology and immunology*, 6th ed. London, Arnold, 1975, Vol. 2, pp. 2075, 2258.

35. **Velimirovic, B.** The geographical distribution of the human disease due to *V. parahaemolyticus*. *Zentralblatt für Bakteriologie, Parasitenkunde, Infektionskrankheiten und Hygiene*, I Abt., **227**: 385–397 (1972).

36. **Bech, K. et al.** *Yersinia enterocolitica* infection and thyroid diseases. *Acta endocrinologica*, **84**: 87 (1977).

37. **Lassen, J.** *Yersinia enterocolitica* in drinking water. *Scandinavian journal of infectious diseases*, **4**: 125–127 (1972).

38. **Mollaret, H.H. et al.** *In: Contributions to microbiology and immunology*. Basle, Karger, 1979, Vol. 5, pp. 174–184.

39. **Gilbert, R.J.** *Bacillus cereus* gastroenteritis. *In:* Riemann, H. & Bryan, F.L., ed. *Foodborne infection and intoxication*, 2nd ed. London, Academic Press, 1979.

40. **Bezdenezhnykh, I.S. & Nikiforov, V.H.** Epidemiological analysis of anthrax in Sverdlovsk. *Žurnal microbiologii, epidemiologii, immunologii*, 1 May 1980, pp. 111–113.

41. **Bachmann, P. et al.** Isolation of viruses from the organs of freshly slaughtered animals. *In: Proceedings of the World Congress on Foodborne Infections and Intoxications, Berlin, 29 June–3 July 1980.* Berlin (West), Robert von Ostertag Institute, 1982, pp. 269–271.

42. **Danner, K. & Mayre, A.** Virus persistence during the processing of foodstuffs of animal origin. *In: Proceedings of the World Congress on Foodborne Infections and Intoxications, Berlin, 29 June–3 July 1980.* Berlin (West), Robert von Ostertag Institute, 1982, pp. 888–895.

43. **Gilbert, R.J. et al.** Scombrotoxic fish poisoning: features of the first 50 incidents to be reported in Britain. *British medical journal*, **281**: 71–72 (1969).

44. **Aires, P.I.** Fish poisoning risk associated with food other than meat, poultry and shellfish. *Health and hygiene*, **3**: 11–26 (1979).

45. **Bourée, P. et al.** A propos d'une épidémie de trichinose dans la banlieue parisienne. *Bulletin de la Société de Pathologie exotique*, **69**: 177–178 (1976).
46. **Steele, J.H.** Trichinosis: a world problem with extensive sylvatic reservoirs. *In: Wildlife diseases.* New York, Plenum, 1976, pp. 565–584.
47. **Canestri-Trotti, G. & Gramenzi, F.** Trichinosi. *Bollettino epidemiologico nazionale*, No. 1–3, p. 33 (1982).
48. **Bommer, W. et al.** Outbreak of trichinellosis in a youth centre of Niedersachsen by air-dried imported camel meat. *In: Proceedings of the World Congress on Foodborne Infections and Intoxications, Berlin, 29 June–3 July 1980.* Berlin (West), Robert von Ostertag Institute, 1982, pp. 441–445.
49. **Velimirovic, B.** Food habits and their influence on foodborne disease. *In: Proceedings of the World Congress on Foodborne Infections and Intoxications, Berlin, 29 June–3 July 1980.* Berlin (West), Robert von Ostertag Institute, 1982, pp. 87–101.
50. **England, R.** More myths in international health planning. *American journal of public health*, **68**: 153–159 (1978).
51. **Bryan, F.L.** Factors contributing to foodborne outbreaks. *Journal of food practices*, **41**: 816–827 (1978).
52. **Müller, E.H.** Probleme der Speiseeis-Überwachung aus hygienischer Sicht. *Offentliche Gesundheitswesen*, **42**: 612–617 (1980).

6

Bacterial pathology

H.H. Mollaret[a]

Three factors always make it difficult to assess an epidemic situation.

1. The volatile nature of the situation itself, which can only be discerned *a posteriori*, when in most cases it is too late to identify all the parameters responsible for the change that has occurred. One is then generally limited to a recording of the fact, without being in a position to provide any explanation.

2. The extreme difficulty of distinguishing between the actual situation and the human factors that play a part in its assessment or, more simply, the observation: the quality of the clinical, epidemiological and biological data possessed by the medical practitioners; the technical level of the laboratories carrying out the biological diagnosis; and the diversity of medical attitudes about recourse to the laboratory to establish the diagnosis, the search for the latter all too often giving way to the immediate introduction of blind antibiotic therapy.

3. The date of the first isolation in a given region of a pathogenic bacterium previously unknown in that same region does not at present allow any conclusion to be drawn as to the actual date of its introduction. This reservation, though obvious, is frequently omitted in assessments of epidemic situations. A number of exceptional observations have shown that often a long period of time (30 years in the case of *Yersinia enterocolitica* and *Legionella pneumophila*, one year in the case of *Pseudomonas pseudomallei*) has elapsed between the introduction of a bacterial species in a region and its emergence in pathology. The role of human factors is fundamental here, influencing as they do the information on the disease and the development of appropriate diagnostic techniques and systematic screening. In short, the recognition of or failure to recognize the disease depends finally on the quality of these purely human factors.

The major problem is essentially one of data, which are still inadequate, imprecise and fragmentary. Of all the fields of pathology, that of

[a]Institut Pasteur, Paris, France.

infectious diseases is undoubtedly the one about which we are most poorly informed. The first reason for this deficiency lies in the lack of basic data, i.e. the failure of practitioners to notify infectious diseases. Many reasons have been cited for this: indifference, scepticism, excessive workload, fear of triggering restrictive measures, etc. In fact, physicians fail to declare infectious diseases because they are not sufficiently aware of the importance of doing so and particularly because they do not feel personally concerned. So long as notification remains just another administrative procedure for the practitioner, without his receiving in return the share of the information to which he is entitled, much of the data will be lost. Data should not be the confidential property of administrations only; they are obtained from the practitioners and should be returned to them to inform them of the situation.

Next, what has to be notified? We shall examine below the extent to which infectious pathology as it presents itself to the practitioner differs from infectious pathology as it is taught and classified. Here we may say that notification as it currently exists takes account of only a very small proportion of infection generally.

The actual procedures of notification need to be examined. As far as causes of death are concerned, cases of diabetes, cirrhosis, leukaemia, cancer, etc. are listed in the ICD chapter corresponding to the original disorder and not under the heading "infection". Infection, which is the main cause of death in intensive care units, is not reflected in the statistics, being replaced by the original reason for hospitalization. In the field of rheumatology, which accounts for 15% of consultations in Western Europe, cases of so-called "reactive" arthritis are notified as "rheumatic disease" and not listed according to the bacterial agents responsible for them.

The value of the notifications received gives rise to serious reservations. In outpatient practice, less than 2% of patients with "infections" are the subject of laboratory tests and over half of the examinations prescribed are the "standard" ones of cytobacteriological tests of the urine, which in the majority of cases are of no value in establishing or confirming the diagnosis. More specific tests, such as blood tests and especially stool tests, are still carried out only in exceptional circumstances in urban areas.

Another information gap concerns the anthropozoonoses; it arises from the customary lack of communication between physicians and veterinarians, who come under different ministries and administrative structures. Anthropozoonoses, while a common feature of the two fields of medicine, remain administratively separate. The primary role of national reference centres and of WHO collaborating centres should be to link the two sources of information.

A final difficulty lies in the difference between infectious pathology as it is described and taught and as it presents in reality; the contents of a medical textbook or a list of notifiable diseases is remote from what the practitioner actually encounters daily. For one case of typhoid fever, or scarlet fever, or a typical pneumonia, there are many poorly definable, unclassifiable, but real infections of the upper respiratory tract that qualify for immediate antibiotic therapy. A survey in France in 1980 on reasons for consultations shows the following proportions (certain syndromes such as diarrhoea have been excluded because of the lack of a precise etiology):

upper respiratory tract infections	15.84%
lower respiratory tract infections	7.04%
urinary tract infections (women)	1.62%
fevers with rash	1.47%
genital infections (women)	1.32%
skin infections	0.62%
otorhinolaryngological infections	0.51%
urinary tract infections (men)	0.46%
genital infections (men)	0.18%
bone infections	0.03%
infected wounds	0.03%
typhoid fever	0.03%

These figures show that infection, which in 1960 was said to have fallen to seventh place among the causes of death, now constitutes over a quarter of the reasons for consultation. They also show that, even though there has certainly been a regression in the major pathological entities, infection proper is gaining ground.

Reappearance of infections that have largely regressed over the last 30 years

Pneumococcal, meningococcal and group A streptococcal infections have reappeared, their distribution and advance being unconnected with the emergence of resistant strains and unexplainable. The same is true of tuberculosis, the regular decline of which has been marked by two pauses in Western Europe, probably in connection with the high incidence of this disease among Asian immigrants in 1960 and immigrants from East Africa in 1970. The situation is similar for syphilis, gonorrhoea and, generally speaking, all sexually transmitted diseases, which mark a worldwide recrudescence.

The reappearance or increased frequency of certain infections may be accompanied by changes in their clinical picture. This is so for gonococcal and meningococcal diseases. The discovery of *Neisseria gonorrhoeae* in the otorhinolaryngological region, exceptional before 1960, has become sufficiently frequent in the last ten years for some authorities to recommend systematic pharyngeal swabbing in any test for the presence of gonococci. This new form of gonococcal infection, linked chiefly with orogenital and sometimes mouth-to-mouth transmission, manifests itself clinically in a third of cases in the form of tonsillitis, parotitis, stomatitis and ulcers of the tongue. It is also transmitted by asymptomatic vectors, with epidemiologically serious consequences.

N. meningitidis, whose habitat was until recently limited strictly to the rhinopharynx, is now beginning to be isolated from the urethra and the rectum. This extension of the areas capable of being colonized by the gonococcus and the meningococcus (the frequency varying according to the sex and the homosexual or heterosexual character of the patient, with some seasonal character as regards the meningococcus) should henceforth make obligatory full bacterial identification of any *Neisseria* of whatever origin and systematic search for possible β-lactamase production. This recrudescence of gonococcal infection in clinically different forms has been accompanied, since 1976, by the appearance of two types of β-lactamase-producing strains, the first originating in South-East Asia and later found on the west coast of the United States, the second originating in West Africa; they have now been isolated in Belgium, France, the Netherlands, Poland, Scandinavia, Switzerland and the United Kingdom. The potential hazard of these strains is twofold. First, the South-East Asian strains carry three plasmids that give rise to two pathways of spread and resistance, the one being sexual, the other strain-to-strain transmission. Further, the hypothesis has been put forward that one of these plasmids has been acquired from *Haemophilus influenzae*, an opportunistic bacterium of the pharynx. In theory there is nothing to prevent this gonococcal resistance from being transmitted to the meningococcus, and the fact that the two *Neisseria* have recently been colonizing identical territory may well facilitate this.

The frequency and clinical picture of pasteurellosis have also changed. Before the First World War, in general milder forms predominated over serious forms; since the Second World War, after undergoing an appreciable diminution between the wars, pasteurellosis has recurred in a new form, the so-called "inoculation pasteurellosis" following a bite. It would be tempting to link this recrudescence in its new clinical form with the steady increase in the number of domestic dogs and cats that are most often responsible for the inoculation bite. But there are some discordant aspects, such as the fact that this type of pasteurellosis is rare among veterinarians, who are the first to be exposed to bites.

Geographical spread of certain bacterial infections

Infection spreads in two ways: by the extension of the areas of distribution of existing infections, and by the importation of previously absent infections. Three examples may be taken as typical of the first type of spread: tularaemia, leptospirosis and brucellosis.

Tularaemia, bacteriologically demonstrated in the USSR in 1928 (although some clinical documents testify to its existence since 1897), was next found in Norway in 1929 and Sweden in 1931. Its westward progress was marked by the first isolations in Turkey in 1935, in Austria in the same year (several suspected cases since 1917), in Czechoslovakia in 1936, in Romania in 1938, and in France in 1945. Despite the diversity of animal species involved in its cycle (hare, lemming, vole, hamster, etc.) and the different modes of human contamination (by water, by direct contact with the animal, or through the bites of ticks or insects) the disease retains a remarkable unity of anatomical and clinical features in both man and animals.

The regular geographical spread of leptospirosis in Europe is accompanied by a loosening of the preferential relationships between certain serological groups and certain animal species. Thus *Leptospira canicola*, initially found in dogs, is being more and more frequently isolated from pigs, cattle and horses, while inversely *L. icterohaemorrhagiae* accounts for up to one third of the strains isolated in dogs. *L. bataviae*, introduced into the Italian ricefields between 1934 and 1936, is now present throughout Europe. Although some associations, such as that between *Microtus* and *L. grippotyphosa*, remain very stable, they do not prevent this form of leptospirosis from spreading to other animal species, nor do they prevent an increase in the frequency of *L. pomona* isolations in *Microtus*.

Generally speaking, under the influence of changes in the ecological conditions favouring an increase in the opportunities of transmission between feral hosts and domestic animals, the enzootic cycle of the leptospirae is intensifying and diversifying and the number of species affected is growing, as is the area of spread of the disease. Although this general area is increasing in size, the incidence is not uniform; there is a tendency for leptospirosis to be found more in urban areas, in connexion with the development and centralization in and around cities of abattoirs, docks, food industries, etc., all of which attract the rodent hosts.

Brucellosis has experienced the same geographical spread through Europe as leptospirosis since the beginning of the century, with the same tendency towards an increase in the number of species affected and the same loosening on the part of each *Brucella* species of its initial affinity for a given animal species.

Pseudomonas pseudomallei and *Plesiomonas shigelloides* are two examples of imported pathogenic bacteria. Although the date (before 1966) and the mode of introduction of melioidosis into Spain are not known, its introduction into France can be dated accurately (1974), since in all probability two pandas sent from China to Paris were the intermediaries. *P. pseudomallei* was isolated a year later during an epizootic at the Botanical Gardens of the Natural History Museum, Paris. From there the infection spread to stud farms in the Paris region by unidentified means (possibly via manure, rodents or pigeons). *P. pseudomallei* has so far been isolated almost always from horses in some 15 locations in France (only two indigenous human cases are known).

Plesiomonas shigelloides was known for some 30 years as a diarrhoeal agent in tropical and subtropical areas, especially on the coasts of the Pacific and Indian Oceans. Since 1953 it has been isolated in Czechoslovakia, France, the Federal Republic of Germany, Italy, the United Kingdom and Yugoslavia. However, it has not yet been possible to ascertain whether each case was imported by a traveller or was related to an infection already existing in Europe.

Alongside these imported diseases, the present situation with regard to typhoid fever and paratyphoid A fever should be considered. The dramatic regression of indigenous European cases has been accompanied by an increase in the number of cases imported by returning travellers;

95% of *Salmonella paratyphi* A strains isolated in the United Kingdom originate outside Europe. Of *S. typhi* strains, 90% of those isolated in the United Kingdom and 75% of those isolated in France are likewise from outside Europe. Importation occurs in all countries of Europe in varying proportions.

Similar changes may be observed with regard to bacillary dysentery: in the United Kingdom the number of notified cases has fallen by 90% in the past 20 years, mainly owing to the growing rarity of *Shigella sonnei*. At the same time, the importation of *Sh. flexneri* has led to changes in the age groups affected and in the seasonal nature of these infections.

Human anthrax, whose regression in Western Europe has followed that of anthrax in animals, is tending to become an imported disease; most cases in the past 30 years or so have been caused by the handling of animal products originating in enzootic areas in the Middle and Near East and Asia. Human anthrax, which was initially found in rural areas, its spread reflecting that of the disease in herbivores, is being succeeded by urban or industrial anthrax, which is localized at the points of arrival (ports, docks) or where infected wool, skins or carcases are treated.

Appearance of serious infections caused by known bacteria until recently regarded as non-pathogenic

In the front line of these appears the inoffensive *Bacillus prodigiosus*, now known as *Serratia marcescens*, a type of saprophyte that has become pathogenic and all the more formidable in that it is often multiresistant. A number of other species or genera of bacteria have acquired or are in the process of acquiring the same pathogenic potential. On the basis of the literature, and especially in the light of the list of strains sent to the Institut Pasteur in Paris for identification, the following species may be mentioned.

- Group B streptococci, known for almost a century, the incidence of which in cases of septicaemia and meningitis in neonates has, for some 20 years, shown a tendency to approximate that of *Listeria*. At present they are the main bacterial agents in serious forms of neonatal infection.

- *Gemella haemolysans*, isolated for the first time in 1938, and long considered to be a simple saprophyte of the mucosa, is now known to cause endocarditis.

- Two normal parasites of the buccal cavity, *Actinobacillus actinomycetes comitans*, known since 1912, and *Eikenella corrodens*, known since 1948, have been isolated in cases of septicaemia, meningitis and suppuration.

- Certain bacteria that have a plant environment, such as *Erwinia* spp. and especially *Agrobacterium tumefaciens*, classically regarded strictly as a plant pathogen, have been isolated by blood culture.

260

- *Aeromonas* (*A. hydrophilia*, *A. sobria*), originally isolated by blood culture in immunodepressed subjects, has been isolated during focal or intestinal infection in subjects who show no apparent signs of ill health.

- Reference should also be made to *Flavobacterium*, *Corynebacterium vaginale*, *Pseudomonas cepecia*, *Moraxella*, certain types of *Kingella*, certain types of *Achromobacterium*, *Cardiobacterium hominis* and *Brevibacterium*, which are being encountered more and more frequently as superinfectants or as agents responsible for endocarditis or septicaemia.

This list is not exhaustive; it includes only species that are being isolated with abnormal frequency in man during serious illness. These microorganisms are the pathogens of tomorrow. Whether they were initially saprophytic bacteria in water, soil or plants, their pathogenic advance is difficult to explain; it shows that the inventory of pathogenic bacteria will never be finally completed and that new agents of infection, if not new diseases, will continue to make their appearance. It also shows that, apart from hospital infections and medical procedures such as catheterization, tracheotomy, endoscopy and immunosuppression that have made certain species of bacteria pathogenic (staphylococci, *Bacillus pyocyaneus*, *Klebsiella*, *Enterobacter*, etc., the Gram-positive kinds that predominated around 1930 having been rapidly overtaken by the Gram-negative kinds) there are other factors, as yet unknown, which allow other formerly non-pathogenic groups of bacteria to become implanted in apparently healthy people.

Appearance of new pathological forms resulting from recently identified pathogenic bacteria

Examples of these are *Campylobacter* enteritis, *Vibrio parahaemolyticus* infections and, in veterinary pathology, infectious metritis in Equidae, which appeared in the United Kingdom in 1977 and whose recently identified agent, *Haemophilus equigenitalis*, has been found in France, the Federal Republic of Germany and elsewhere. Two infections in particular are of interest in this respect: legionnaires' disease and yersiniosis.

The spectactular discovery of *Legionella pneumophila* in the United States in 1977 is noteworthy for the fact that an early example had already been preserved in store for 30 years as a "rickettsia-like" agent and that, several years prior to the episode in Philadelphia in July 1976, other outbreaks of legionnaires' disease had already occurred, as *a posteriori* studies have demonstrated in the United States (Washington DC, 1965; Pontiac, 1968; James River, 1973; Philadelphia, 1974) and in Spain (Benidorm, 1973). It is also noteworthy that, in connexion with the episode in Philadelphia, attention was alerted both by its mass character (221 cases of serious lung disease, 34 deaths) and by the statistical services of the Department of Public Health, which noted an excess number of 26 deaths between 27 July and 16 August 1976 (the Congress of the American Legion was held from 21 to 24 July) compared with the usual mortality for the age group in question.

It should be emphasized that, as soon as European laboratories were in possession of the diagnostic techniques, the existence of legionnaires' disease was immediately recognized in Austria, Denmark, France, the Federal Republic of Germany, Italy, the Netherlands, Portugal, Spain, Sweden and the United Kingdom. A notable feature is ecological; as the investigations showed, *L. pneumophila* is a common bacterium of the natural environment. Before it was discovered, an analysis of cases of lung disease occurring in 1965 in Washington DC had raised the question of the air at an excavation site; we are now aware of the role of aerosols caused by air-conditioning systems. Legionnaires' disease is a typical example of a new disease caused by a bacterium in the external environment that has been given its chance by human activity to cause an epidemic.

Yersinia enterocolitica infection, now found throughout Europe, is another example. While the disease has appeared in man with some frequency in Western Europe from 1965 onwards, microbial strains had already been collected under various names ("unidentified micro-organism", "*Bacterium enterocoliticum*") in the United States since 1923, in Denmark before 1932, in Switzerland in 1948; they were only recognized as authentic *Y. enterocolitica* in 1956. Once again there is a gap of some 30 years between bacteriological proof of the existence of this *Yersinia* in Europe and its appearance in human pathology.

An analysis of various parameters enables us to put forward the following explanation for this clinical emergence of *Y. enterocolitica* infection in France. Whereas almost all pathogenic bacteria have an optimum growth temperature of between 20°C and 40°C, *Yersinia* — in particular *Y. enterocolitica* — is capable of reproducing at temperatures of between 4°C and 10°C. At these temperatures the growth of almost all other bacterial species is inhibited, and *Y. enterocolitica* is the only one to continue reproducing. This feature is used to advantage in the laboratory to make preferential isolations of *Y. enterocolitica* from stools or from samples of water, soil and food.

Another characteristic is the variability of the pathogenic potential of *Y. enterocolitica* according to the incubation temperature. When innoculated into the peritoneum of the mouse, a strain cultivated previously at 37°C is rapidly eliminated, whereas the same strain continues to reproduce if it has been previously cultivated at 25°C. Thus, cold favours both the reproduction and the pathogenicity of *Y. enterocolitica*.

In the years that preceded the appearance of infection in man — an infection contracted via the digestive tract — three important changes took place in France in food and eating habits.

1. Food safes, which were exposed to the ambient temperature, were gradually replaced by refrigerators, in which the temperature of between 4°C and 10°C favours the reproduction and pathogenicity of *Y. entero-*

colitica. In 1954 only 7% of French households had refrigerators; the proportion rose to 8.4% in 1957, then shot up to 26.8% in 1960, 37.1% in 1962, and 91.3% in 1977.

2. The items of food most regularly and massively infected by the *Y. enterocolitica* present in the soil are vegetables, especially carrots, tomatoes, lettuces, radishes, parsley and mushrooms, i.e. vegetables that are often consumed raw. Various surveys have shown a count of between 10^2 and 10^3 *Y. enterocolitica* per gram of grated carrot or sliced tomato. Investigations among statistical organizations and consumer associations, together with an analysis of menus, have shown that these raw vegetables became fully established as part of the French diet from 1960 onwards.

3. Collective feeding, which makes considerable use of these raw vegetables, sometimes simply as a decoration on meals, and involves food items being kept at temperatures of between 4°C and 10°C during storage and transport, increased in France from 6 million meals per week in 1956 to 16 million in 1971 and is still rising.

Human exposure to infection via the digestive tract by the *Y. enterocolitica* present in the soil remained slight before these three factors had assumed practical significance. Their combination in the last few decades has provided *Y. enterocolitica* with conditions favourable to their cryophilic characteristics and has resulted in contacts between man and the bacteria being raised to a level sufficient for the latter to reveal their pathogenic potential.

Yersiniosis, too, is an example of an "ethological" disease, a new disease whose appearance is directly connected with changes in man's behaviour that place him in close contact with certain bacteria in his environment.

Pathological manifestations are developing under similar conditions in those animal species subjected to the new industrial rearing procedures. The manifestations include enterotoxaemia in cattle caused by *Clostridium perfringens*, staphylococcal or colibacillary mastitis in cows, and ovine listeriosis connected with silage.

The failure of antibiotic therapy

Although antibiotics have brought about a transformation in the prognosis for tuberculous meningitis, pneumonic plague and endocarditis (to name only their more outstanding successes) antibiotic therapy has nevertheless not led to the disappearance of infection. The causes of its failure are known. One is prescribing without valid indications, a precise clinical diagnosis or a proper bacteriological investigation. According to surveys such prescriptions could amount to as many as 80% in some hospital sectors and 30% in urban areas. Another cause is a badly chosen antibiotic that may be inactive against the organism responsible or fail to reach the actual site of infection. According to a recent French survey, 20% of all treatments of severe urinary infection in women are carried

263

out without a cytobacteriological test, or involve an antibiotic whose active ingredient does not pass into the urine or is not active against the organisms usually found.

The causes of these failures are strictly human. Since miracle drugs have given rise to such high hopes, the use of antibiotics has favoured all kinds of relaxation in the practice of hygiene and asepsis. The ever-increasing prescription of antibiotics or sulfonamides for cerebrospinal meningitis or for healthy carriers of staphylococci, streptococci or pathogenic enterobacteria has ultimately proved useless, and has led to the widespread appearance of increasingly resistant strains. From 1960 long-term umbrella therapy with antibiotics has also proved ineffective. Its justification was found in the growing overestimation of the potential risk of infection after ever more complex surgery, with increasingly lengthy operations, more and more sophisticated resuscitation procedures increasing the pathways of entry of organisms, the extension of indications for immunodepressant therapies, etc. It has also contributed to the selection and dissemination of resistant strains.

The main effect of poorly conducted antibiotic therapy, and especially of the administration of antibiotics for preventive purposes, would seem to have been to upset the microbial flora and exert selective pressure on certain species. For 20 years there has been a steady general increase in the number of infections involving Gram-negative bacilli in Europe; it goes hand in hand with a regular growth in their resistance to certain antibiotics or with an increase in the number of resistance factors. In 1973 bacteria appeared — principally *Proteus*, *Providentia*, *Pseudomonas* and *Moraxella* — that were resistant to all the antibiotics on the market. There is an increasingly large number of cases in which no antibiotic is active or in which the only antibiotics still active do not reach the focus of infection or are contraindicated.

It has therefore become an urgent task to lay down a prescribing policy for antibiotics in communities, to evaluate the degree to which they will be effective, and particularly to reduce the volume of haphazard supposedly prophylactic antibiotic therapy in order to restrict its selection pressure. It is imperative to return to a rational infection prevention policy based on effective hygiene and asepsis, and to seek new methods of vaccination against Gram-negative bacilli. Finally, it is essential to reorient bacteriological research towards medical bacteriology, to improve methods of detecting and isolating bacteria in pathological products, and to establish methods of detecting early antibodies. The pathology of infection of the future depends on such action.

The future of
viral pathology

N.R. Grist[a]

The host–parasite balance on which the future trends of infections depend is conditioned by many factors and many variations in the host and parasite populations and in their shared environment, of which herd immunity is only one. Changes in the viruses are possible but unpredictable; they include the antigenic shift and drift of influenza viruses, the emergence of neurovirulent variants of enteroviruses, and the theoretical possibility that a human virus might appear with severe pandemic potentialities analogous to the canine parvovirus that emerged recently. Previously unknown viruses continue to be discovered or imported, but the likelihood that hitherto unrecognized major pathogens remain to be found is diminishing with time. Host factors already vary greatly within and between countries; they include socioeconomic changes, population movements, immigration from other continents, changes in lifestyle and culture and in acceptance or rejection of conventional standards and of science and medicine, promiscuity, drug abuse, and the effects of technological and medical advances. Population density, age structure and urban crowding are classically important factors. Geographical and climatic factors are also relevant. In addition to slow natural changes in the environment there are major effects from deliberate or accidental intervention by man, effects such as increasing pollution and changes in agriculture and the production and distribution of food. This complex situation prevents firm predictions from being made, and it is uncertain that past and recent trends, as assessed by more or less incomplete and imperfect epidemiological surveillance, will continue.

Influenza and other respiratory virus infections

Acute respiratory infections are recognized as a major cause of mortality and morbidity in all parts of the world, especially affecting the very young

---

[a]Ruchill Hospital, Glasgow, Scotland.

and the very old. They remain essentially unconquered even in developed countries (1–4). Most of these diseases are caused by viruses, the large number of which, with their numerous antigenic types and variations, limit the scope of control by immunization. Few viruses as yet are susceptible to antiviral agents, which are not yet ready for routine use in the community. Transmission of infection is by the respiratory route, sometimes by direct or indirect contact, and the high prevalence of these viruses in all except the smallest and most isolated population groups militates against effective prevention and control except, incompletely, by improved social conditions and housing, reduced crowding, and relief of malnutrition and other predisposing factors (5).

Influenza
Influenza C, mainly a minor infection of children, seems unimportant. Influenza B shows antigenic drift; it infects mainly schoolchildren, but sometimes causes outbreaks, mainly local, or epidemics also involving older persons. It is increasingly reported as a possible cause of Reye's syndrome. Influenza A presents the major epidemic and potential pandemic threat because of the tendency to both drift and shift in its antigenic makeup. Antigenic shift is attributable to genetic interactions with strains from other host species. Major epidemics cause not only high morbidity with disruption of community life but also high mortality, especially in the oldest age groups, much of which is classified as pneumonia, bronchitis, cardiac failure, etc. Cold weather and overcrowding are well known predisposing factors. Neither inactivated nor attenuated vaccines have proved sufficiently effective for general use, though they can benefit selected high-risk groups. Improved vaccines and antiviral agents would be valuable, but the prospects seem poor of developing prophylactics that are effective at the community level. Caution is required in the use of the vaccines, which have possible adverse effects that may include the generation of dangerous recombinants of live vaccine viruses with virulent circulating strains. The danger of influenza will remain for many years, probably decades, and justifies continued epidemiological surveillance and research. Meanwhile, the reduction of influenza depends on improved conditions and the elimination of predisposing factors.

Paramyxoviruses
Respiratory syncytial virus (RSV) is a major cause of severe bronchiolitis, pneumonia and other respiratory infections in infants and young children. It is also the cause of reinfection with minor illness in later life and of a few severe illnesses in the elderly or predisposed. RSV is endemic in large crowded populations and causes annual epidemics in temperate zones, mainly in winter. After an initial disaster with inactivated vaccine, attempts to develop an effective vaccine are in progress, but the need to stimulate immunity early in infancy to protect the most vulnerable group at risk is a problem, and the incompleteness of immunity after natural

infection makes success doubtful. Antiviral agents may offer more hope but are not yet effective.

The paramyxoviruses include the mumps virus, as well as parainfluenza types 1–4. The latter cause a range of upper, middle and lower respiratory infections in children, mainly below the age of 5 years, and some mainly minor upper respiratory illness in adults. Reinfections occur. Neither effective vaccines nor useful antiviral agents have yet been developed. Since no significant change in the pattern of infection with paramyxoviruses is likely in the next few decades, the main hope must lie in improving living conditions and nutrition for disadvantaged population groups. Mumps is an important cause of neurological disease (6) and in some countries is becoming an infection of older children and adults, with an increased risk of complications such as orchitis. Opinions vary on the value of the mumps vaccine now available (7).

Adenoviruses

These occur in numerous antigenic types. Some cause infection early in life and persist in latent form, with intermittent reactivation and release of virus into the respiratory secretions and faeces. Others cause acute respiratory infections in childhood or in later life, with subsequent immunity. In addition to a range of respiratory illnesses, a few severe, the eyes may be affected, sometimes in outbreaks or epidemics of iatrogenic origin or in heavy industries with a high incidence of eye injury. Epidemic keratoconjunctivitis can be controlled by improved hygiene and avoidance of the spread of infection by contaminated fingers or instruments, but this is not readily achieved and maintained in industry or even in busy clinics. Newly characterized fastidious adenoviruses may be important causes of diarrhoea in children (8–10). The faecal–oral route is important in children, the respiratory route in adults. Bivalent live virus vaccine in enteric-coated capsules is effective against the main adenovirus causing respiratory disease in military recruits in the United States, but its potential oncogenicity makes this vaccine unacceptable for general use. No effective antiviral agent is available, and the limited contribution of adenoviruses to the totality of respiratory disease (perhaps 5%) makes the search for one not worth while.

Coronaviruses

Little is known about these viruses, which are very difficult to cultivate and study. They cause some relatively sharp upper respiratory illnesses. Transmission is by the respiratory route and reinfections are fairly common.

Picornaviruses

The very numerous types of rhinovirus in this group are the most frequent cause of the common cold and of some lower respiratory infections in infants and in adults with chronic bronchitis. Transmission is by both the respiratory route and contact, particularly among children and others in close proximity.

More than 20 of the numerous types of enteroviruses can also cause a small percentage of colds and other respiratory illnesses, including some pneumonias in infants. Transmission likewise is by the respiratory route and by direct or indirect contact (including the faecal–oral route). Prevention of these infections by vaccines is impracticable because of the more than 100 types involved, and effective antiviral agents are not yet available.

Poliovirus and other enteroviruses

More than 70 antigenic types of enterovirus are recognized. They are widespread in the world and circulate particularly among young children under conditions of poor hygiene and overcrowding, especially in summer and autumn in temperate and cold countries. The faecal–oral route of transmission predominates, directly from person to person via contaminated food or water, but respiratory transmission can be important in developed countries with good hygiene. Homotypic post-infective immunity to the disease is good, but transient minor reinfections can occur. Most infections are silent or cause only minor illness, but a variety of serious and occasionally life-threatening diseases can be caused. The importance of the viruses as causes of cardiac disease is increasingly recognized (*11*).

Polioviruses

These viruses may infect most children in most of the world unless they are protected by immunization or there is sufficient herd immunity. They sometimes cause neurological illness, often complicated by a paralysis that may be fatal or permanently crippling. Both inactivated and live attenuated vaccines are widely used and have brought this potentially epidemic disease under control in most of Europe. Maintenance of control requires maintenance of the immunization programme, since the viruses circulate actively in the crowded populations of the developing countries with which Europeans are in contact by travel. Inadequate coverage by vaccination, including refusal of vaccination by religious or other cultural groups, quickly results in the recurrence of paralytic poliomyelitis, as has been shown in the Netherlands and Sweden. Provided that effective vaccines continue to be available and are fully utilized, the downward trend of poliomyelitis in Europe over the past 30 years should continue until extinction of this disease. If economic or sociocultural pressures weaken the immunization and monitoring programme, paralytic poliomyelitis will recur and present a problem in the future.

Other enteroviruses

A few other types can sporadically cause paralysis or occasional outbreaks of paralytic disease (e.g. coxsackievirus A7 and enterovirus 71), but none poses the major or continuing threat of the polioviruses (*11*). With socioeconomic improvement and advances in hygiene the rate of circulation of enteroviruses in childhood falls. As shown by the history of poliomyelitis, a growing population of relatively non-immune children and even adults then accumulates and provides an increasing opportunity for periodic epidemic spread. It is already noticeable that enteroviruses that recur in larger epidemics at longer intervals are those that cause a higher proportion of infections in older age groups (*11*). Epidemics of coxsackievirus, echovirus, and other enterovirus infections are thus a growing problem for the future. Sporadic infections may also occur when non-immune persons visit areas where there is a high prevalence of enterovirus infection, including anywhere where traveller's diarrhoea is a serious hazard. In addition to viral meningitis and non-specific fevers, the illnesses caused include acute cardiac disease, particularly associated with coxsackieviruses (*12*), epidemic myalgia, foot-and-mouth disease, and enteroviral haemorrhagic conjunctivitis caused by coxsackievirus A24 or enterovirus 70, which became pandemic after 1969. Diabetes mellitus and certain chronic cardiovascular and neurological diseases are among the possible complications and late sequelae. As the proportion of non-immune adults increases, infants born without passive immunity become vulnerable to sporadic infections or institutional outbreaks of severe neonatal disease caused by echovirus 11 or other enteroviruses; this was noted as an emergent problem in the United Kingdom in 1978 (*13*).

The different socioeconomic, hygienic and housing standards of different countries and of different groups within the same area or city provide rich opportunities for the transfer of infection between groups and for occasional outbreaks or epidemics involving the older age groups. Since vaccination against the numerous types of virus is impracticable, this unstable epidemiological balance will require careful surveillance until and unless an antiviral agent effective against a broad spectrum of enteroviruses becomes available. Improved living conditions and health education to reduce the transmission of these viruses will be important. The pollution of water supplies with sewage containing enteroviruses presents a potential hazard that merits careful monitoring.

Viral hepatitis

Hepatitis A
This is for practical purposes another enterovirus infection with similar epidemiological characteristics, including spread from person to person directly or by the faecal–oral route via contaminated food, water or molluscs. In countries of Northern Europe with good standards of hygiene most children and even young adults are not immune and are thus at risk when visiting endemic areas unless passively protected by immunoglobulin. In developing countries the distribution of reported cases is shifting from childhood to older ages as socioeconomic and hygienic conditions improve (*14*). As with enteroviruses, this will provide future opportunities for epidemics in adults. Notification data and laboratory-confirmed cases will need careful watching over the next few

decades of epidemiological instability. The inactivated vaccines now under development may be important aids to controlling hepatitis A.

Hepatitis B
Hepatitis B is an entirely different infection caused by a virus that spreads by the transfer of infected blood or, occasionally, other body fluids from carriers or acute cases (often during the presymptomatic stage) into the tissues of non-immune persons, usually directly by apparent or inapparent parenteral routes including intimate personal contact. In addition to acute disease the infection can cause serious subacute, relapsing, and chronic hepatitis and multisystem diseases including hepatocellular carcinoma, of which it appears to be a major cause (15,16). The carrier and acute infection rates are lower in Europe than in many other parts of the world, higher in the age group 20–40 years but with a shift to younger age groups in many countries, reflecting intravenous drug abuse trends. Drug abuse and homosexual practices, especially among males, cause most of the acute infection in many countries of Europe. Opportunities for iatrogenic infection are provided by many dental and surgical procedures (including acupuncture) and by recent advances in medical technology involving the transfer of blood and immunosuppression, e.g. in renal dialysis units. There is also a risk to health care workers and clinical laboratory staff (17). Recognition of the factors involved and improvements in procedures have proved capable of reducing these risks to very low levels in well organized units. Immigration from countries with a high prevalence of infection and carriage presents a risk to recipient countries which has not in fact proved to be important, although some infections have been caused in, for instance, members of non-immune families adopting carrier children from endemic areas. The evolving pattern of hepatitis B infection is therefore complex and depends on many, largely sociological factors. Continuing surveillance is required and improvement of procedures found to favour the spread of infection. Vaccines, already shown to be safe and effective, provide the opportunity to protect high-risk groups and perhaps reduce vertical infection from mother to child, but much depends on the cost of the vaccines and on the interest and willingness of drug addicts and other population groups to cooperate in control measures. The vast world reservoir of carriers guarantees that hepatitis B will remain a problem for the foreseeable future, but much cheaper vaccines are likely to become available within a few decades.

Non-A non-B hepatitis
This form of hepatitis is as yet a problem of uncertain magnitude in Europe. Several causal agents are concerned, one or more transmitted by contaminated water and epidemiologically resembling hepatitis A, others transmitted parenterally like hepatitis B. The latter now cause most cases of post-transfusion hepatitis when hepatitis B virus has been effectively excluded from blood supplies. The epidemiological trends of this infection would be expected to follow those of hepatitis A and B, respectively, but unmodified by the influence of vaccines. The problem is ill-defined at

present, since no specific tests are available to identify cases, but the disease appears to be less serious than hepatitis A or B, except for cases with high mortality in pregnant women in North Africa. Vigilance is required to detect outbreaks affecting travellers, drug addicts and other groups.

Measles

Measles persists in large populations, with periodic epidemics. It dies out in remote, thinly populated areas, which then become vulnerable to epidemics affecting many age groups if infection is introduced from outside. The virus persists in some individuals after recovery from the acute disease and may cause late sequelae such as subacute sclerosing panencephalitis. Measles vaccines confer good and lasting herd immunity, which is potentially sufficient to eliminate measles from large areas, as shown by recent experience in the United States. Acceptance of the vaccine is variable and incomplete (about 50% in the United Kingdom at present), insufficient to influence herd immunity markedly and to control measles in inadequately protected populations. Control requires a greater acceptance of vaccine than at present by the populations of larger areas of Europe than single countries. The cost and acceptability of the vaccine will therefore condition the future trend of measles in Europe. The eradication of measles by vaccination is theoretically possible and would be a worthy objective, but constant vigilance would be required in case of reimportation.

Rubella

Rubella is less infectious than measles, most infections occurring in childhood. Since a varying proportion of adults are non-immune, however, some cases involve adults. The special importance of this is that, unless protected by previous infection or immunization, pregnant women may be affected by this minor illness, which will imperil the health of their unborn children. Improved hygiene and living conditions reduce the transmission of rubella by the airborne route and so an increasing proportion of adults remain non-immune. Control therefore depends on vaccination, either selectively for the female population or else covering both sexes from childhood in order to increase herd immunity and prevent epidemics. It is too early to judge which of these strategies is more effective, but neither will suffice unless the uptake of vaccine is higher than at present; once again cost, acceptability, and health education are important. Sustained surveillance with laboratory support is required to monitor the trends.

Herpesviruses

Varicella–zoster
The primary infection (varicella) is very highly infectious by the airborne

route. Reactivation as zoster releases much less virus, mainly from the local lesions, and rarely transmits infection. A few adults remain non-immune. Improving conditions and effective isolation of cases of chicken-pox should reduce its incidence and shift the age distribution upwards. Illness is more severe in adults and in immunosuppressed persons. Vaccines may become available but will require evaluation, including cost. Several antiviral agents influence infections by members of the herpesvirus group, and therapy for varicella–zoster may become available in the next decade or so.

Herpes simplex
Type 1 infection, a common primary infection of children recurring usually as circumoral or gingivostomal lesions, is transmitted by direct contact. Antibody surveys confirm the reduced prevalence in higher socioeconomic groups, and the trend of this infection should be towards a rising age incidence of primary infections, a few of which are associated with severe encephalitis.

Type 2 infection is spread largely as a sexually transmitted disease, causing acute and recurrent genital lesions. Its incidence is rising in sexually permissive societies, and there is concern about its possible long-term oncogenicity. Genital lesions may also arise from type 1 herpesvirus infection.

Both these herpesviruses attract growing attention. Both cause increasing trouble by reactivation in patients under immunosuppression. Reasonably effective antiviral agents are available, but vaccines appear to be unlikely in the near future.

Epstein-Barr virus
This is spread mainly by intimate mucosal contact, especially in teenagers and young adults in developed countries, but also as a common infection of children in conditions of crowding and poor hygiene. Its interest lies in its effects on the immune system and its possible long-term oncogenicity. As living conditions improve, the age incidence will rise with more symptomatic disease. Infectious mononucleosis has become common in higher socio-economic groups in Europe.

Cytomegalovirus
This likewise spreads mainly by intimate contact and is a common infec-tion of young children in crowded conditions of poor hygiene, though many adults remain susceptible in developed countries. Like rubella, the virus presents a threat to unborn children, and the safety and effective-ness of the vaccines under development are uncertain. Antiviral therapy is not yet satisfactory but is expected to progress during the coming decades, which will be important for immunosuppressed patients, in whom cytomegalovirus can cause severe problems by reactivation or by primary infection from transfused blood. A rising age incidence is to be expected for this infection, which is attracting increasing concern.

272

Zoonoses

Rabies is the indigenous viral zoonosis of most serious concern. Improved vaccine makes both pre-exposure and post-exposure prophylaxis more effective, but the long-term trend of rabies depends on unknown ecological factors and on the success or failure of new control methods being applied and developed. Increased travel and the popularity of camping and field activities enhance the chances of exposure to rabies-infected animals both in Europe and in other regions. The advance of rabies across Europe may be reversed, but eradication of rabies (or of the other viral zoonoses considered here) is most unlikely.

Tick-borne encephalitis is a disease that mainly reflects the interaction of man with infected vectors in appropriate habitats. Increased camping and weekending in infested woodland and moorland areas favour human exposure to the tick vectors. Occupational exposure in rural areas is often important as a cause of Central European tick-borne encephalitis, which has shown recent activity with severe complications and deaths.

Knowledge of other arboviruses is incomplete in Europe, but West Nile fever virus is prevalent in some areas of South-East Europe, causing encephalitis and meningitis. Other areas of Southern Europe where the climate and terrain favour the mosquito vectors are also potentially receptive to this and other arboviruses, with the possibility of epidemic spread from time to time. A proportion of febrile illness among tourists in these areas is caused by arboviruses and the situation merits careful surveillance.

Lymphocytic choriomeningitis, an arenavirus of rodents, is rarely recognized in most European countries but has recently shown increasing activity in Southern Europe. Haemorrhagic fever with renal syndrome is becoming better understood. Sporadic cases occur in at least six countries in Europe, and the disease seems able to spread. Exposure to Lassa fever, Marburg-Ebola, monkeypox, yellow fever and other arboviruses occurs mainly as a result of travel, though there are rare instances of imported infected animals (*18*). There is no risk of general spread to the population.

Other and recently discovered viruses

Electron microscopy has unmasked a large group of incompletely characterized and largely unrelated viruses present in faeces, often in very large numbers, particularly in persons with diarrhoeal disease but also in symptomless excretors (*19*). The best known are the rotaviruses, which are able to cause infantile gastroenteritis as well as some cases of diarrhoea in adults. Astroviruses, caliciviruses, orbiviruses, Norwalk agent and its relatives, and a miscellany of unclassified "small round viruses" show various degrees of etiological relationship to diarrhoeal or vomiting illnesses or both, and the antigenically new fastidious adenoviruses, are also good candidates as important causes of diarrhoea (*8–10*). Much remains to be learned about the epidemiology of these viruses, but at present it seems reasonable to regard them as probably similar to known enteroviruses and likely to follow the same trends, good hygiene and sanitation being important modifying influences.

Human parvoviruses have also been recognized, serological evidence suggesting a high prevalence in many populations. So far their main importance is in relation to immunosuppressed persons, but much remains to be learned about their epidemiology and significance in diseases of the urinary tract and of the blood, particularly in view of the recent linkage of the infection with hypoplastic crises in children with sickle-cell diseases (20).

Polyomaviruses and reoviruses have no public health significance at present, but may have unsuspected late effects.

The role of slow viruses in chronic and degenerative diseases is a challenge for research and may be increasingly relevant to the health of aging populations. Creutzfeldt-Jakob disease can be transmitted by tissue transplantation, and precautions are recommended to avoid the transmission from potentially infected blood or cerebrospinal fluid (21).

*　　　*　　　*

Socioeconomic improvement remains the major weapon for reducing the incidence and severity of many infections, but it can no longer be taken for granted that this trend will continue indefinitely. Improvements in housing and in personal and community hygiene are capable of reducing the incidence of infections and of postponing infections until older ages, particularly with diseases transmitted by the faecal–oral route, but this may result in larger epidemics at longer intervals involving a higher proportion of adults, in whom the clinical manifestations are often more severe. Improved nutrition may reduce the severity of many respiratory infections in infancy, although the basic epidemiology of respiratory infections is unlikely to be greatly changed by socioeconomic advances.

Sociocultural factors and changing patterns of behaviour and attitude are increasingly important. They can increase the vulnerability of populations to outbreaks of classical infections, which became rarer during the first half of the century.

Mixing populations with different forms of herd immunity and other different epidemiological characteristics can create problems, e.g. within a country or city receiving immigrants from areas with a higher prevalence of infections (though these problems are often greater for the immigrants), or in relation to travellers with low immunity visiting countries with a higher prevalence of infection.[a] Increasing long-distance tourism merits careful surveillance (22).

New dangers and new high-risk groups will continue to appear, some secondary to the development of new medical procedures, others as paradoxical consequences of improved conditions, the postponement of infections until later life, and the decreased immunity of childbearing women and thus reduction in the extent of passively transferred immunity

---

[a]*Prevention of the inter-country spread of infectious diseases:* report on a conference. Unpublished WHO document EURO 1002, Copenhagen, 1974.

274

to newborn babies and increased susceptibility to prenatal infections. Viruses of low virulence, such as rubella, hepatitis B and cytomegalovirus, are increasingly recognized as important causes of infections of medical and public health importance.

A poorly explored area of growing interest for the next few decades concerns the role of viruses as causes of immunopathological, neoplastic and chronic diseases. Many viruses of low virulence not recognized as important at present may prove to be significant causes or co-factors in chronic, degenerative and neoplastic diseases, particularly in aging populations.

Herd immunity can also be influenced by vaccines against some important infections, notably poliomyelitis (which should be controllable throughout Europe) and measles (which might be eradicable from most of Europe). More effective control of rubella to prevent damaging prenatal infections requires greater use of existing vaccines. Hepatitis B vaccine should be very valuable for selected risk groups, but the optimal use of a future hepatitis A vaccine remains to be worked out.

It is clear that continuing and improving surveillance of infections by modern methods will remain essential for monitoring known problems and the effectiveness of control programmes, and also for detecting the new problems that will inevitably continue to arise.[a] Planners and administrators can be seriously misled by traditional morbidity and mortality notification systems designed for past eras, which conceal the realities of new and increasing infections in the modern world (23).

References

1. **Cockburn, W.C. & Assaad, F.H.** Some observations on the communicable diseases as public health problems. *Bulletin of the World Health Organization*, **49**: 1–12 (1973).
2. **Cockburn, W.C.** The importance of infection of the respiratory tract. *Journal of infection*, **1**(Suppl. 2): 3–8 (1979).
3. WHO Technical Report Series, No. 642, 1980 (*Viral respiratory diseases:* report of a WHO Scientific Group).
4. **Lennette, E.H.** Viral respiratory diseases: vaccines and antivirals. *Bulletin of the World Health Organization*, **59**: 305–324 (1981).
5. **Miller, D.L.** Acute respiratory infections: short-term interventions and long-term strategy. *WHO Chronicle*, **32**: 286–290 (1978).
6. **Assaad, F.H. et al.** Neurological diseases associated with viral and *Mycoplasma pneumoniae* infections. *Bulletin of the World Health Organization*, **58**: 297–311 (1980).
7. **Wiedermann, G. & Ambrosch, F.** Costs and benefits of measles and mumps immunization in Austria. *Bulletin of the World Health Organization*, **57**: 625–629 (1979).

[a]*Communicable diseases: methods of surveillance:* report on a seminar. Unpublished WHO document EURO 3872, Copenhagen, 1969.

8. **Brandt, C.D. et al.** Comparative epidemiology of two rotavirus serotypes and other viral agents associated with viral gastroenteritis. *American journal of epidemiology*, **110**: 243–254 (1979).

9. **Johansson, M.E. et al.** Direct identification of enteric adenovirus, a candidate new serotype, associated with infantile gastroenteritis. *Journal of clinical microbiology*, **12**: 95–100 (1980).

10. **Kidd, A.H. & Madeley, C.R.** *In vitro* growth of some fastidious adenoviruses from stool specimens. *Journal of clinical pathology*, **34**: 213–216 (1981).

11. **Grist, N.R. et al.** Enteroviruses in human disease. *Progress in medical virology*, **24**: 114–157 (1978).

12. **Grist, N.R.** Coxsackie virus infections of the heart. *In:* Waterson, A.P., ed. *Recent advances in clinical virology*. Edinburgh, Churchill Livingstone, 1977, Vol. 1, pp. 141–150.

13. **Galbraith, N.S. et al.** Changing patterns of communicable disease in England and Wales. Part 1: Newly recognised diseases. *British medical journal*, **281**: 427–430 (1980).

14. **McCollum, R.W. & Zuckerman, A.J.** Viral hepatitis: report on a WHO informal consultation. *Journal of medical virology*, **8**: 1–29 (1981).

15. **Szmuness, W.** Hepatocellular carcinoma and hepatitis B virus: evidence for a causal association. *Progress in medical virology*, **24**: 40–69 (1978).

16. **Beasley, R.P. et al.** Hepatocellular carcinoma and hepatitis B virus. *Lancet*, **2**: 1129–1132 (1981).

17. **Grist, N.R.** The significance of hepatitis in the public health care system. *In:* Sherlock, S. & Krugman, S., ed. *Proceedings of the European Symposium on Hepatitis B*. Rahway, Merck, Sharp & Dohme, 1981.

18. **Simpson, D.I.H.** Viral haemorrhagic fevers of man. *Bulletin of the World Health Organization*, **56**: 819–832 (1978).

19. **WHO Scientific Working Group**. Rotavirus and other viral diarrhoeas. *Bulletin of the World Health Organization*, **58**: 183–198 (1980).

20. **Pattison, J.R. et al.** Parvovirus infections and hypoplastic crisis in sickle-celled anaemia. *Lancet*, **1**: 664–665 (1981).

21. *Advisory Group on the Management of Patients with Spongiform Encephalopathy (Creuztfeldt-Jakob Disease (CJD)):* report to the Chief Medical Officers of the Department of Health and Social Security, the Scottish Home and Health Department and the Welsh Office. London, H.M. Stationery Office, 1981.

22. **Reid, D. et al.** Infection and travel: the experience of package tourists and other travellers. *Journal of infection*, **2**: 365–375 (1980).

23. **Grist, N.R.** Realities of infection in the eighties, 1: England and Wales. *Communicable diseases (Scotland) weekly reports*, No. 81/16, ix-xi (1981).

Changes in outlook: communicable as opposed to infectious disease

B. Velimirovic

From Girolamo Fracastoro's book *De contagione et contagiosis morbis*, published in 1546, comes the notion of transmission of disease and of infection and the postulate of disease germs, well before the germ theory became established. "Contagion is an infection that passes from one thing to another", he wrote, distinguishing "contagion that infects by contact only, contagion that infects by fomites and contagion at a distance". In the second part of his book he lists as contagious fevers phthisis, rabies, syphilis, leprosy and scabies.[a] The expression "contagious" is still not infrequently used, but has been largely replaced by the current "transmissible" or "communicable", based on Koch's postulates. These said that the agent must be present in every case of the disease under appropriate circumstances, that it should occur in no other disease as a non-pathogenic agent, and that it must be isolated from the body in pure culture, repeatedly passed, and induce the disease afresh. However, it became progressively apparent with the advent of virology at the beginning of this century that these postulates do not satisfy all infectious processes adequately — they do not allow for asymptomatic carriers, the impossibility of propagating viruses on lifeless media, and the fact that other factors or co-factors might be necessary to produce disease. The

---

[a]The theory of contagion gradually replaced the miasmatic theory, which had been supported by empirical observation of air full of "miasmas" associated with such unhealthy areas as swamps, whence the name malaria. Miasmatic theory was contested by proponents of "contagium vivum" and "pathologia animata" from the seventeenth to the nineteenth centuries, who associated scabies with "animalculi" and typhus with lice in the eighteenth century and, less clearly, plague with rodents. The theory was put to rest by Koch in 1882. The communicability of certain diseases has been known or suspected since Greco-Roman times.

concept of antibody production had to be introduced as immunological proof of the presence of infection, and reluctantly the notion had also to be admitted that the same clinical picture could often be produced by a variety of different agents and that many bacterial and viral diseases are not contagious in the ordinary sense.

The term "communicable diseases" is based on experience of a mixture of classical epidemic diseases, some already known to Hippocrates. The communicability of these diseases was described by Fracastoro and explained scientifically towards the mid-nineteenth century in the germ theory by Henle (1840), Pasteur (1877) and Koch (1878), and by others at the beginning of the twentieth century. Their codification was based on tradition and knowledge at a time when dramatic acute infections dominated the field, and this is the engram for most health administrators, many public health specialists and some desk epidemiologists. The ICD displaces a great number of truly infectious diseases — diseases caused by bacteria, viruses, mycoplasmas and chlamydia that are mainly manifested in specific organs, although many are also able to cause generalized infections. This kind of classification, limited to traditional categories oriented towards communicability and contagiousness instead of towards disease states caused by microorganisms and their consequences, while perhaps still justifiable 40 years or more ago, is today incomplete or misleading.

Thus, long before host factors, including socioeconomic variables, started to be taken into account, the whole field of infection was saddled with the situation of centuries ago. Lately the classical infections have come to be considered as a sign of underdevelopment, implying perhaps shame or guilt and thus better not talked about. The conclusions drawn from the decline of the classical acute communicable diseases have been overemphasized, while the changes in the spectrum of infection have not been fully appreciated. Respiratory infections, sexually transmitted diseases, salmonelloses and opportunistic infections have not been reduced by rising living standards and development, but in many ways have taken advantage of them. Population density, urbanization, travel, changes in lifestyle, age-related factors and therapeutic technology have changed the picture of infection. Infections cannot be adequately studied today or understood and controlled without taking into account, along with the pathogenic agents, the social ecology and environment in which the host lives. This is a truism to anybody involved in infectious disease control. It is indeed in this field that attention was first paid to those factors long before it became the fashion to do so in every single field of the health sciences. Thus they need no emphasis here.

One of the many important factors militating for reassessment, and not only a semantic reassessment, of communicable diseases is the emergence of bacterial strains in hospitals that are resistant to antibiotics, often to a number of antibiotics. This happens either as chromosomal mutation caused by antibiotic selection pressure, resulting in an increased proportion of resistant organisms, or by the transfer of accessory extra-chromosomal genetic elements (plasmids) that carry the genetic determi-

278

nants for antibiotic resistance (R-factor-mediated resistance). In Japan in 1959, it was discovered that some plasmids can be transferred not only from one cell to another but also between different species. The number of drug-resistant strains of obligate, facultative and opportunistic pathogens has increased in the last decade all over the world, but it is not known whether there are significant regional differences in the prevalence of bacterial strains resistant to different antibiotics or how rapidly such resistance disappears (Annex 5).

Information on the incidence of R factors in the normal flora of healthy people not seeking medical attention is scarce, and in most European countries not available at all, nor is there integrated epidemiological surveillance and systematic monitoring of resistance trends in the world (an antibiotic resistance register was established in Scotland in 1978 and computer programs started in Czechoslovakia and France); there are a large number of studies on bacterial antibiotic resistance from individual hospitals, but without wider epidemiological analysis and international comparison of data. The problems raised by this phenomenon are best seen in the spread of R-factor-mediated resistance between patients and personnel and a rapid rise in hospital infection of surgical wounds and of the urinary and respiratory tract, and an increase in generalized infection with septicaemia. It is now becoming apparent that resistance has eroded the beneficial results of antibiotic therapy and made a number of formerly highly active antibiotics useless, so that new antibiotics are constantly being required for a "succession of temporary respites in an otherwise deteriorating situation"(1). The indiscriminate use of antibiotics in hospitals and in feeding livestock has been the chief reason for the increase of R-factor-mediated resistance. However, resistance may also occur without antibiotic treatment by colonization of the environment by the R factor. Every resistant isolate in a patient may be regarded as part of some epidemic.

Not only is there an increased risk to patients of death or prolonged illness but there is also a constant need for new and more expensive antibiotics, which already account in many hospitals for over 50% of total costs for drugs. This makes antibiotic resistance an explicit epidemiological problem requiring the attention of many disciplines, including clinicians, microbiologists, epidemiologists and people working in public health and in the control of infectious diseases. The urgency of the situation cannot be sufficiently emphasized to the health administrators concerned not only in defining antibiotic policy but also in setting priorities for research and planning the health services in general.

A recent study from Norway (2), a country with one of the highest standards of health care, should be mentioned as indicative of the magnitude of the problem. The prevalence rate of infections among hospitalized patients in 15 Norwegian hospitals on 28 November 1979 was 17%, and of hospital infections 9%. Hospital infections were most frequent in haematology and intensive care departments (23% and 22% respectively), least frequent in ophthalmology and psychiatry (2%). Urinary tract infections played a major role both overall (33.5%) and in hospital infections (41.9%). In community-acquired infections alone lower respiratory tract infections were slightly more common than urinary tract infections (26.6% as against 24.1%).[a]

The problem of coping with change is wider than that of coping with the increase of infections caused by opportunistic pathogens and anti-biotic resistance. Dubos (3) writes:

> The point at issue is that the microbial diseases which account for the greatest morbidity in our communities today are completely different in their origin and manifestation from those which are so effectively dealt with by modern techniques. ... The sciences concerned with microbial diseases have developed almost exclusively from the study of acute or semi-acute infectious processes caused by virulent micro-organisms acquired through exposure to an exogenous source of infection. In contrast, the microbial diseases most common in our communities today arise from the activities of micro-organisms that are ubiquitous in the environment, persist in the body without causing any obvious harm under ordinary circumstances, and exert pathological effects only when the infected person is under conditions of physiological stress.

The appearance of hospital infections has drawn more attention to endogenous infections and the pathogens that colonize different organs. Facultative pathogens cause generalized disease mostly in persons with resistance to infection reduced by other severe diseases, in the newborn, or in patients when introduced into tissues or a normally sterile body area by specific procedures. Among them are Gram-positive cocci (*Staphylococcus aureus* and other staphylococci, *Streptococcus* groups A, C and G, enterococci, other non-haemolytic cocci), anaerobic bacilli, clostridia, Gram-negative aerobic bacilli (*Escherichia coli*, *Aerobacter*, *Pseudomonas aeruginosa* and other *Pseudomonas* types, *Proteus*, *Serratia*, *Klebsiella*, *Enterobacter*), opportunistic pathogens, *Listeria*, anonymous mycobacteria, fungi and yeasts (*Candida*, *Nocardia*, *Histoplasma*), the protozoan *Pneumocystis carinii*, and others.

Persistent infections

In addition to the acute diseases caused by known classical microbial agents in the absence of specific immunity, endogenous infections and various other phenomena require a brief mention. It came as a surprise to discover that even such classical pathogens as *Rickettsia prowazeki*, e.g. in Brill-Zinsser disease, can persist for 10–20 years or more in the lymph nodes or the reticuloendothelial system after the original infection, and

---

[a]The whole important issue of hospital-acquired infections has not been discussed here because it has been dealt with recently in several working group reports, e.g. **Parker, M.T.**, ed. *Hospital-acquired infections: guidelines to laboratory methods.* Copenhagen, WHO Regional Office for Europe, 1978 (WHO Regional Publications, European Series No. 4). WHO began in 1983 a major study to determine the scale of common factors in, and differences between, hospital infections in various regions of the world.

produce a second infection less severe but with the rickettsiae circulating in the blood. Equally surprising was the latency over years of the spirochaete *Treponema pertenue* causing yaws. The existence of long-persisting forms of *Plasmodium vivax*, postulated for a long time, has only recently become accepted. This persistence for years of an agent that the organism is unable to eliminate, and which is able to retain its pathogenicity, was previously known in the case of *Entamoeba histolytica*, of some bacteria such as *Salmonella typhi*, *Mycobacterium tuberculosis* and *M. leprae*, of parasites such as *P. malariae*, and more recently of *Toxoplasma gondii*.

There is also evidence of an important group of persisting viruses, causing chronic, latent and slow infections. The viruses are hidden, intracellular, and often located in macrophages, and the mechanisms of persistence are as yet ill defined.

Chronic infections are those where the virus multiplies normally but the organism is unable to eliminate it. The virus persists in the tissues and an equilibrium is formed between the host and the pathogen. This may lead to a manifest illness if the defence mechanisms fail, as for example when there is an immune deficiency (possibly genetic) or the host is under immunosuppressive drugs. Sometimes they might lead to a malignant transformation. Such is the case for hepatitis B, in which the antigen may persist for many years in the organism, even in the absence of viraemia; a link has been shown with primary liver cell cancer. Other examples are cytomegalovirus, which is shed in urine and milk, remains in leucocytes in about 5% of normal people, and is transmitted by blood transfusion; and the Epstein-Barr lymphotropic herpesvirus of infectious mononucleosis, in which prolonged illness and serological evidence indicate persistent infection. The EB virus has also been linked with nasopharyngeal carcinoma and lymphoid tumours of the Burkitt type. Similar persistence has been observed in animals, leading to infections in man, e.g. lymphocytic choriomeningitis, the newly isolated papovavirus BK in humans with renal transplants, and the JC virus recently isolated from the human brain in progressive leucoencephalitis (4). Chronic infection can lead to glomerulonephritis of the autoimmune type by deposition of immune complexes in the kidney.

In latent infections there is no multiplication of the virus after the first acute illness but, when the equilibrium between the agent and the host is disturbed, rapid multiplication occurs and causes manifest disease. Examples are: the herpes simplex virus type 1, in which the virus persists in the trigeminal ganglia, a common cause of meningoencephalitis and eye disease, a main cause of corneal blindness; herpes genitalis (HSV-type 2) in which the virus persists in the sacral ganglia and may be associated with cervical cancer; and varicella, in which the virus persists in a non-infectious state in the sensitive trigeminal ganglia, the dorsal root ganglia and the spinal neurons, causing herpes zoster in later life. The illness may be triggered by a temporary natural decrease in immunity following infection, menstruation, ultraviolet irradiation, etc., or after therapeutically induced immunosuppression.

Slow virus infection is a process in which the virus or some specific forms of it persist over months or years, evolving slowly and leading eventually to death. Several diseases of this type exist in animals, where the phenomenon was first observed, caused by unconventional viruses such as scrapie[a] in sheep. Examples in man are presenile dementia and Creutzfeldt-Jakob disease, which have a universal distribution, and kuru, which is of no relevance in Europe but is of great theoretical and scientific interest. These viruses do not produce inflammatory or immune reactions but multiply in the nervous system, progress slowly, and are always fatal. They are suspected to be viroids, pathogenic molecules of nucleic acid of small size first observed in plants in 1969 and probably a new type of pathogenic agent. They are highly resistant to heat, β-propiolactone, formol, and ultraviolet and ionizing radiation (5).

Creutzfeldt-Jakob disease, a spongiform encephalopathy demonstrated within families, but also in neurosurgeons, nurses and pathologists, is a catastrophic but sporadic and very rare disease of the nervous system (0.1–0.5 per million population) of unknown etiology and without great public health importance. A survey in France, however, revealed 170 cases between 1968 and 1977 (some 17 new cases each year, of which 19% were in families). Another survey carried out since 1978 suggests an increase in frequency: 28 new cases each year. No infection of health personnel has been seen so far in France, but cases of accidental transmission do occur that require epidemiological clarification. Progressive rubella panencephalitis and subacute sclerosing panencephalitis are caused by the widely spread rubella and measles viruses. With the latter there is an inflammatory encephalitis, progressive dementia, and a fatal demyelination and degeneration of neurons in a certain number of people, occurring after years of inapparent subacute or chronic phases in which the virus remains masked. The nucleocapsids of the measles virus accumulate on the surface of the neurons, where they do not multiply further but produce antigenic immune reactions. The virus can be demonstrated in the nerve cells by electron microscopy or by immunological tests. The reason this disease occurs as a rare sequela of measles is not clear; it is assumed, but not yet proved, that it is because of the absence of the natural killer-cell interferon system in the tissues and of interference with interferon produced by other viruses. A similar defect in producing interferon is suspected in several other diseases in man: multiple sclerosis, lupus erythematosus and poliomyositis (5). Medical science is only at the beginning of an understanding of the phenomena involved, but it is possible that these diseases may, with the help of immunogenetics, explain some other chronic degenerative diseases (Parkinson's disease, Behçet's disease, chronic encephalitis with epilepsy, Mollaret's meningitis). A cautious evaluation will be needed of an

---

[a]The causal agent of scrapie, a degenerative disease of the central nervous system in sheep and goats and occasionally in man, has recently been discovered. This novel organism, called tentatively a prion to distinguish it from viruses, is a small proteinaceous infectious particle resistant to inactivation by most procedures that modify nucleic acid.

increasing number of isolations of viruses in leukaemia, multiple sclerosis, amyotrophic lateral sclerosis, schizophrenia and Paget's disease. The last word in virology has yet to be said; the period of biochemical advance and molecular biology into which the science of infection has now entered will perhaps provide a means of answering some of the questions that have always puzzled the physician about the persistence and dynamics of infective agents over long periods of time.

Have the major infections changed?

Spontaneous change in the character of infections over time usually means a change in the pathogen itself, i.e. an increase or decrease in virulence, or a change in the relationship between the host and the infective agents. McKeown (6) accepted the latter without elaborating on the mechanisms, except in the case of scarlet fever and perhaps, with some doubt, measles and a few other less clear-cut examples. He concluded that "the reduction of deaths from infectious diseases was not due substantially to change in their character". Later research has demonstrated that changes in the clinical picture of scarlet fever, for example, are linked to variations in the toxigenicity of the strains, the existence of more antigenic types of scarlet fever toxin, and other factors. The answer to the question of change depends essentially on individual views on evolution in general. That issue seems to have been settled, in spite of some "living fossils" whose evolution has not made any notable change. Dubos (3), a microbiologist, believed that "changes have occurred during historical times in the relation between man and various microbial agents of disease, either that the latter undergo fluctuations in their infectibility and pathogenicity, or that the resistance of man to them can fluctuate". He assumed that both mechanisms can operate singly or jointly and that genetic changes in the virulence of viruses or bacteria are possible, as we know from plasmid-mediated transfer of antibiotic resistance and from the changes in the surface proteins (shifts) of influenza A virus. Pathogens can undergo mutations resulting in changes of their characteristics, of their antigenic properties (including their immunological specificity), of their ability to produce toxins, and of their virulence factors if the mutants are selected by favourable conditions in the micro-environment. The influence of genetic factors on susceptibility to infection has been demonstrated in animals under natural epidemic conditions and is used deliberately in selective breeding of laboratory and domestic animals. The same phenomenon has not yet been studied extensively in agents affecting man, because the tools were not available before the advent of genetic techniques in molecular biology. There is a constant interaction between viral and host genomes and the result can be a highly infectious or an attenuated viral progeny.

Examples of spontaneous changes in the severity of epidemics are plentiful in the history of medicine but are insufficiently documented. By "spontaneous" is meant that the changes cannot be attributed either to

283

socioeconomic changes such as better nutrition, famine or the improvement of environmental or other conditions, to exhaustion of the pool of susceptible persons, or to an increase in herd immunity. Spontaneous change is thought to have happened in the past: the disappearance of plague after the big epidemics of the time of Justinian, in the Middle Ages and in the seventeenth century; the complete disappearance of the English sweating sickness, which appeared in 1485, vanished without trace in 1551 and is still a mystery; and the decline in severity of syphilis from a rapid and often fatal disease in the fifteenth and sixteenth centuries to the frequently mild, slowly progressive disease of more recent times. It is difficult to assess the situation existing in past centuries, but the change in the severity of scarlet fever seems better documented. A mild disease from 1604 to 1631, becoming severe from 1634 to 1672 and rare around 1700, it developed again into a disease with a very high mortality in children in the nineteenth century, accounting for 4–6% of deaths at all ages; it then started to decline in numbers and severity towards the end of the century. Measles, formerly a rather mild disease, changed its character about 1800. By about 1900 scarlet fever was of less importance than measles, which reached a peak by about 1915 and has fallen ever since. Diphtheria increased in prevalence and severity in the middle of the nineteenth century and declined thereafter before the introduction of antitoxin in 1894. There may perhaps have been a change in toxin production due to lysogenic conversion. Since then, with increasing vaccination coverage in the twentieth century, it has all but disappeared in Europe (3) although nontoxigenic strains continue to circulate.

What exactly happened may remain in the domain of speculation, but it is now known that mutation and thus virulence are a consequence of small changes in the genome of bacteria and viruses, and genetic susceptibility is better understood. Through genetic recombination and reassortment viruses have the potential to convert benign bacteria into virulent pathogens. The influenza virus also, for example, has the potential to resist the natural selection pressure exerted by the host response. Monoclonal antibody techniques, fine structural analysis of changes in viral surface polypeptides and polynucleotides, DNA sequencing, RNA segment separation, and oligonucleotide mapping have provided powerful new sensitive epidemiological tools for understanding the diversity of immune responses, virulence and pathogenicity. The influence of herd immunity is well documented in a number of diseases, such as tuberculosis and leprosy; so is the selective adaptation by genetic polymorphism to selection pressure in immunity against malaria from *Plasmodium falciparum* in the African environment. Fluctuations such as the present increase in scarlet fever in some European countries of over 100%, after almost 20 years of apparent absence, is particularly interesting, since the prevalence of streptococcus A in the environment, the percentage of carriers, and the susceptibility of streptococcus A to penicillin do not seem to have changed. However, there are about 80 types of streptococci with three different erythrogenic toxins carried by a temperate phage, and changes in their respective importance occur constantly. Even minor changes in the M protein that coats group A haemolytic streptococci can lead to significant changes in virulence. There are also indications at present of an increasing frequency of infection by group B streptococci, at least in some geographical areas of Europe, and of *Streptococcus mulleri* infections causing encephalitis, meningitis and hospital infections. Disregarding the various possible mechanisms involved in changes of pathogens and the nature of the infections, which we cannot yet assess or are just beginning to understand, such as mutation in the gene of thymidine kinase and shifts and drifts in the influenza viruses, it is obvious that a system for the assessment of these long-term changes is required. Even the present picture, based as it is on fragmentary data and empirical observations, might be quite different from that assumed to have existed a few decades ago. For example, since 1953 dengue fever has changed its character and developed into a severe haemorrhagic illness in children between 6 months and 15 years of age, first in South-East Asia and then in some countries of the Western Pacific and the Caribbean area. The reason for the change, presumably related to immunity, is as yet not clear. It may be related to an increased number and density of susceptible people, an increased number and density and a wider distribution of the vector *Aedes aegypti*, a logarithmic increase in the turnover of infection, changes in the intrinsic virulence of the virus, or a hypersensitivity reaction triggered by sequential infection with two different serotypes during a critical period. There is no firm evidence at this stage in favour of any of these hypotheses.

To sum up, the question of changes in pathogens will be solved only after the epidemiologicial data have been assessed, along with the results of long-term monitoring and molecular characterization of the disease agents.

Cautious optimism

The changes in and the decline of infections in modern times have been induced mainly by therapy, which has eliminated most of the mortality, shortened or stopped infection and reduced morbidity, curtailed the chronic stage, and reduced the sequelae of many of the classical infections. Prophylactic immunization combined with epidemiological surveillance and containment of transmission has reduced the morbidity of infections or, in the case of smallpox, for the first time in history entirely eliminated a communicable disease. Improved socioeconomic conditions, but also changes in the biological environment and occupational categories, have reduced — although not entirely eliminated — exposure to major infections and vectors and to animal hosts and reservoirs that are the source of infection in man. Thus the prognosis for many major infections is favourable. It remains to be seen how this will balance out against the challenge of importation, the appearance of pathogens with altered or new biological properties, or of new strains, the emergence of opportunistic and facultative pathogens, the resistance of vectors, and the increase of risk from age-related and other demographic factors and changes in lifestyle. Infections are still associated in the mind of many health professionals with great plagues and epidemics decimating cities and villages. This concept, associated with the notion of "magic bullets" and immunoprophylaxis and immunotherapy (which society expects for every remaining infectious disease) is today in Europe of little relevance. Instead, there will be many smaller problems of different kinds cropping up: persistent infections not ordinarily transmissible from man to man, such as endogenous infections; infections transmissible from person to person by asymptomatic carriers; infections not transmissible in the usual way but requiring a vector; infections resulting from treatment such as blood transfusion and immunosuppression; and diseases with a clear infectious pattern suspected to be viral but without demonstrated etiology.

Research in immunology has made tremendous progress in recent years in clarifying the complexity and consequences of immune reactions. For example, a hypothesis has been put forward that hepatitis B virus is not primarily cytopathogenic and causes damage to the liver cells only when in combination with a cellular immune reaction. This opens up new vistas not only in infection but also in other fields, such as synergism and mutagenesis in cancer, and in relation to the advance identification of persons at risk because of their anticipated response to infections. The association of Kaposi's sarcoma with various opportunistic infections, *Pneumocystis carinii* pneumonia in AIDS, and the reactivation of cytomegalovirus (7) (whose immunodepressing capacity is well known) are examples of the type of challenge to be met in the future. This brings the question of lifestyles not yet studied systematically within the context of infections.[a] Infection is, simply stated, an invasion of the tissues of the body by microorganisms, which up to now have been studied mainly from the point of view of their identification and clinical manifestation. However, rapid progress in biochemistry, molecular biology and genetic engineering will transfer the study of infection to a different level, that of understanding the mechanisms involved, the relationships between pathogens and organisms, and the reasons why invasion occurs; this in turn will open up new perspectives for control. In terms of age-related changes and the specific risks of infection in the elderly, research is starting on chemotactic mechanisms, the age-conditioned functioning of macrophages and neutrophils, alterations of mucosal surfaces, and the changes involved in colonization by pathogens. Increased attention to the epidemiology of infection and timely diagnosis, so often lacking, may reduce the mortality of the aged significantly and distinguish chronic

---

[a]Infections may be acquired, for example, from animals kept in the house. The number of households with pet animals in the Federal Republic of Germany increased from 19 million in 1956 to 24 million in 1981.

conditions not accessible to intervention from those where an increased quality of life is possible.

Where do we stand now?

Looking back on the past 30 years or so, and in the light of our present incomplete assessment of the possibilities, what are the present trends of infection in Europe? Galbraith (8), analysing the changing patterns of some communicable diseases in England and Wales, divided them tentatively into three groups: newly recognized diseases, disappearing or declining diseases, and increasing diseases. This division is probably generally applicable to some other developed countries in Europe. We have modified this classification and added two additional groups: diseases that seem to be stationary and diseases where the situation is uncertain and no judgement on trends is feasible. In the absence of hard data this expanded listing of selected diseases is only an impression derived from the very incomplete official notifications and published papers from the whole of Europe. It cannot fit any particular country exactly, has thus only a very rough orientation value, and needs to be constantly readjusted.

Newly recognized infectious diseases
Cytomegalovirus infections, *Campylobacter* enteritis, non-A non-B hepatitis, yersiniosis, legionnaires' disease, mycoplasma infections, primary amoebic meningoencephalitis, viral haemorrhagic fevers, neonatal necrotizing enterocolitis caused by *Clostridium difficile*, staphylococcal toxic shock syndrome, rotavirus and Norwalk agent infections, haemorrhagic fever with renal syndrome, newly recognized infections with low-grade opportunistic pathogens (appearing particularly as hospital infections), chlamydial infections, probably Kawasaki disease (if this proves to be infectious) and AIDS.

Disappearing and declining diseases
Diphtheria, poliomyelitis, typhus and taeniasis (*Taenia solium*) have almost disappeared. Declining are dysentery as an autochthonous disease in Northern Europe, tetanus in younger generations, tuberculosis, anthrax, brucellosis (in some countries only), autochthonous typhoid fever, hepatitis A (in many countries), measles, rubella and pertussis (in countries that vaccinate), some rickettsioses, trachoma, amoebiasis, ancylostomiasis, ascariasis, trichinosis and trichiuriasis.

Infectious and parasitic diseases on the increase
Salmonellosis and other foodborne infections, sexually transmitted diseases, particularly herpesvirus 2, non-gonorrhoeal urethritis, pelvic inflammatory diseases, diseases due to human papillomavirus (condylomata), *Clostridium perfringens* infections, mononucleosis, hepatitis B, ornithosis (in several countries), rabies (in wild animals), subacute

287

bacterial endocarditis, streptococcal septicaemia and osteomyelitis, streptococcal pharyngitis, pneumococcal pneumonia, hospital enterovirus infections. Parotitis has shown an increase in the last few years (within an overall decline), imported leprosy, imported cholera, toxoplasmosis, pediculosis, scabies, giardiasis, hymenolepiasis, trichomoniasis, isosporiasis, imported parasitic diseases, and imported malaria and dysentery. There are indications in most countries of an increase in scarlet fever since the mid 1970s, and group B streptococcal infections are probably increasing.

Stationary infections
Respiratory infections (various types of bacterial pneumonia, influenza, bacterial and viral meningitis), syncytial virus infections, dysentery (in most countries), otitis, leptospirosis, echinococcosis, infections caused by *Taenia saginata*. Tick-borne meningoencephalitis is probably stationary, although it is claimed to be spreading where ecological conditions are favourable.

Infections of uncertain situation
There have been increasing reports of botulism in several countries in the last few years, but the numbers are too small to permit a judgement on the trends. The situation of rubella and varicella is uncertain at present because of the wide fluctuations from year to year; the situation of leishmaniasis (in areas where the vectors exist), listeriosis, and pneumocystosis is also uncertain.

*   *   *

In the decades between 1950 and 1970 the near disappearance in Europe of a number of classical communicable diseases and the considerable reduction of many others as a result of medical and environmental achievements (any dogmatic statement about which was the most important cause has to be avoided) led to the optimistic assumption by many health administrators that infections in general were no longer a problem. That assumption no longer exists with the realization that some diseases have shown particular persistence or a tendency to return, and that others — foodborne diseases such as salmonellosis and hospital and respiratory infections — are tending to increase or persist, particularly in the developed countries. Changes in lifestyle and medical technology, a changed demographic structure, and many other factors that interfere with immunity will certainly alter the incidence of different diseases and bring fresh challenges. Instead of dramatic acute conditions, infection will assume greater prominence as a complication to other diseases and involve the more demanding task of elucidating the various aspects of bacterial allergy, the consequences of bacterial toxins, immunity diseases, immune responses to viral antigens, their effects on the patient, and their role as co-factors in chronic disease.

At the technical discussions on national and global surveillance of communicable diseases held at the Twenty-first World Health Assembly in Geneva in May 1968, epidemiological surveillance was defined as the exercise of continuous scrutiny of and watchfulness over the distribution and spread of infections and factors related thereto, of sufficient accuracy and completeness to be pertinent to effective control.[a] That definition is still valid. There is a need to determine continuously the nature of the factors responsible for the occurrence and distribution of diseases, the risk factors for the individual and the community, the time changes in the pattern of disease, the determinants of those changes and, as far as possible, future developments in order to devise approaches to intervention and test already existing or new control tools and strategies. For this, goodwill, a system of assessment of the validity of data, international exchange of data, use of the same standards for surveillance, and improvement of field laboratory techniques are a precondition to proper geographical and historical perspective. Until they are achieved, a precise comparison between countries will remain difficult. This is not to decry comparisons of trends, which are valuable.

Perhaps Europe, so richly endowed, will find a better way of assessing regional trends flexibly and comprehensively, without overloading the primary health care organization and the individuals involved. Infections can and, we hope, will progressively come to represent a smaller part in the overall picture of pathology in Europe, but it is a part that still needs to be defined. The importance of infections must be viewed not in terms of numbers alone but also in terms of the risks involved for public health, the volume of effort necessary to maintain complete or partial freedom from them, the collateral costs, and the readiness of society to tolerate even a small number of diseases, many of which are controllable or theoretically preventable. The recurrent costs of maintaining freedom from major infections will remain and probably, until better tools are available, even increase in the future. Man will probably never be free from the threat of bacterial and viral infections and "complacency will lead with certainty to recrudescence of problems" (9). A vast range of immensely adaptable pathogenic microorganisms will continue to circulate in nature as they have done for millions of years; they have evolved from non-pathogenic bacteria, and it is reasonable to assume that this process will continue in the human environment. Most of them can now be successfully controlled and, perhaps one day in the future, some may even be eradicated. We cannot say how they will evolve in the future or what chances they have of attacking man, who cannot, in his daily routine, live in a sterile environment; nor can we venture to predict the future response of natural, enhanced or decreased immunity mechanisms or the ecological effect. We need not be pessimistic, but optimism should not preclude carefulness.

What is now called for is renewed interest and emphasis on infections rather than on the classical communicable diseases, a more realistic and continuous monitoring of the changes in pathogens and diseases and of

---

[a]Unpublished WHO document A 21/Technical Discussions/5, Geneva, 1968.

the progress achieved in their control, a reassessment of their relationship to the complex environmental and ecological situation, an updating of and improvement in epidemiological surveillance, a better use of laboratory diagnosis, and a fuller collaboration with other related disciplines. Only if these are assured can a more complete understanding and evaluation be envisaged of the risks and challenges posed by microorganisms and of strategies to deal with them, in the context of the total health-oriented effort and within the social, economic, ecological and biological framework of the European Region as an integral part of a single world.

References

1. **Johnsson, M.** On the persistence of R-factors in the gram-negative flora of the human infections. *Scandinavian journal of infectious diseases*, **10**: 3 (1974).
2. **Horig, B. et al.** A prevalence survey of infections among hospitalized patients in Norway. *MIPH Annals*, **4**: 49–60 (1981).
3. **Dubos, R.** *Man adapting*, 7th ed. New Haven, Yale University Press, 1971, p. 164.
4. **Padgett, L. et al.** Cultivation of papova-like virus from human brain with progressive leukoencephalopathy. *Lancet*, **1**: 1257–1260 (1971).
5. **Girard, M. & Hirth, L.** Virologie générale et moléculaire. Paris, Doin, 1980.
6. **McKeown, T.** *The role of medicine: dream, mirage or nemesis?* London, Nuffield Provincial Hospitals Trust, 1976.
7. Epidemiological aspects of current outbreak of Kaposi's sarcoma and opportunistic infections. *New England journal of medicine*, **306**: 248–252 (1982).
8. **Galbraith, N.S. et al.** Changing patterns of communicable disease in England and Wales. Part 1: Newly recognised diseases. *British medical journal*, **281**: 427 (1980); Part 2: Disappearing and declining diseases, 489 (1980); Part 3: Increasing infectious diseases, 546 (1980).
9. **Hanlon, J.** *Principles of public health administration*, 5th ed. Saint Louis, Mosby, 1969.

Annex 1

INFECTIOUS AND PARASITIC DISEASES
IN THE NINTH REVISION OF THE INTERNATIONAL
CLASSIFICATION OF DISEASES

In ICD-9, infectious and parasitic diseases appear in two broad groups:

— mainly general infectious and parasitic diseases

— mainly local infectious and parasitic diseases.

The first group appears in Chapter I: *Infectious and parasitic diseases* (categories 001–139). The second group appears in chapters other than Chapter'I, as follows:[a]

Chapter III: *Endocrine system*
Acute thyroiditis, 245.0
Abscess of thymus, 254.1

Chapter VI: *Nervous system and sense organs*
Nervous system
Meningitis, 320.0–320.3, 320.4*–320.7*, 320.8, 320.9, 321.0*–321.8*, 322
Encephalitis, myelitis, encephalomyelitis, 323.0*–323.4*, 323.5, 323.6*, 323.8, 323.9
Intracranial abscess, 324(*)
Intracranial phlebitis and phlebothrombosis, 325
Sequelae of intracranial infection, 326
Post-herpetic trigeminal neuralgia, 350.0*
Acute infective polyneuritis, 357.0
Secondary polyneuropathy, 357.4*

Eye
Eye globe, 360.0, 360.1, 363.0(*), 363.1(*), 363.2, 364.0(*), 364.1(*), 364.3, 370.0, 370.1*, 370.2, 370.3(*), 370.4(*), 370.5(*), 370.8, 370.9
Eye adnexa, 372.0(*), 372.1(*), 372.2, 372.3(*), 373.0, 373.1, 373.4*–373.6*, 375.0, 375.3, 375.4, 376.0, 376.1(*)
Optic neuritis, 377.3(*)

---

[a]Conventional signs used:
- — includes intermediate category numbers
- * indicates that all the diagnostic terms included within the category number are primarily classified to categories in Chapter I: 001–139
- (*) indicates that some of the diagnostic terms included within the category number are primarily coded to categories in Chapter I: 001–139.

Ear
External otitis, 380.0, 380.1(*), 380.2
Otitis media, 382(*)
Mastoiditis, 383(*)
Myringitis, 384.0–384.2
Otitis interna, 386.3

Chapter VII: *Circulatory system*
Acute rheumatic fever, 390–392
Chronic rheumatic heart diseases, 393–398
Acute pericarditis, 420(*)
Acute and subacute endocarditis, 421(*)
Acute myocarditis, 422(*)
Cardiomyopathy, 425.6*, 425.8*
Phlebitis and thrombophlebitis, 451

Chapter VIII: *Respiratory system*
Common cold, 460
Other acute upper respiratory infections, 461–465
Acute bronchitis and bronchiolitis, 466
Chronic upper respiratory infections, 472–476
Pneumonia, 480–483, 484*, 485, 486
Influenza, 487
Chronic and unspecified bronchitis, 490, 491.0, 491.1, 491.8, 491.9
Other respiratory infections, 510, 511, 513, 517*, 519.2

Chapter IX: *Digestive system*
Mouth infections, 522.0, 522.4–522.7, 523.0–523.4, 527.2, 528.0–528.3, 529.0
Oesophagitis, 530.1
Acute gastritis, 535.0
Appendicitis, 540–542
Anal and rectal abscess, 566
Peritonitis, 567(*)
Liver and biliary tract, 572.0, 572.1, 573.1*, 573.2*, 575.0, 575.1, part of 576.1
Pancreatitis, 577.0(*), 577.1

Chapter X: *Genitourinary system*
Urinary infections, 590, 595, 597, 598.0(*), 599.0
Male genital infections, 601(*), 604(*), 607.1, 607.2, 608.0
Mastitis, 611.0
Gynaecological infections, 614(*)–616(*)

Chapter XI: *Pregnancy, childbirth, puerperium*
Infected abortion, 634.0, 635.0, 636.0, 637.0
General infections complicating pregnancy, childbirth and the puerperium, 647
Major puerperal infections, 670
Venous complications, 671.2–671.5
Infections of the breast associated with childbirth, 675

Chapter XII: *Skin and subcutaneous tissue*
    Furuncle, 680
    Cellulitis, 681, 682
    Acute lymphadenitis, 683
    Impetigo, 684
    Other local infections of skin and subcutaneous tissue, 686
    Pemphigus, 694.4
    Folliculitis, 704.8
    Acne, 706.0, 706.1

Chapter XIII: *Musculoskeletal system and connective tissue*
    Pyogenic arthritis, 711.0, 711.9
    Arthropathies associated with general infections, 711.1*–711.8*
    Synovitis, 727.0(*), 727.3(*)
    Infective myositis, 728.0(*)
    Bone infections, 730(*)

Chapter XV: *Perinatal period*
    Congenital pneumonia, 770.0
    Perinatal infections, 771

Chapter XVII: *Injury and poisoning*
It is difficult if not impossible to identify infections following injury. In many of the categories a fourth digit appears to indicate a complication.

Examples:
    For fractures, the qualifying term "open" indicates: compound, infected, with foreign body
    Compound dislocation includes: infected, open, with foreign body
    Complicated wound includes: delayed healing, delayed treatment, foreign body, major infection

The only explicit ones are:
    Post-traumatic wound infection, not elsewhere classified, 958.3
    Infection complicating prosthetic device, 996.6
    Postoperative infection, 998.5

Categories of ICD-9 supplementary classifications having some relation to infectious diseases
    Failure of sterile precautions during procedure, E872
    Administration of contaminated substance (blood, other fluid, drug, etc.), E875
    Contact with or exposure to communicable diseases, V01
    Carrier or suspected carrier of infectious diseases, V02
    Need for prophylactic vaccination or inoculation, V03–V06
    Need for other prophylactic measures, V07
    Personal history of infectious and parasitic diseases, V12.0

WHO COLLABORATING CENTRES
IN THE FIELD OF INFECTIONS AND VECTOR CONTROL

A WHO collaborating centre is an institution, or a department or laboratory in an institution, or a group of reference, research and training facilities in different institutions, designated by WHO to form part of an international and inter-institutional collaborative network in support of its programme. Together with institutions of internationally recognized high scientific and technical standing, institutions with an expanding ability to fulfil a function or range of functions related to WHO's programme may also qualify for designation as WHO collaborating centres.

A WHO collaborating centre participates in cooperative programmes supported by WHO at the country, intercountry, regional, interregional and global level. It also contributes to increasing the capability of countries by providing information, services, research and training in support of national health development.

The functions performed by WHO collaborating centres, severally or collectively, may include the following:

— information synthesis and dissemination

— standardization of terminology and nomenclature; technologies; diagnostic, therapeutic and prophylactic substances; methods; and procedures

— provision of reference and other services

— participation in collaborative research developed under WHO's leadership, including the planning, implementation, monitoring and evaluation of research

— training and research training

— coordination of activities carried out by several centres on the same subject.

WHO headquarters or a regional office selects the centres for designation in consultation with the national authorities concerned. The centres are designated for an initial period of three years and redesignation for the same or a shorter period is reviewed every three years, depending on the requirements of the programme.

Europe has the largest number of collaborating centres serving either regional or global needs. The distribution of the centres is uneven and the full potentialities of institutions theoretically suitable for collaboration in specific regional research in support of WHO's regional programme have not yet been exploited. There is great interest on the part of the institutions but administrative difficulties have so far not been overcome.

A list of the collaborating centres in the European Region is given at the end of this annex.[a]

National cooperating institutions
In agreement with the national authorities concerned, WHO may use any institution in a country that is able and willing to participate in collaborative activities, even though it does not qualify as a WHO collaborating centre. Such an institution is formally recognized as a national cooperating institution, and is so designated by the national authorities concerned in an agreement with WHO specifying the tasks to be performed by the institution and the institution's entitlement to WHO support. National cooperating institutions are authorized by their respective governments to maintain direct working relations with WHO and with WHO collaborating centres.

WHO's agreement to the designation of a national cooperating institution is furnished by the Regional Director. Working relationships with the institution are developed at whichever operational level — regional or global — WHO is called upon to cooperate. Their most useful function so far has been in the global monitoring of circulating influenza strains and types. However, they have had little contact with the WHO Regional Office and again full use of their collaborative potential has not as yet been made. There are 47 centres concerned with enterobacteria, 45 with influenza, 26 with streptococci and staphylococci, 13 with hepatitis, 9 with meningococci, 7 with vibrios and one each with leptospirosis and interferon.

---

[a]Additional collaborating centres recently designated or in the process of being designated are situated at Bondy, France (medical entomology), Lyon (legionellosis), Paris (comparative immunology; Expanded Programme on Immunization), Hanover (defined laboratory animals), Munich (viral hepatitis), Rome (epidemiological surveillance), Nijmegen (malaria), Lund, Sweden (sexually transmitted diseases), Stockholm (legionellosis), Alma-Ata, USSR (vector biology and control), Leningrad (mycology), Moscow (Expanded Programme on Immunization; vector biology and control; virology; virus biologicals), Sukhumi, USSR (defined laboratory animals), Brighton (schistosomiasis) and London (acute respiratory diseases; onchocerciasis and leishmaniasis).

WHO collaborating centres in the European Region

Country	Title of centre	Institution
Virus diseases		
Belgium	Reference and research on viruses	Department of Microbiology and Virology Prince Leopold Department of Tropical Medicine Antwerp
Czechoslovakia	Reference and research on arboviruses	Institute of Virology Slovak Academy of Sciences Bratislava
	Reference and research on rickettsiae	Department of Rickettsiae Institute of Virology Slovak Academy of Sciences Bratislava
	Reference and research on viruses	Department of Microbiology and Epidemiology Institute of Hygiene and Epidemiology Prague
	Rapid laboratory viral diagnosis	Institute of Sera and Vaccines Prague-Vinohrady
Denmark	Reference and research on viruses	Ornithosis Department State Serum Institute Copenhagen
France	Reference and research on arboviruses	Section for Viral Ecology Pasteur Institute Paris
	Reference and research on viruses	Virology Laboratory Claude Bernard University Lyon
Hungary	Viruses	Division of Epidemiology and Microbiology National Institute of Hygiene Budapest
Romania	Viruses	Stefan S. Nicolau Institute of Virology Bucharest
Sweden	Reference and research on viruses	National Bacteriological Laboratory Stockholm
Switzerland	Viruses	Institute of Medical Microbiology St Gallen

USSR	Viruses	Laboratory of Mycoplasmas
		Gamaleja Institute of Epidemiology
		  and Microbiology
		Academy of Medical Sciences of
		  the USSR
		Moscow

	Reference and
	  research on viruses
		Ivanovskij Institute of Virology
		Academy of Medical Sciences of
		  the USSR
		Moscow

	Viruses	Department of Arboviruses Ivanovskij Institute of Virology Academy of Medical Sciences of the USSR Moscow

	Reference and
	  research on
	  arboviruses
		Institute of Poliomyelitis and Viral
		  Encephalitides
		Academy of Medical Sciences of
		  the USSR
		Moscow

	Reference and
	  research on viruses
		Institute of Poliomyelitis and Viral
		  Encephalitides
		Academy of Medical Sciences of
		  the USSR
		Moscow

	Reference and
	  research on viruses
	  (special pathogens)
		Institute of Poliomyelitis and Viral
		  Encephalitides
		Academy of Medical Sciences of
		  the USSR
		Moscow

	Reference and
	  research on viral
	  hepatitis
		Institute of Poliomyelitis and Viral
		  Encephalitides
		Academy of Medical Sciences of
		  the USSR
		Moscow

	Reference and
	  research on
	  rickettsiae
		Laboratory of Rickettsial Ecology
		Gamaleja Institute of Epidemiology
		  and Microbiology
		Academy of Medical Sciences of
		  the USSR
		Moscow

United Kingdom	Reference and
	  research on viral
	  hepatitis
		London School of Hygiene and
		  Tropical Medicine
		London

	Reference and
	  research on
	  influenza
		Division of Virology
		National Institute for Medical
		  Research
		Medical Research Council
		London

	Reference and research on viruses	Common Cold Research Unit National Institute for Medical Research Medical Research Council Harvard Hospital Salisbury
	Viruses	Virus Reference Laboratory Central Public Health Laboratory London
	Reference and research on influenza	Virus Reference Laboratory Central Public Health Laboratory London
	Reference and research on viruses (special pathogens)	Special Pathogens Reference Laboratory Centre for Applied Microbiology and Research Public Health Laboratory Service Salisbury
	Reference and research on rapid laboratory viral diagnosis	Division of Microbiological Reagents and Quality Control Central Public Health Laboratory London
Yugoslavia	Viruses	Department of Virology Andrija Štampar School of Public Health University of Zagreb Zagreb

Bacterial diseases

Czechoslovakia	Reference and research on streptococci	Streptococcus Reference Laboratory Institute of Hygiene and Epidemiology Prague
Denmark	Reference and research on pneumococci	Pneumococcal Laboratory State Serum Institute Copenhagen
France	Reference and research on meningococci	Institut de Médecine tropicale Service de Santé des Armées Marseille-Armées
Romania	Reference and research on diphtheria	Department of Diphtheria Dr I. Cantacuzino Institute Bucharest

USSR	Reference and research on pertussis	Laboratory of Research on Respiratory Infections Gamaleja Institute of Epidemiology and Microbiology Academy of Medical Sciences of the USSR Moscow
	Reference and research on plague	Plague Research Institute of the Caucasus and Transcaucasia Stavropol
United Kingdom	Reference and research on hospital infections	Division of Hospital Infections Central Public Health Laboratory London
Yugoslavia	Reference and research on bacterial vaccines and immunization programmes	Institute of Immunology Zagreb

Tuberculosis

Czechoslovakia	Tuberculosis chemotherapy	Second Tuberculosis Clinic Charles University Prague
	Standardization of laboratory procedures for the diagnosis of mycobacterial diseases and for bacteriological research	Department of Tuberculosis Microbiology Institute of Hygiene and Epidemiology Prague
Denmark	Worldwide reference for BCG seed lots and for coordination of control of BCG products	BCG Department State Serum Institute Copenhagen
United Kingdom	Tuberculosis chemotherapy and its application	Tuberculosis and Chest Diseases Unit, and Unit for Laboratory Studies of Tuberculosis Medical Research Council London

Leprosy

| Belgium | Epidemiology of leprosy | Department of Epidemiology School of Public Health Université Catholique de Louvain Brussels |
| United Kingdom | Reference and research on *Mycobacterium leprae* | Laboratory for Leprosy and Mycobacterial Research National Institute for Medical Research Medical Research Council London |

Venereal diseases and treponematoses

Denmark	Reference and research on treponematoses	Treponematoses Department State Serum Institute Copenhagen
	Reference and research on gonococci	Neisseria Department State Serum Institute Copenhagen
France	Reference and research on endemic treponematoses	Laboratory of Serology and Experimental Chemotherapy Paris
	Reference and research on sexually transmitted diseases	Alfred Fournier Institute Paris

Veterinary public health

Czechoslovakia	Epidemiology of leptospirosis	Institute of Epidemiology Faculty of Medicine Komensky University Bratislava
	Research and training in veterinary public health	Institute of Veterinary Research Brno-Medlanky
Denmark	Animal mycoplasmas (with FAO)	Institute of Medical Microbiology Medical Faculty University of Aarhus Aarhus
	Reference and research on toxoplasmosis (with FAO)	Department of Toxoplasmosis and Viral Diseases State Serum Institute Copenhagen

300

France	Reference and research on rabies	Rabies Laboratory Pasteur Institute Paris
	Yersinia pseudotuberculosis and *Y. enterocolitica* infections	Bacterial Ecology Unit Pasteur Institute Paris
	Epidemiology of leptospiroses (with FAO)	Leptospiroses Laboratory Pasteur Institute Paris
Germany, Federal Republic of	Research and training in veterinary public health	School of Veterinary Medicine Hanover
	Neurological zoonoses	Institute of Medical Virology and Immunology University of Essen Essen
	Collection and evaluation of data on comparative virology	Institute for Veterinary Microbiology, Infections and Epidemic Medicine Ludwig Maximilians University Munich
	Rabies surveillance and research	Rabies Laboratory Federal Research Institute for Animal Virus Diseases Tübingen
	Research and training in food hygiene and zoonoses (with FAO)	Robert von Ostertag Institute of Veterinary Medicine Berlin (West)
Netherlands	Reference and research on leptospirosis (with FAO)	Royal Tropical Institute Amsterdam
USSR	Reference and research on rabies	Rabies Prophylaxis Laboratory Institute of Poliomyelitis and Viral Encephalitides Academy of Medical Sciences of the USSR Moscow
	Reference and research on brucellosis	Brucellosis Laboratory Gamaleja Institute of Epidemiology and Microbiology Academy of Medical Sciences of the USSR Moscow

	Epidemiology of leptospirosis	Leptospirosis Laboratory Gamaleja Institute of Epidemiology and Microbiology Academy of Medical Sciences of the USSR Moscow
	Defined laboratory animals	Research Laboratory for Experimental Biological Models Academy of Medical Sciences of the USSR Moscow
	Zoonoses	Central Research Institute of Epidemiology Moscow
United Kingdom	Reference and research on brucellosis (with FAO)	Diseases of Breeding Department Central Veterinary Laboratory Weybridge
	Reference and research on leptospirosis	Leptospirosis Reference Laboratory Public Health Laboratory Service London
	Defined laboratory animals	Laboratory Animals Centre Medical Research Council Laboratories Carshalton
	Comparative oncology	Department of Clinical Veterinary Medicine School of Veterinary Medicine University of Cambridge Cambridge

Diarrhoeal diseases

Belgium	*Campylobacter jejuni*	Department of Microbiology and Infectious Diseases Saint-Pierre University Hospital Brussels
Denmark	Reference and research on *Escherichia* and *Klebsiella*	Coli Department State Serum Institute Copenhagen
France	Reference and research on salmonellae	Salmonellae Laboratory Pasteur Institute Paris

302

Hungary	Reference and research on bacterial vaccines	Institute for Human Serobacteriological Production Budapest
United Kingdom	Phage-typing and resistance of enterobacteriaceae	Division of Enteric Pathogens Central Public Health Laboratory London
	Human rotavirus	Regional Virus Laboratory East Birmingham Hospital Birmingham
	Environmental and epidemiological aspects of diarrhoeal diseases	Ross Institute of Hygiene and Tropical Medicine London

Smallpox

France	Poxvirus research	Virus Section National Laboratory for Public Health Paris
Netherlands	Smallpox vaccine	Virus and Rickettsial Disease Laboratory National Institute of Public Health Bilthoven
USSR	Smallpox and other poxvirus infections	Laboratory of Viral Vesicular Infections Research Institute of Virus Preparations Moscow
United Kingdom	Characterization of variola and related poxviruses	Department of Virology Wright-Fleming Institute of Microbiology St Mary's Hospital Medical School London

Research promotion and development

Belgium	Monitoring advances in the biomedical sciences	International Institute for Cellular and Molecular Pathology Brussels

Prevention of blindness

Denmark	Chlamydiae	Ornithosis Department State Serum Institute Copenhagen

303

USSR	Prevention of blindness caused by infectious eye diseases	Department of Viral and Allergic Eye Diseases Helmoltz Research Institute of Ophthalmology Moscow
United Kingdom	Prevention of blindness	Department of Preventive Ophthalmology University of London London

Vector biology and control

Czechoslovakia	Biological control of arthropod vectors of disease	Department of Insect Pathology Institute of Entomology Czechoslovak Academy of Sciences Prague
Denmark	Insecticide resistance-*Musca domestica*	Insect Control Section Danish Pest Infestation Laboratory Lyngby
	Applied malacology	Danish Bilharziasis Laboratory Copenhagen
France	Studies on viruses of insects	Research Station of Cytopathology Faculty of Sciences Montpellier University St Christol
	Entomopathogenic sporulating bacteria for vector control	Laboratory for Bacteriological Control of Insects Paris
	Vector biology	Laboratory for Bacteriological Control of Insects Paris
	Serological techniques	University of Grenoble Grenoble
Germany, Federal Republic of	Vector control	Department of Entomology Bernhard Nocht Institute of Naval and Tropical Diseases Hamburg
Italy	Cytogenetic studies on malaria vectors	Institute of Parasitology Faculty of Medicine University of Rome Rome

304

USSR	Evaluating safety and development of specifications for public health insecticides	All-Union Scientific Research Institute for Disinfection and Sterilization Moscow
	Vector biology and control	Marcinovskij Institute of Medical Parasitology and Tropical Medicine Moscow
United Kingdom	Evaluating and testing new insecticides	Division of Chemical Control Research Centre for Overseas Pest Research Porton Down, Salisbury
	Insecticide resistance and cytotaxonomic, biochemical and genetic applied research on major vector species, especially mosquitos	Department of Entomology London School of Hygiene and Tropical Medicine London
	Evaluation and testing of new insecticides	Toxicology Research Unit Medical Research Council Laboratories Carshalton
	Evaluation and development of pesticide application equipment in Europe	Overseas Spraying Machinery Centre Imperial College Field Station Imperial College of Science and Technology University of London Ascot

VACCINATION SCHEDULES IN EUROPEAN COUNTRIES

Age	Vaccine
ALBANIA	
At birth	BCG
2 months	OPV (trivalent)
3 months	DPT
4 months	OPV (trivalent), DPT
5 months	DPT
6 months	OPV (trivalent)
9 months	Measles
11–14 months	DPT
18 months	OPV (trivalent)
3 years	DPT
6 years	BCG
6–7 years	DT
7 years	OPV (trivalent)
10–12 years	Diphtheria
12 years	Tetanus
ALGERIA	
At birth	BCG
3 months	OPV (trivalent), DPT
4 months	OPV (trivalent), DPT
5 months	OPV (trivalent), DPT
9–12 months	Measles
17 months	OPV (trivalent), DPT
5 years	OPV (trivalent), DPT, BCG
AUSTRIA	
First week	BCG
3 months	DPT
4 months	DPT, OPV (trivalent) or DT
5 months	DPT
6 months	OPV (trivalent)
8 months	OPV (trivalent)
14 months	Measles, mumps
18 months	DT
7 years	DT, OPV (trivalent)
13 years	Rubella (girls)
14 years	Tetanus, BCG (in non-reactors)
15 years	OPV (trivalent)

BELGIUM

3 months	DPT, OPV (trivalent)
4 months	DPT
5 months	DPT, OPV (trivalent)
13–14 months	DPT, OPV (trivalent)
15 months	Measles, or measles and mumps
6 years	DT, OPV (trivalent)
11–12 years	Rubella (girls)
15–16 years	Tetanus

BULGARIA

First 2 months	BCG
2 months	OPV (trivalent)
3 months	DPT
4 months	DPT
5 months	DPT
6 months	OPV (trivalent)
10 months	Measles
11–12 months	OPV (trivalent)
12 months	Mumps
13–24 months	2 doses of OPV (trivalent), DPT
2 years	OPV (trivalent)
4 years	DPT
6 years	OPV (trivalent)
7 years	DPT
12 years	DT

CZECHOSLOVAKIA

4 days–6 weeks	BCG
3 months	DPT
5 months	DPT
10–12 months	DPT
During first year	OPV (monovalent, type 1), followed one month later by OPV (bivalent, types 2 and 3)
13 months	Measles
17 months–2 years	Measles
3 years	DPT
First year of school	DPT
Second year of school	OPV (trivalent)
Third year of school	DT
12–13 years	Rubella (girls)
School age	BCG (in non-reactors)

DENMARK

5 weeks	Pertussis
9 weeks	Pertussis
5 months	Di-T-Pol (diphtheria, tetanus, trivalent inactivated poliomyelitis)
6 months	Di-T-Pol
10 months	Pertussis
15 months	Di-T-Pol
2 years	OPV (trivalent)
3 years	OPV (trivalent)
4 years	OPV (trivalent)
7 years	BCG (in non-reactors)

FRANCE

	Schedule A	Schedule B
First month	BCG	BCG
3 months	DPT	Pertussis
6 months	OPV (trivalent)	DT, inactivated poliomyelitis (trivalent)
1 year	DPT, OPV (trivalent)	Inactivated poliomyelitis (trivalent), pertussis
2 years		DT
4 years	DT	DT
6 years	DT, OPV (trivalent)	DT, inactivated poliomyelitis (trivalent)
11 years	OPV (trivalent)	DT, inactivated poliomyelitis (trivalent)

GERMAN DEMOCRATIC REPUBLIC

First week	BCG
2 months	OPV (monovalent, type 1)
3 months	DPT, OPV (type 2)
4 months	DPT, OPV (type 3)
5 months	DPT
13 months	Measles
1 year	OPV (trivalent)
2 years	DPT
7 years	OPV (trivalent)
15 years	Tetanus
School age	BCG (in non-reactors)

FEDERAL REPUBLIC OF GERMANY

	Schedule A	Schedule B
3 months	DT, OPV (trivalent)	DPT, OPV (trivalent)
or 4 months		or DPT
5 months	DT, OPV (trivalent)	DPT, OPV (trivalent)
2 years	Measles, DPT (or DT), OPV (trivalent)	
6–7 years	Diphtheria	
10 years	Tetanus, OPV (trivalent)	
11–15 years	Rubella (girls)	

GREECE

3 months	DPT, OPV (trivalent)
4 months	DPT, OPV (trivalent)
5 months	DPT, OPV (trivalent)
1 year	DPT, OPV (trivalent)
14–18 months	Measles (optional)
3 years	DPT, OPV (trivalent)
6 years	DT, BCG (in non-reactors)
10 years	Tetanus or DT (if Schick test positive)
12–14 years	Mumps (boys), rubella (girls)

HUNGARY

3–42 days	BCG
3 months	DPT
4 months	DPT
5 months	DPT
6 months	BCG (in non-reactors)
During first year	OPV (monovalent, in series 1, 3, 2)
14 months	Measles
During second year	OPV (monovalent, in series 1, 3, 2)
During third year	OPV (monovalent, in series 1, 3, 2)
36 months	DPT
6–7 years	DPT
7–8 years	BCG (in non-reactors)
11–12 years	DT
13–14 years	BCG (in non-reactors)
16–18 years	BCG (in non-reactors, except those vaccinated at 13–14 years)

ICELAND

3 months	DPT
4 months	DPT
5 months	DPT, poliomyelitis
6 months	Poliomyelitis
1 year	DPT, poliomyelitis
13 months	Measles
4 years	Poliomyelitis
6 years	DT
9 years	Poliomyelitis

IRELAND

At birth	BCG (urban areas)
3 months	DPT, OPV (trivalent)
4–5 months	DPT, OPV (trivalent)
8–11 months	DPT, OPV (trivalent)
13 months	Measles
4–6 years	DT
6–7 years	OPV (trivalent)
12–14 years	BCG (in non-reactors), rubella (girls)

ITALY

3 months	OPV (trivalent), DT
4–5 months	OPV (trivalent), DT
10–12 months	OPV (trivalent), DT
15–18 months	Measles
3 years	OPV (trivalent)
6 years	DT
12–13 years	Rubella (girls), mumps (boys)
14 years	Tetanus

LUXEMBOURG

First week	BCG
3 months	DPT, OPV (trivalent)
4 months	DPT
5 months	OPV (trivalent)
1 year	DPT, OPV (trivalent), measles
2 years	DPT
6 years	DT
12 years	OPV (trivalent), BCG (in non-reactors), rubella (girls with no antibodies)

MALTA

3 months	DPT, OPV (trivalent)
4–5 months	DPT, OPV (trivalent)
8–11 months	DPT, OPV (trivalent)
4–6 years	DT, OPV (trivalent)
12–14 years	BCG (in non-reactors)
10–13 years	Rubella (girls)

MOROCCO

Urban areas

At birth	BCG
3 months	DPT, OPV (trivalent)
4 months	DPT, OPV (trivalent)
5 months	DPT, OPV (trivalent)
9 months	Measles

Rural areas

3–5 months	DPT, OPV (trivalent), BCG
6–8 months	DPT, OPV (trivalent)
9 months – over	DPT, OPV (trivalent), measles

NETHERLANDS

3 months	DPT, inactivated poliomyelitis (trivalent)
4 months	DPT, inactivated poliomyelitis (trivalent)
5 months	DPT, inactivated poliomyelitis (trivalent)
11–14 months	DPT, inactivated poliomyelitis (trivalent)
14 months	Measles
4 years	DT, inactivated poliomyelitis (trivalent)
9 years	DT, inactivated poliomyelitis (trivalent)
11 years	Rubella (girls)

NORWAY

3 months	DPT
4 months	DPT
5 months	DPT
6 months	Inactivated poliomyelitis
7 months	Inactivated poliomyelitis
15 months	Measles
16 months	Inactivated poliomyelitis
17 months	DPT
7 years	Inactivated poliomyelitis
12 years	DT
13–15 years	Rubella (girls)
16 years	Inactivated poliomyelitis, BCG (in non-reactors)

POLAND

4–15 days	BCG
3 months	DPT, OPV (trivalent)
4–5 months	DPT, OPV (trivalent)
6 months	DPT, OPV (trivalent)
11–12 months	BCG (children with no scars)
13–15 months	Measles
18–24 months	DPT, OPV (trivalent)
6–7 years	BCG (in non-reactors), DT, OPV (trivalent)
14 years	BCG (in non-reactors), DT
18 years	BCG (in non-reactors)

PORTUGAL

First week	BCG
3 months	DPT, OPV (trivalent)
5 months	DPT, OPV (trivalent)
12 months	OPV (trivalent)
1 year	DPT, OPV (trivalent), measles
5–7 years	DPT, OPV (trivalent), BCG (in non-reactors)
10–12 years	Tetanus, OPV (trivalent), BCG (in non-reactors)

ROMANIA

4–60 days	BCG
3 months	DPT
4 months	DPT
5 months	DPT
11 months	DPT
1½–12½ months	1 dose OPV (monovalent) type 1, 2 doses OPV (trivalent)
9–21 months	Measles
15½–22 months	OPV (trivalent)
29 months	DPT
6–7 years	BCG (in non-reactors)
9 years	OPV (trivalent)
13–14 years	DT, BCG (in non-reactors)
17–19 years	BCG (in non-reactors)

SPAIN

0–12 months	BCG
3 months	DPT, OPV (trivalent)
4 months	DPT, OPV (trivalent)
5 months	DPT, OPV (trivalent)
12 months	Measles
18 months	DPT, OPV (trivalent)
6 years	DT, OPV (trivalent), BCG
10 years	Tetanus, OPV (trivalent)
14 years	Tetanus, OPV (trivalent)
12–14 years	Rubella (girls)

SWEDEN

2–3 months	DT
4–5 months	DT
6 months	DT
9–10 months	Inactivated poliomyelitis
10–11 months	Inactivated poliomyelitis
18 months	Inactivated poliomyelitis, MMR
6 years	Inactivated poliomyelitis
10 years	DT
12 years	MMR, BCG (in non-reactors)

SWITZERLAND

At birth	BCG
3 months	DPT, OPV (trivalent)
4 months	DPT, OPV (trivalent)
5 months	DPT, OPV (trivalent)
18 months	Measles or MMR, DT, OPV (trivalent)
5–7 years	DT, OPV (trivalent), BCG (in non-reactors)
15 years	DT, OPV (trivalent), BCG (in non-reactors), rubella (girls), mumps (boys)

TURKEY

2–3 months	DPT
3–4 months	DPT
4–5 months	DPT
2 months–3 years	Poliomyelitis 3 times a year × 3 years, monovalent in spring, trivalent in autumn and winter
1 year	DPT
15 months	Measles
3–8 years	TDT (typhoid – diphtheria – tetanus)

USSR

5–7 months	BCG
3 months	OPV (trivalent), DPT
4–5 months	OPV (trivalent), DPT
6–7 months	OPV (trivalent), DPT
15–18 months	Measles, mumps
1–2 years	OPV (trivalent), 2 doses DPT
2–3 years	2 doses OPV (trivalent)
6 years	DT
7 years	BCG
11–12 years	BCG
16 years	Tetanus

UNITED KINGDOM

3 months	DPT, OPV (trivalent)
4–5 months	DPT, OPV (trivalent)
8–11 months	DPT, OPV (trivalent)
2 years	Measles
4–6 years	DT, OPV (trivalent)
13 years	OPV (trivalent)
10–13 years	BCG (in non-reactors), rubella (girls)

312

YUGOSLAVIA

3 months	DPT, OPV (trivalent)
4 months	OPV (trivalent)
5 months	OPV (trivalent)
5–7 months	DPT
9–11 months	DPT
13 months	Measles
1 year	DPT, OPV (trivalent)
2–4 years	DPT
3 years	OPV (trivalent)
6 years	DT, OPV (trivalent)
13 years	DT, OPV (trivalent)

THE RISING COST OF ANTIMICROBIAL THERAPY

The rising cost of antimicrobial drugs can be illustrated by the example of the Ulm University Clinics in the Federal Republic of Germany, which in 1980 and 1981 had an average of 964 and 959 beds, respectively. Some 26 000 patients were admitted to the clinics in each of those years, the average length of stay being 11 days. The clinics have a good surveillance scheme, including a computerized resistance profile list for the most important nosocomial infection pathogens.

Table 1. Costs of antimicrobials used in the Ulm University Clinics

Antimicrobial	1980	1981	Difference	
			DM	%
Systemic treatment				
Penicillins	1 052 202	1 146 989	+ 94 787	+ 9.01
Cephalosporins	411 508	648 095	+236 587	+ 57.49
Aminoglycosides	400 953	432 465	+ 31 512	+ 7.86
Tetracyclines	72 112	36 268	− 35 844	− 49.71
Chloramphenicol	4 389	3 601	− 788	− 17.95
Polymycins	97 690	118 245	+ 20 555	+ 21.04
Sulfamethoxazole/trimethoprim	12 470	9 944	− 2 526	− 20.26
Other sulfonamides	411	1 011	+ 600	+145.99
Nitrofurans	3 330	10 713	+ 7 383	+221.71
Antimycotics	44 008	76 410	+ 32 402	+ 73.63
Tuberculostatics	13 405	16 105	+ 2 700	+ 20.14
Others	54 579	102 102	+ 47 523	+ 87.07
Local treatment	42 217	49 465	+ 7 248	+ 17.17
Total	2 209 274	2 651 413	+442 139	+ 20.01

Although there was a decrease in spending on tetracyclines, chloramphenicol and sulfamethoxazole/trimethoprim during that period, the overall costs rose. Cephalosporins were mainly responsible for the rise, followed by penicillins, antimycotics and polymycins. The most expensive group of antimicrobials remained the penicillins, mainly due to the use of the new generation "broad spectrum" forms such as azlocillin, mezlocillin and ticarcillin, followed by the cephalosporins and aminoglycosides. The penicillins also headed the list of the most used group of antimicrobials. The use of some antimicrobials fell in 1981 compared with 1980, namely penicillins (3128 doses fewer), tetracyclines

(17 780), chloramphenicol (130), sulfamethoxazole/trimethoprim (2318), antimycotics (547) and others (3781). At the same time the use of others increased, namely cephalosporins (1436 doses more), aminoglycosides (2919), polymycins (2547), slowly resorbed sufonamides (396), nitrofurans (518) and tuberculostatics (979). Although there was a net fall in the number of doses used in 1981, the overall cost of antimicrobial therapy rose by 20% compared with 1980.

Annex 5

PERCENTAGE DRUG RESISTANCE
IN CLINICALLY IMPORTANT PATHOGENS

Pathogen	Penicillin G	Ampicillin	Oxacillin	Carbenicillin	Mezlocillin	Azlocillin	Ticarcillin	Piperacillin	Erythromycin
Escherichia coli	91.1	20.0	98.9	17.7	12.7	17.1	20.0	19.0	95.9
Proteus mirabilis	21.8	17.4	100.0	9.7	8.1	10.4	8.0	9.0	100.0
Proteus (indole positive)	85.0	79.1	100.0	9.1	10.0	14.6	22.0	29.0	100.0
Enterobacter	94.9	75.0	98.7	30.9	28.6	31.6	30.0	32.0	93.9
Serratia	100.0	95.8	100.0	37.5	31.8	36.4	57.0	57.0	100.0
Citrobacter	100.0	47.1	100.0	11.8	7.1	7.1	25.0	30.0	94.1
Salmonella	11.3	2.5	100.0	1.3	1.3	2.5	—	5.0	100.0
Pseudomonas aeruginosa	99.4	99.4	100.0	15.2	33.8	7.0	11.0	5.0	99.4
Enterococci	0.7	0.7	97.2	0.7	3.1	0.0	0.0	0.0	32.2
Klebsiella pneumoniae	94.7	86.3	100.0	48.3	23.6	25.7	60.0	61.0	97.5
Staphylococcus aureus	72.0	74.0	0.6	0.5	67.0	68.0	5.0	45.0	12.3
Number tested	1 138	763	1 248	237	265	201	1 012	1 012	1 244

Pathogen	Tetracycline	Lincomycin	Chloramphenicol	Co-trimoxazole	Gentamicin	Tobramycin	Sisomicin	Amikacin	Nitrofurantoin	Nalidixic acid
Escherichia coli	27.2	99.4	16.0	12.9	3.1	1.2	1.8	0.0	3.6	2.0
Proteus mirabilis	96.4	100.0	36.8	8.4	7.6	2.1	4.1	1.0	43.9	3.5
Proteus (indole positive)	62.8	100.0	31.0	19.0	6.8	4.5	6.8	0.0	45.5	2.3
Enterobacter	26.3	96.2	28.4	19.8	17.3	6.1	8.5	0.0	7.4	7.4
Serratia	68.0	100.0	52.0	32.0	8.0	0.0	0.0	0.0	48.0	16.7
Citrobacter	11.8	100.0	5.9	17.6	11.8	0.0	0.0	—	0.0	5.9
Salmonella			5.0	3.8	0.0	0.0	0.0		8.8	0.0
Pseudomonas aeruginosa	88.8	100.0	96.4	90.6	10.2	3.4	6.2	3.0	99.4	95.0
Enterococci	68.8	96.5	39.0	88.8	85.7	75.7	58.3	99.3	2.0	99.3
Klebsiella pneumoniae	22.5	100.0	25.8	17.6	10.7	5.7	0.8	0.0	7.3	6.6
Staphylococcus aureus	22.5	1.9	9.9	9.5	9.0	4.5	4.2	0.6	0.3	74.7
Number tested	691	1 230	475	437	234	149	132	266	295	550

317

Pathogen	Cefalotin	Cefazolin	Cefalexin	Cefaclor	Cefamandole	Cefuroxime	Cefoxitin	Cefotaxime	Cefadroxil	Cefacetrile
Streptococcus faecalis (n = 120)	95	89	100	97	19	98	99	97	97	61
Staphylococcus aureus (n = 155)	1	3	24	30	0	3	2	3	0	1
Escherichia coli (n = 214)	13	6	10	10	8	2	2	0	10	9
Proteus mirabilis (n = 119)	9	5	39	9	7	2	0	0	25	20
Pseudomonas aeruginosa (n = 228)	100	100	100	100	99	99	99	15	100	100
Klebsiella pneumoniae (n = 36)	40	35	12	33	35	1	0	0	20	10
Enterobacter species (n = 57)	94	91	89	89	48	42	82	16	99	90
Proteus (indole positive) (n = 49)	96	94	94	94	78	80	2	2	90	82
Serratia (n = 14)	100	99	100	100	97	97	91	86	100	100

Source: **Daschner, F.** *Infektionskontrolle in Klinik und Praxis.* Baden-Baden, Cologne, New York, Witzströh, 1980.

318

Annex 6

MORBIDITY FROM SELECTED GASTROINTESTINAL INFECTIONS IN SOME EUROPEAN COUNTRIES, 1980

Country	Typhoid fever	Paratyphoid fever	Other salmonelloses	Shigellosis	Other bacterial infections	Enteritis	Ill-defined intestinal infections
Austria	28	66		40	1 530	37 209[a]	
Belgium	24	7	584	56	13	77[b]	
Bulgaria	3	—		9 385	8	20[c]	
Czechoslovakia[d]	83	9	12 513	20 793	441	4 209	6 686
Denmark	9	10		53			
Finland	7	20	2 145	210		51 385	
France[e]	951[f]			4 805			
German Democratic Republic	110	15	6 584	1 500		3 937[b]	449 889
Germany, Federal Republic of	352	212	48 606	1 272	865[a]		
Hungary	21	1	7 464	5 519		607[b]	
Norway	16	11	309	160		41[b]	
Poland	103	14	9 243	6 988			
Portugal[e]	586	20		29			
Spain	3 742[f]			4 805			
Switzerland	44	25	3 032	447	2 086		
Turkey[e]	2 402	880		1 086			
United Kingdom	230	104	9 540	2 709	1 316	10 318	

[a] Other forms.
[b] Pathogenic E. coli.
[c] Children under 2 years of age.
[d] 1982 data.
[e] 1981 data.
[f] Includes paratyphoid fever.

319

CASES OF HUMAN ANTHRAX IN EUROPE
REPORTED TO WHO, 1965–1981

Country	Average 1956–1960	1965	1966	1967	1968	1969	1970	1971	1972	1973
Austria	8	0	1	2	1	2	0	0	0	1
Belgium	4.6	5	4	0	4	1	1	0	1	2
Bulgaria	391	152	102	59	57	39	49	36	28	126
Czechoslovakia	10.8	0	4	4	1	1	0	1	1	0
France		1		4	4		1	3	1	0
German Democratic Republic	4.8	2	6	2	1	0	0	1	4	1
Germany, Federal Republic of	19	15	21	8	3	3	2	6	3	3
Greece	136.8	104	79	118	102	93	95	56	42	43
Hungary	27.8	5	8	10	27	4	5	10	4	6
Italy	417.2	218	173	143	153	108	88	83	75	94
Netherlands										
Norway	0.4	0	0	1	0	0	0	0	0	0
Poland	8.8	8	4	5	10	3	3	11	4	3
Portugal	318	51	34	29	37	7	10	10	8	3
Romania	553[a]	184	168	132	150	133	94	95	119	131
Spain		455	353	316	350	311	284	198	220	198
Sweden		0	0	1	0	0	0	0	0	0
Switzerland	24	3	1	0	0	0	0	0	1	1
United Kingdom:										
England & Wales		7	10	19	9	3	5	5	4	3
Northern Ireland		0	1	2	0	0			0	
Scotland		9	2	5	1	8	2	1	1	0
Yugoslavia	331.5[b]	197	204	153	130	105	84	84	54	57
Turkey			1 159	794	849	912	843	669	697

[a] 1956 only.

[b] 4-year average.

Country	Average 1956–1960	1974	1975	1976	1977	1978	1979	1980	1981
Austria	8	1	0	0	0	0	2	0	1
Belgium	4.6	0	1	0	1	1	2	3	2
Bulgaria	391	33	26	23	21	28	16	12	15
Czechoslovakia	10.8	1	0	0	0	1	0	0	0
France		1	3	4	1	0	0	1	0
German Democratic Republic	4.8	0	1	4	1	0	0	0	0
Germany, Federal Republic of	19	4	6	2	4	6	1	2	3
Greece	136.8	55	99	59	26	50	38	14	27
Hungary	27.8	4	0	4	0	0	0	0	0
Italy	417.2	90	98	71	82	64	40	40	
Netherlands							2	0	0
Norway	0.4	0	0	0	0	0	2	0	0
Poland	8.8	4	0	0	3	3	1	0	0
Portugal	318	3	7	9	10	4	3	15	13
Romania	553[a]	96	86	43	36	39	28		37
Spain		235	251	216	222	227	298	289	258
Sweden		0	0	0	0	0	0	0	0
Switzerland	24	0	0	0	1	3	3	5	14
United Kingdom:									
England & Wales		4	4	4	4	0	3	0	0
Northern Ireland							0		
Scotland		3	0	0	1	1	1	0	0
Yugoslavia	331.5[b]	13		49		40	31		
Turkey		526	505	305	798	540	360	369	397

[a] 1956 only.

[b] 4-year average.

PERSONS RESPONSIBLE AT THE NATIONAL LEVEL
FOR THE PREVENTION OF INFECTIOUS DISEASES AND FOR
EPIDEMIOLOGICAL SURVEILLANCE

Responsible Officer at the Regional Office
for Europe of the World Health Organization

Regional Officer for Communicable Diseases
WHO Regional Office for Europe
Scherfigsvej 8
DK-2100 Copenhagen Ø
Denmark

Cables: UNISANTE Copenhagen
Telex: 15348
Telephone: (01) 29 01 11

Albania

Directeur, Direction de l'Hygiène
 et de la Lutte contre les
 Maladies infectieuses
Ministère de la Santé publique
Tirana

Algeria

Médecin-chef de la Section
 d'Epidémiologie
Ministère de la Santé publique
Chemin Mohamed Gacem
Algiers

Telephone: 66 46 98

Austria

Federal Ministry of Health and
 Environmental Protection
Stubenring 1
A-1010 Vienna

Telephone: 7500 ext. 6431
Telex: 11 11 45 or 11 17 80

Belgium

Inspecteur-en-chef-Directeur
Ministère de la Santé publique et
 de la Famille
Quartier Vésale—Bureau 447
Cité administrative de l'Etat
1010 Brussels

Telephone: (02) 564 11 54
Telex: 25768 MUGSP F.B.
Cables: Santé publique Bruxelles

Bulgaria

Directeur, Direction du Control
 d'Etat d'Hygiène et
 d'Epidémiologie
Ministère de la Santé publique
5 Place Lenine
Sofia-1000

Czechoslovakia

Chief, Department of
 Epidemiology of the Czech
 Socialist Republic
Ministry of Health of the CSR
Tr. W. Piecka 98
120 37 Prague 10—Vinohrady

Telephone: 73 54 86
Telex: 121048

Chief, Department of
 Epidemiology
Ministry of Health of the Slovak
 Socialist Republic
Ul. Csl. Armady 6
88305 Bratislava

Telephone: 51758
Telex: 92361

Denmark

Head of Division D
National Board of Health
St. Kongensgade 1
DK-1264 Copenhagen K

Telephone: (01) 14 10 11
Telex: 31316 Serum DK

Chief, Department of
 Epidemiology
State Serum Institute
80 Amager Boulevard
2300 Copenhagen S

Telephone: (01) 95 2817 ext. 2444
Telex: 31316 Serum DK

Finland

Department of Health Promotion
 and Hygiene
National Board of Health
Siltasaarenkatu 12 A
00530 Helsinki 53

Telephone: 190-718511
Telex: 12-1774 NBH

France

Ministère de la Santé
Direction générale de la Santé
Service de la Prévention et de
l'Organization des Soins
Sous-Direction de la Prévention
générale et de l'Environnement
Bureau I.C.
8 Avenue de Ségur
75700 Paris

Telephone: 567 55 44 poste 44-63
783 75 88
Telex: Santé SEC 250011 F

German Democratic Republic

Deputy Chief, Division of Hygiene
Ministry of Public Health
Rathausstrasse 3
1020 Berlin

Telephone: 235 5811
235 5812
235 5813
235 5814
Telex: 114765/114766

Germany, Federal Republic of

Chief, Section for Communicable
Diseases Control
Federal Ministry for Youth, Family
Affairs and Health
Postfach 20 0490
5300 Bonn Bad Godesberg

Telephone: 0228/3381
Telex: 088 55 17 or 088 54 37

Greece

Professeur de l'Université
d'Athènes
Chef de Service de Maladies
infectieuses à l'Université
d'Athènes
Hôpital Ag. Sophie
Athens

Hungary

Chief, Department of
Epidemiology
Ministry of Health of the
Hungarian People's Republic
Postafiok 1
Arany János u. 6–8
1361 Budapest V

Telephone: 126-889
Telex: 224337 Eü.Min.H.

Iceland

Director General of Health
(Landlaeknir)
Skrifstofa Landlaeknis
Arnarhvali
Reykjavik

Telephone: 96 27555
Cables: Foreign Secretary

Ireland

Deputy Chief Medical Officer
Department of Health
Custom House
Dublin 1

Telephone: 742961
Telex: 4894

Italy

Chief, Infectious Diseases
Department
Ministry of Health
Via Liszt 34
00144 Rome

Telephone: 5923501
Telex: 610453 or 613169

Director
Communicable Diseases
Epidemiological Unit
Istituto Superiore di Sanità
Viale Regina Elena 299
00141 Rome

Telephone: (06) 4954617

Luxembourg

Médecin-Inspecteur
Inspection sanitaire
4 rue Auguste Lumière
1950-Luxembourg

Telephone: 4 0801 poste 92
Telex: 2546 SANTE LU

Malta

Senior Medical Officer
Department of Health
15 Merchants Street
Valletta

Telephone: 28823 or 24071
Telex: 100 MOD MLT
Cables: Health Malta

Monaco

Direction de l'Action sanitaire et
  sociale
Ministère d'Etat
Monaco

Telephone: 30 19 21

Morocco

Chef de la Division de
  l'Epidémiologie
Ministère de la Santé publique
335 Avenue Mohammed V
Rabat

Telex: 0407-31642 sante

Netherlands

Head, Division of Infectious
  Diseases
Department of the Chief Medical
  Officer of Health
P.O. Box 439
2260 AK Leidschendam

Telephone: 070-20 92 60 ext. 2097
Telex: 32 362 v m nl or 32 347 v m nl

Norway

Division of Hygiene and
  Epidemiology
P.O. Box 8128 Dep
Oslo 1

Telephone: (02) 11 84 12
Telex: 17241 NSBDPN
Cables: Helsedirektoren

National Institute of Public Health
Infectious Diseases Control
  Department
Postuttak
Oslo 1

Telephone: (02) 356020
Cables: SIFF, Oslo

Poland

Chief, Epidemiological
  Department
National Institute of Hygiene
24 Chocimska Street
00-791 Warsaw

Telephone: 49 74 84

Portugal

Service de la Prophylaxie
Direction générale de la Santé
Alameda D. Afonso Henriques 45
1056 Lisbon

Telephone: 57 55 03
Cables: Direcçao Geral de Saude

Romania

Rue Ilfov Nr. 6 Sect. 5
Bucharest

Telephone: 13 68 43
Telex: 11468

Spain

Sub-Director General de Vigilancia
    Epidemiológica
Ministerio de Sanidad y Consumo
Paseo del Prado 20
Madrid 14

Telephone: (91) 239 82 31 or
           (91) 230 34 01
Telex: 44014 or 22608

Sweden

Department of Epidemiology
National Bacteriological
    Laboratory
105 21 Stockholm

Telephone: (08) 730 00 80
Telex: 11911 SBL S

Switzerland

Chef de la Section des Maladies
    transmissibles
Office fédéral de la Santé publique
Case postale 2644
3001 Berne

Telephone: (031) 61 95 45
Telex: 33 880
Cables: FEDHYGIENE BERNE

Turkey

Public Health Service
Ministry of Health and Social
    Assistance
Ankara

Telephone: 250686
Cables: Ministry Health, Ankara

USSR

Chief, Main Board of Quarantine
    Diseases
Ministry of Health of the USSR
3 Rahmanovskij pereulok
Moscow

Telephone: 221 34 81

United Kingdom

Senior Principal Medical Officer
Department of Health and Social
    Security
Alexander Fleming House
Elephant and Castle
London SE1 6BY

Telephone: (01) 407 5522
           ext. 6882/6888
Telex: 22106

Scottish Home and Health
    Department
St Andrew's House
Edinburgh EH1 3DE

Telephone: (031) 556 8501
           ext. 2362

Yugoslavia

Senior Adviser
Epidemiological Surveillance of
    Communicable Diseases
SIV II
Bulevar Avnoj-a 104
11070 Belgrade

Telephone: 5551480
Telex: 11062 YU SIV

Senior Adviser at the Federal
    Committee for Labour, Health
    and Social Welfare
SIV II
Bulevar Avnoj-a 104
11070 Belgrade

Telephone: 64 22 91
Telex: 062-11062yu siv
            ZDRAVKOM BELGRADE

Annex 9

DEMOGRAPHIC DATA ON THE COUNTRIES OF THE WHO EUROPEAN REGION

Country	Population estimate mid-1981 (millions)	Birth rate	Death rate	Rate of natural increase (annual, per cent)	Number of years to double population	Population projection for 2000 (millions)
Albania	2.8	29	7	2.2	32	3.9
Algeria	19.3	46	14	3.2	22	36.2
Austria	7.5	11	12	−0.1	—	7.3
Belgium	9.9	13	11	0.1	578	9.9
Bulgaria	8.9	16	10	0.5	139	9.6
Czechoslovakia	15.4	18	12	0.6	110	17.2
Denmark	5.1	12	11	0.1	770	5.1
Finland	4.8	13	9	0.4	169	4.9
France	53.9	14	10	0.4	178	56.4
German Democratic Republic	16.7	14	14	0.0	6 930	16.6
Germany, Federal Republic of	61.3	10	12	−0.2	—	57.5
Greece	9.6	16	9	0.7	96	10.6
Hungary	10.7	15	13	0.2	315	11.2
Iceland	0.2	19	6	1.2	57	0.3
Ireland	3.4	20	10	1.0	69	4.1
Italy	57.2	12	9	0.2	289	57.4
Luxembourg	0.4	11	11	0.0	3 465	0.3
Malta	0.3	17	9	0.8	90	0.4
Morocco	21.8	43	14	3.0	23	37.7
Netherlands	14.2	12	8	0.4	154	14.9
Norway	4.1	13	10	0.3	258	4.1
Poland	36.0	20	9	1.0	67	41.0
Portugal	10.0	15	8	0.7	105	11.5
Romania	22.4	18	10	0.9	79	25.7
Spain	37.8	16	8	0.8	83	43.5
Sweden	8.3	12	11	0.1	1 155	8.0
Switzerland	6.3	12	9	0.3	267	6.2
Turkey	46.2	32	10	2.2	32	69.0
USSR	268.0	18	10	0.8	86	310.0
United Kingdom	55.9	13	12	0.1	693	57.1
Yugoslavia	22.5	17	8	0.9	81	25.7

Country	Infant mortality rate	Population under 15 years (per cent)	Population over 64 years (per cent)	Life expectancy at birth (years)	Urban population (per cent)	Per capita gross national product (US $)
Albania	—	38	5	69	37	840
Algeria	127	48	4	56	61	1 580
Austria	15	21	15	72	54	8 620
Belgium	12	22	14	73	95	10 890
Bulgaria	22	22	11	72	64	3 690
Czechoslovakia	19	23	12	70	67	5 290
Denmark	9	20	14	74	84	11 900
Finland	8	21	11	72	62	8 260
France	10	23	14	73	78	9 940
German Democratic Republic	13	21	16	72	77	6 430
Germany, Federal Republic of	15	20	15	72	92	11 730
Greece	19	23	13	73	65	3 890
Hungary	24	21	13	70	54	3 850
Iceland	11	29	10	76	88	10 490
Ireland	15	31	11	73	58	4 230
Italy	15	22	13	73	69	5 240
Luxembourg	13	18	13	71	68	12 820
Malta	16	24	11	70	94	2 640
Morocco	133	47	4	55	40	740
Netherlands	8	23	11	75	88	10 240
Norway	9	23	14	75	44	10 710
Poland	22	24	10	71	57	3 830
Portugal	39	27	10	70	30	2 160
Romania	30	25	10	70	48	1 900
Spain	13	26	11	73	74	4 340
Sweden	7	20	16	75	83	11 920
Switzerland	9	21	13	75	58	14 240
Turkey	125	39	4	61	47	1 330
USSR	36	26	9	69	65	4 110
United Kingdom	13	22	14	73	76	6 340
Yugoslavia	32	25	8	69	42	2 430

Source: 1981 world population data sheet of the Population Reference Bureau, Inc.

Annex 10

THE SPECTACULAR INCREASE OF AIDS IN EUROPE

Table 1. The incidence of AIDS in Europe,
up until October 1983

Country	Year of diagnosis						Total
	Before 1979	1979	1980	1981	1982	1983	
Austria						7	7
Belgium			2	4	8	24	38
Czechoslovakia					1	1	2
Denmark			1	2	4	6	13
Finland						2	2
France	6	1	5	5	30	47	94
German Democratic Republic							0
Germany, Federal Republic of	1	1			7	33	42
Greece							0
Hungary							0
Ireland						2	2
Italy	1				2		3
Luxembourg							0
Netherlands					3	9	12
Norway						2	2
Poland							0
Spain				1	1	4	6
Sweden					1	3	4
Switzerland			2	3	5	7	17
USSR							0
United Kingdom				2	5	17	24
Yugoslavia							0
Total	8	2	10	17	67	164	268[a]

[a]Includes 59 African cases (see Table 2) as well as 8 from Haiti, one from the United States and one from Nicaragua.

Table 2. African patients with AIDS in Europe up until October 1983

	Country of residence				
Country of origin	Czechoslovakia	Belgium	France	Switzerland	Total
Zaire	1	31	9	4	45
Congo			4	1	5
Mali			2		2
Gabon			2		2
Rwanda		2			2
Burundi		1			1
Chad		1			1
Cameroon			1		1
Total	1	35	18	5	59